...ONT CENTER
...NTON AVENUE
...TE 300
...TER, NY 14604

...NT CENTER
...NTON AVENUE
SUITE 300
ROCHESTER, NY 14604

GRIEF
AS A FAMILY PROCESS
A Developmental Approach
to Clinical Practice

ESTER R. SHAPIRO

THE GUILFORD PRESS
New York   London

© 1994 The Guilford Press
A Division of Guilford Publications, Inc.
72 Spring Street, New York, NY 10012

Printed in the United States of America

This book is printed on acid-free paper.

Last digit is print number: 9 8 7 6 5 4 3 2

Library of Congress Cataloging-in-Publication Data

Shapiro, Ester R.
    Grief as a family process : a developmental approach to clinical
practice / Ester R. Shapiro.
        p. cm.
    Includes bibliographical references and index.
    ISBN 0-89862-196-8
    1. Bereavement—Psychological aspects. 2. Family—Psychological
aspects. 3. Family—Mental health. 4. Grief therapy. I. Title.
RC455.4.L67S373 1994
155.9'37—dc20   94-18297
                                                              CIP

ACKNOWLEDGMENTS

This book first took form as I listened to my grandparents' stories about
the traumatic family deaths that occurred during their childhoods in
Poland before World War I and before they all made their way, at various
stages of their own family life cycles, to Cuba and eventually to
Miami. I subsequently became a devoted student of a culturally and
historically based approach to family development as a means of understanding the enduring resonance of these stories in our shared lives.
My Cuban-Jewish extended family taught me not to immigrate alone,
and so I am grateful to my sisters, Rachel and Miriam, for their warm
presence in cold Boston and for their inexhaustible capacity to help
me process our shared family "business."

No book results from one person's efforts, but is instead the
cummulative result of many supportive resources. I have been fortunate to be surrounded by family, friends, colleagues, and clients who
share my commitment to understanding individual lives in the family
context—I am indebted to all of them. There are many I cannot name,
because of space constraints and concern for privacy, to whom I also
gratefully give thanks.

When I began work on a model of family development as a graduate student at the University of Massachusetts at Amherst, I was fortunate to collaborate with the following faculty and graduate students,
now colleagues, who shared my interest in the influences of family
and culture on individual experience. Stuart Golan, in making his own
transition from community psychologist to family therapist, initiated
a one-year seminar on family development which brought together
Paul Lipman, an interpersonal psychoanalyst, with developmentally
oriented family systems thinkers. Stuart's untimely death in 1990 made
it impossible for me to show him just how far down the path he initiated I have been able to travel. Alice Rossi, a sociologist with an extraordinary interdisciplinary reach, put together a series of seminars in
life studies which placed the particularities of women's lives fully in a
social and historical family context. Alexandra Kaplan, a feminist clinical psychologist, supervised research on the barriers to women's full
development that were given theoretical voice as well as practical

responses. Harold Jarmon, whose own clinical psychology career spanned the child guidance and family systems approaches, remained committed to clinical teaching within a humanistic, relational, and developmental frame. Many of my fellow graduate students in the program, including Ann Greif, Ed Yeats, Mona Fishbein, and Maryanne Sedney, continue to be supportive colleagues. Castellano Turner, true to his African-Caribbean roots, supported a vibrant community of Latino students that includes Guillermo Bernal, Ana Isabel Alvarez, Lillian Comas-Diaz, Julia Ramos McKay, Maria Lourdes Mattel, and Iris Zavala who have remained part of the collegiate community that sustains my work.

In Boston, my colleguial network has been rich with contacts in the child therapy, family therapy, psychoanalytic, and cross-cultural communities. I was fortunate to be at Judge Baker Children's Center as a postdoctoral fellow when Sandra Sutherland Fox founded the Family Support Center for grieving families. An extremely talented and committed group of supervisors and trainees participated in the Center between October 1979, when it opened, and May 1985, when it closed for lack of funding; they included Al Poussaint, Esther Gross, Regina Yando, Gabrielle Brenninkmeyer, John Baker, and Maryanne Sedney. The group provided a safe haven from our often overwhelming emotional responses to our work with traumatically bereaved families. Al Poussaint and Esther Gross initially collaborated with me on a version of this manuscript. I hope that the final product fairly reflects each of their distinctive capacities to balance a respectful, empathic response to children and families with a healthy dose of brain power and humor. Sandra Fox's work has continued through the Good Grief Program which provides death education counseling to schools and communities, and whose current director is Maria Trazzi.

Colleagues at the Latino and Portuguese clinical teams at Cambridge Hospital, the contextual therapy group of Boston, the Massachusetts Association for Psychoanalytic Psychology, the Massachusetts Institute for Psychoanalysis, the psychology department and clinical doctoral program at the University of Massachusetts, Boston, and the multicultural training program in clinical psychology at Boston City Hospital, all have provided me with supportive intellectual homes with diverse perspectives but a shared vision that committed clinical practice requires the constant challenge of our cherished personal, intellectual, and social assumptions.

Many people read portions of the manuscript in draft form and made invaluable comments: Esther Gross, Al Poussaint, Ana Margarita Cebollero, Rachel Shapiro, Miren Uriarte, Jodie Kliman, Hillel Levine, Robert Weiss, Celia Falicov, Ed Yeats, Suzanne Loughlin Yeats, Ann

Greif, and Randy Howe. A number of these readers offered comments not only as supportive colleagues and friends but also from their own experience of personal losses. It was always especially reassuring to be told that the perspectives in this book resonated with their own experiences of death, grief, and growth.

I owe a special thanks to my husband, Alan West, whose literary sensibility and love of ideas has greatly enhanced my work. My editor at The Guilford Press, Sharon Panulla, production editor David Lasky, and copy-editor Toby Troffkin helped make every stage of work on the book both personally and professionally rewarding. Their contributions to the clarity of the ideas and the accessibility of the writing have been enormous and much appreciated.

Finally, I would like to thank the individuals and families with whom I worked over the years, beginning with the bereavement support group I co-led at UMass Amherst with then graduate student Denise Gelinas as my supervisor. From the beginning of my work at the Family Support Center, I talked with individuals and families about what aspects of grieving they might want to share with others. I found families to be extraordinarily generous and committed to sharing their hard won personal experience with me and with others. They have taught me everything I know about grief, and I am deeply grateful. In the interests of protecting the privacy of these individuals and families, most of the case reports are written as composites of different families. All names are pseudonymous, and identifying details are substantially altered. Gail Kaplan, who bravely agreed to collaborate with me on the full telling of her grief experience in Chapter 4, "A Widow's Story," deserves a coauthorship which she can only receive pseudonymously in order to safeguard her privacy.

CONTENTS

PART I: OVERVIEW

1. Introduction   3

Grief as Cultural Criticism, 3
How to Read This Book, 7

2. A Systemic Developmental Approach   9
to Family Bereavement

Grief and Its Family Choreography, 9
Answering Nancy's Question, 12
A Systemic Developmental Framework for Family
     Bereavement, 17

PART II: INDIVIDUAL GRIEF IN SYSTEMIC CONTEXT

3. Grief in Adulthood   21

Adult Bereavement as a Systemic Developmental
     Process, 21
Models of Adult Bereavement, 25
Relational Aspects of Grief, 39
Summary, 42

4. A Widow's Story: The Systemic Developmental   44
Experience of Grief in Adulthood

This is How It Happened: A Moment Frozen
     in Time, 44
The Beginning of Therapy, 50
The First-Year Anniversary: Restoring the Flow
     of Time, 55
Transformations of Self as Transformations
     of Relatedness: Couples' Therapy with the Dead, 56
Changing Image of the Dead: Making Way
     for a New Form of Relating, 62
Rediscovering Aspects of the Complex Self: New Life
     after Grief, 67

5. Bereavement in Childhood: Child Grief   71
   as a Systemic Developmental Process

   Theoretical Attempts to Understand Bereavement
      in Childhood, 72
   Theories Informing a Systemic Developmental
      Approach to Child Bereavement, 74
   Vulnerabilities in the Caretaking Environment, 78
   Summary, 85

6. The Stories of Grieving Children: Weaving Grief   87
   and Coping into the Developmental Fabric

   Bereavement in Infancy, 87
   Bereavement and the Preschool Child, 98
   Bereavement and the School-Age Child, 105
   Bereavement in Adolescence, 113
   Conclusion: Child Grief in a Family
      Developmental Context, 119

PART III: GRIEVING FAMILIES
AND THEIR SHARED DEVELOPMENT

7. Family Systems Theory and Models of   125
   Family Bereavement

   Family Systems Theory: Basic Concepts, 125
   Bereavement in the Family Systems Literature, 128
   Summary: Family Therapy Approaches to
      Bereavement, 138

8. Family Development and Adaptation   141
   to the Crisis of Grief

   Relocating "Pathological Grief" in its Normal
      Developmental Context, 141
   Principles of Family Development, 146
   Strategies for Managing Developmental Stress:
      Controlling the Rate of Discontinuity and Change, 153
   Summary, 158

9. Helping Bereaved Families: Enhancing Strategies   159
   for Stable Reorganization

   A Grieving Family's First Priority: Establishing
      Emotional Equilibrium, 159
   Triangulation of the Dead, 164
   The Grieving Child's Increased Burden
      of Family Responsibility, 168

Family Bereavement and Differentiation of Self, 170
Symptoms in Individual Family Members as
   Communications of Shared Adaptation, 177
Coconstructing a New Family Narrative, 180
Conclusion: Preserving the Capacity for Ongoing
   Family Development after a Death, 183

10. The Death of a Child: Its Impact on Adult and Family Development   185

The Death of a Child as a Crisis of Adult
   Development, 185
Parental Grief and the Collapse of Adult Life
   Structure, 190
Early Adolescence as a Developmental Challenge to a
   Grieving Family's Postbereavement Adaptation, 201
Conclusion: The Adult and Family Developmental
   Impact of the Death of a Child, 211

PART IV: CULTURAL AND SOCIAL FACTORS IN FAMILY BEREAVEMENT

11. The Sociocultural Context of Grief   217

The Sociocultural Perspective in Clinical Work, 219
Applying a Sociocultural Perspective to Grief
   Practices in the United States, 231
Limitations of the Mental Health Field's Own
   Assumptions, 236

12. The Interweaving of Cultural Background and Family Developmental History: The Story of a Daughter's Grief   240

Background, 240
Attachment beyond the Grave: Renegotiating the
   Balance between Self-Assertion and Family Loyalty, 241
Discussion, 246
Conclusion: Expanding Our Culture-Bound Notions
   of Family Bereavement, 249

13. The Circumstances of the Death and the Structure of Grief   252

A Violent Death: The Murder of Rafael Gomez, 252
Stressors Specific to the Circumstances
   of the Death, 254
Death and the Meaning-Making Process, 264

Trauma and Bereavement, 267
Conclusion, 273

PART V: CONCLUSION

14. **Family Development and Grief Therapy**   277

References   287

Index   303

PART I

OVERVIEW

CHAPTER 1

Introduction

GRIEF AS CULTURAL CRITICISM

Death is an essential force in the cycle of life, though our North American culture, which promotes high-technology medicine and engineering solutions, often hides it from view. We presume all our natural enemies can be defeated, even death. A great deal has been written about our culture's paradoxical preoccupation with death in the years since publication of Becker's *Denial of Death* and Kübler-Ross's *Death and Dying*. Without the spiritual continuity of ancestral wisdom concerning the eternal cycles of life and death, we are left overburdened with the need to restore personal control over death and dying. The astonishing popularity of *Final Exit*, the 1992 best-seller by Humphry supporting the right of terminal patients to end their own lives on their own terms, reflects the recent recognition that high-technology medicine, when taken to extremes, deprives terminally ill patients of the right to determine the quality of their own lives at the end of life.

Yet these critical writings, which urge more direct cultural confrontation with the reality of death, have focused on the individual's struggle with the terrible finality of personal mortality and on the restoration of the individual's control over the conditions of his or her own death. In contrast to the experiences of dying patients, the deeply painful experiences of family members who survive the death of a loved one have received far less of our cultural attention. Gail Kaplan, a widow with two young children whose grief experience I describe in depth in Chapter 3, observes that almost everyone she meets talks to her as if he or she has taken "Grief 101" and is an expert on the stages of grief. Yet most people she encounters who have not directly experienced the death of a close family member find it almost impossible to tolerate the depth of her pain or to acknowledge death's radical reverberations in every aspect of her life.

The bereaved often feel profoundly isolated in this culture, in ways that are only too well exemplified by those who have experienced a relative's terminal hospitalization. Most of the people who die in this country die in hospitals, and during a terminal medical crisis their families are often deeply involved with hospital staff, including doctors, nurses, and social workers. Yet once a hospital patient dies, family members are no longer in any way entitled to services; the patient who created the link between hospital and family is gone, taking with him or her the vital administrative and financial connection that justifies family support services. Ironically, the intensive medical attention our hospitals pay to the dying patient often ultimately contributes to a sense of disconnection and isolation on the part of family members. Most physicians and nurses acknowledge that they are in the business of saving lives, a pursuit that makes death their enemy; once death has gained a victory, they want to put their own sense of failure and loss behind them and go on to the next battle with death. Family survivors present the medical staff with the discomforting reminder that death wins its own inevitable victories.

In a culture that emphasizes the accomplishments of independence rather than connection and celebrates the myth of personal mastery over all adversity, the experience of grief, which exposes our deep attachments, our human interdependence, and our true vulnerability in the hands of fate, is as unwelcome as death itself. Our culture, which fragments more and more irreparably the communal and intergenerational ties that bind us to one another, abandons family survivors of a loved one's death to a crisis of loss and a crisis of personal meaning. If we deny the enduring, intimate presence of death in the cycle of life, we are at a terrible disadvantage when death in fact intrudes on our lives. When someone we love dies, we are forced to rebuild both our shattered web of life-sustaining relationships and our shattered assumptions, which turn out to be self-protective myths, about our personal independence and control, about the modern miracle of death held properly at a distance. Death demands the creation of culturally shared customs and beliefs that address the many transformations it catalyzes in our view both of the departed one and of ourselves. Death reveals the public and private structures and meanings through which we organize, make sense of, and arrange our lives, from the sociocultural through the familial to the private and psychological. Every culture finds its own way to address these profound human dilemmas and conveys its beliefs about the natural cycle of birth, death, grief, and renewal that underlies our shared, interdependent lives. Death teaches us a great deal about how we live, sometimes more than we want to know.

I start our conversation here because in facing death we—and you, the clinicians and grief counselors who are the intended readers of this book—are first and foremost human beings who struggle within our own cultural assumptions to live meaningful lives while facing the possibility of loss and the certainty of death. If we can begin with the acknowledgment of our own human vulnerability as we encounter death, if we can consider the devastation the death of someone we love has brought, or might yet bring, to our own lives, we are very much closer to bringing real understanding and true comfort to the bereaved whose lives we join as family, friends, colleagues, and therapists. Our self-awareness when facing the challenging work of grief therapy constitutes the only deterrent against our almost inevitable attempts, both personal and professional, to bring quick resolution to the slow, complex process of healing.

In surviving the death of a close, loved family member we are unavoidably required to face death. Death forces us to dissolve and re-create the deepest human bonds that form us, from the organization of the countless daily acts that represent the inextricably interdependent nature of our lives to the emotional reverberations of these acts. We live, die, grieve, and survive within a family context in which our enduring bonds to those who came before and those who come after us need to be recognized and included. We have grown accustomed in this culture to limiting our intimate acquaintance with death, to sheltering ourselves from the potential fragility of life. When our customary bubble of denial is punctured by death, we try as quickly as possible to make sense of the event so as to maintain our personal sense of control and stability. As long as the death is not that of a close family member or friend, we are able to achieve the distance necessary to explain to ourselves why this disaster could not and will not happen to us.

My work with bereaved families has made the reality of death and its emotional aftermath a far more intimately known, accessible experience to me. My own appreciation of life and of our life-affirming bonds with others has been deeply enriched by my intimately joining these families in their agonizing encounter with loss and in their emergence from grief into the next phase of their shared family experience. In this process I have come to question how we in our culture run our family and emotional lives and how we in the mental health professions transmit these personal and cultural assumptions through the medium of our work as therapists. I think this self-questioning and life review is an inevitable—sometimes burdensome, often beneficial—consequence of close encounters with death and grief.

Our assumptions about grief in the mental health fields accurately reflect those of the wider culture, including the belief that grief is a private crisis of individuals that in its normal states hovers dangerously close to psychopathology. Practitioners committed to working with grieving families are most likely to approach bereavement as a crisis in the individual lives of children or adults. Grief is less commonly understood in terms of its impact on family interrelatedness and least often considered in terms of its impact on the development of the family unit. Most grief counselors and therapists appreciate that children and adults grieve differently in ways that are developmentally determined. Yet adult and child grief experiences are more frequently viewed in isolation, and their interrelationship—the impact of the grieving parent on a grieving child and the impact of a child's grief on a parenting adult's ability to cope—is not always recognized. Prevailing models and assumptions in both the mental health culture and our wider North American culture emphasize the health of the isolated individual rather than that of families and communities.

In this book I offer a model of family development as a framework for understanding grief within its naturally occurring place in an intergenerational family life cycle. From this family developmental perspective, grief will be seen as a shared developmental process that involves the dissolution and reconstruction of a collaborative family identity in response to a new reality, the physical absence of a vital member of the interdependent family. This family developmental model attends to both the interior (private or subjective) experiences of grief and the systemic interweaving of grief reactions in the family, community, and culture. The theoretical model of family development has provided the foundation for my clinical understanding of how best to enhance the family life cycle circumstances for shared growth and change under the highly stressful circumstances typical of family bereavement.

My work toward a clinical and theoretical understanding of family bereavement has been disturbing, disrupting, and also extraordinarily enriching for me. It is harder to deny the reality of death when we work with families who know from agonizing experience that none of us is invulnerable. We become familiar with the random, unexpected ways illness, accident, and violence can strike at the most peaceful and stable lives. We lose our illusion of magical protection from such events. Yet work with the bereaved, the heightened awareness of the impact and presence of death, can help us appreciate life as a gift not to be taken for granted. It can further help us rediscover our own intergenerational histories, inevitably bound as they are with the eternal cycles of birth, rejoicing, death, grief, affirmation, and renewal.

As a Cuban Jew whose eastern European family immigrated to

Cuba in my grandparent's generation and then left Cuba for Miami after Castro came to power, my own experience with multiple immigrations and their enduring intergenerational consequences has also guided my understanding of grief and its impact on development. So much were my own experiences filtered through the lens of the relational realities my grandparents and their Jewish ancestors created in their attempts to cope with overwhelming losses that I have had to regard events in their lives as if they were my own in order to make sense of my own multiple cultures and identities (Shapiro, 1994). My lifelong attempts to understand my own family's traumatic bereavement history and the enduring impact on the family of the upheavals and losses in my grandparent's lives have informed my current work on grief as a family developmental process that reverberates for many generations through its effects on the family's adaptive responses and subsequent reorganizations. My own and my family's experience with multiple politically motivated immigrations has enabled me, as a Jewish Cuban-American, to deeply appreciate the impact of political, historical, and cultural events in constructing the context for our own experience of loss, grief, adjustment, and renewal. I recognize in every moment of our shared family lives the enduring presence of past losses out of which we will continue to weave our shared family futures.

HOW TO READ THIS BOOK

This book is written for those professionals who provide bereavement counseling or therapy to children, adults, and/or families. The goal of the book is to introduce readers from a variety of theoretical and clinical practice perspectives to an integrative, systemic developmental model of grief. For grief counselors and therapists accustomed to working with individual children or adults, the book provides a review of new work in the fields of family systems and relational developmental perspectives that can expand their understanding of individual grief in a family context and grief as an interdependent developmental process. For family therapists who work with grieving families, the book includes developmental perspectives on both child and adult grief that are ordinarily not part of the family therapist's systemically informed understanding of bereavement. In order to make a wide variety of technical literatures accessible to all readers, I introduce the different theoretical sources for a systemic model in as simple a language as possible. I also rely heavily on clinical case descriptions to demonstrate the practical application of an integrative, systemic developmental model.

A systemic developmental approach that simultaneously considers individual, family, and cultural dimensions presents the writer and
reader with the problem of where best to begin. The family developmental model carefully considers the subjective experience of individual grief while appreciating the coconstruction of grief in family
and sociocultural contexts over the course of the family life cycle. Part
I, Overview, consists of two chapters, this introduction (Chapter 1)
and an overview of the systemic developmental approach to family
bereavement (Chapter 2). In Part II, Individual Grief in Systemic Context, four chapters describe the experiences and developmental implications of grief for adults (Chapters 3 and 4) and children (Chapters 5 and 6). These chapters use the systemic developmental model
to critique existing, individually oriented bereavement literatures and
also highlight new relationship oriented approaches compatible with
a family systemic approach to grief. Theoretical reviews of the adult
(Chapter 3) and child (Chapter 5) bereavement literatures are followed
by chapters that elaborate the treatment implications of this approach
through case examples. Chapter 4 offers an in-depth view of Gail
Kaplan's grief experience and its impact on her development as it
evolved during three years of weekly therapy after the death of her
husband. Chapter 6 offers case examples of children at different ages
and stages of development from infancy to adolescence. The clinical
examples of children's grief draw on the earlier review of adult grief
so as to increase one's understanding of how a bereaved adult's needs
impact on the parenting processes so crucial to a grieving child's
developmental outcome.

Part III, Grieving Families and Their Shared Development, consists of four chapters: Chapter 7 discusses family systems; Chapter 8
discusses family developmental approaches to grief; Chapter 9 describes through case examples different family strategies for stability
after a death; and Chapter 10 describes the impact of the death of a
child on parental and family development.

Part IV, Cultural and Social Factors in Family Bereavement, con-
tains three chapters on cultural and social factors in bereavement,
including a theoretical overview on the sociocultural context of grief
(Chapter 11), an in-depth clinical example of grief work involving a
Puerto Rican woman whose mother died of cancer (Chapter 12), and
a theoretical review with case vignettes of the circumstances of the
death as they affect a family's grief (Chapter 13). The concluding chapter (Chapter 14) provides an overview of the treatment implications
of the systemic developmental approach in enhancing the developmental outcomes for grieving children, adults, and families.

CHAPTER 2

A Systemic Developmental Approach to Family Bereavement

GRIEF AND ITS FAMILY CHOREOGRAPHY

I was on my way back to Boston from a conference and on the plane sat next to Nancy, a woman in her early fifties who was also traveling alone. As we talked about our lives and work—Nancy was a teacher at a private school—I mentioned that I was writing a book on family bereavement. Her face filled with intense emotion as she told me that her husband, Paul, had died suddenly and unexpectedly 15 years ago, leaving her with three young children at home, ages 3, 7, and 10. By most measures of grief outcome, Nancy and her children would be considered a well-functioning family that had never required psychotherapy in completing a successful recovery from grief. Yet 15 years later they were still working through the implications of the death of father and husband for their shared lives. While the acute pain and disruption of death and grief were well behind them, the enduring emotions of loss were immediately, vividly accessible, as if Paul had died yesterday. The little I said about my approach to family bereavement reassured Nancy that I would not consider her family disturbed for continuing to struggle with the implications of their loss in their ongoing family lives. Eager to talk about her experience, Nancy asked me if I would mind reviewing her family's grief reaction with her. During the remainder of the flight she related their still unfolding family story.

Why is Nancy's story important to our understanding of grief as a family developmental process? When a parent or sibling dies with young children still at home, the gradual, expectable ebb and flow of change over the course of the family life cycle is radically altered. The family is challenged to absorb the reality of the death, with its many emotional and practical implications, into the already demanding work of growing up together as a family. Nancy and her family illustrate well the persistent developmental impact of death and grief as loss and bereavement both redirect the course of family development and become interwoven with the family's developmental tasks, even for those who succeed in reestablishing family life after a member's death. Nancy's story introduces a systemic developmental model of bereavement that suggests how practitioners might best support the ongoing growth of grieving families. Grief is at heart a family process, and it is within that process that the injury to an interdependent sense of self can best be understood—and healed.

Nancy had felt absolutely shattered and numbed with shock at the first news of her husband's death. With the advances of modern medicine we no longer expect the death of young children and young parents. Nancy and Paul had done practical financial planning, like purchasing life insurance for Paul, but without in any way emotionally connecting such planning with the reality of death. Nothing in her life as a stay-at-home wife and mother, depending so completely on patterns of shared support established over the course of courtship, marriage, and early parenting, had prepared Nancy for the total disintegration of her psychological integrity and the collapse of her daily family life. She was now left alone to parent her three children, all of whom had suffered the agonizing blow of a father's death. In spite of her own and her children's enormous anguish, Nancy had to mobilize immediately to maintain the integrity and continuity of the family as best she could.

As a young widow whose husband had died unexpectedly and who had young children still at home, Nancy was in one of the highest-risk categories for complicated bereavement (Beckwith et al., 1990; Glick, Weiss, & Parkes, 1974; Parkes & Weiss, 1983). She was fortunate to have had sufficient financial resources to enable the family to stay in their home and to keep their daily lives relatively stable. Social supports, economic resources, and stability in the home and caretaking environment are protective factors associated with better outcome for grieving families (Ben-Sira, 1983; Osterweis, Solomon, & Green, 1984; Parkes & Weiss, 1983; Raphael, 1983; Sanders, 1989; Vachon et al., 1982). Nancy had earned a college degree in teaching and was able to return to a previously established career. Although she needed the income from her part-time job, she also appreciated it as an opportunity to make a fresh start among her peers. Because her family life, always a source of great joy and pleasure, now also served as a constant reminder of her grief and loss, she valued the new demands and relationships that came with her job, which allowed her to leave her grief momentarily behind her.

Nancy's three children differed in their responses to their father's death in ways that seemed, at the same time, personally characteristic, age related, and attuned to the needs of other family members. Her oldest child, 10-year-old Cara, had been the most hidden about her grief, so much so that it was sometimes easy to forget how deeply affected she was. Cara's heightened emotional vulnerability had been well hidden under the "don't worry, I'm fine" demeanor so typical of elementary-school-age children who are bereaved. Shortly after her father's death, Cara insisted that she could perfectly well handle a trip to visit friends of the family in Florida. But when she began to experience separation anxiety that bordered on panic, she had to turn around and come back. The separation from her family provided Cara with her first opportunity to express her displaced grief. As she told me about this incident, Nancy asked herself whether she had perhaps been too ready to accept Cara's reassurances that she was perfectly fine. Why didn't she anticipate Cara's vulnerability at such a substantial separation? Did she perhaps have reasons of her own for seeing Cara as well adjusted?

Seven-year-old Ron had become quieter than usual and worried about Nancy's whereabouts immediately after his father's death. However, he made few references to his father and appeared to adjust quickly to Nancy's new work schedule.

In contrast to his two older siblings, 3-year-old Mark had been unrestrained in his questions about his father's death and in his direct statements that he missed him. While Mark would refer to his father spontaneously and openly, other family members were often afraid to do so; it was as if they were afraid they might disturb their fragile emotional stability with too great an upsurge of their grief. Nancy had tried to respond to Mark's questions as openly and as fully as her emotional tolerance would allow, given her preoccupation with her own loss. She wondered now if her need to put her own grief aside had eventually silenced Mark's initially open expressions of grief and the questions he asked about his father's life and death.

Looking back, Nancy realized how preoccupied she and the children had been with coping well and going on with their lives. She worried that perhaps they had achieved this successful coping with their new life circumstances at the expense of sharing their deepest grief with one another. "Why do families find it so hard to share their grief?" Nancy asked me.

ANSWERING NANCY'S QUESTION

Nancy's question is a complex and fundamentally important one for grieving families and those of us who wish to help them. In order to answer her question, we need to appreciate the impact of death and grief on family development. Grief is a deeply shared family developmental transition, involving a crisis of attachment and a crisis of identity for family members, both of which have to be incorporated into the ongoing flow of family development. Both the management of our intense emotions and the organization of a personal identity are achieved through a collaborative, mutually responsive family developmental process throughout the family life cycle. In this collaborative developmental process, a balance of change and stability provides the essential foundation for a healthy, growth-promoting adaptation to and integration of changing life circumstances. Death interrupts the normal flow of family developmental time and redirects the course of family development. In response to the massive discontinuity precipitated by death and grief, families struggle to absorb and integrate their losses so as to reestablish the stability necessary to restore the flow of developmental time and resume ongoing family development.

From a family developmental perspective, relationships are the constituent elements of self. When death interrupted her marital bond, the transformations in Nancy's sense of self as wife and mother had to include the reality both of the loss and of Paul's enduring psychological and spiritual importance as husband and father in the radically restructured family. When death interrupted the father–child bond for Nancy's three children, they continued to need their father to support their ongoing development; now they needed him as an enduring psychological and spiritual presence who could accompany them and grow with them over the course of their development. Parenting is the crucial pivot point around which intergenerational processes of family bereavement are organized, since the surviving spouse's developmental work in reconstructing a sense of self as spouse and parent creates the family expectations that children use to guide their own grief reactions.

Grief counselors often emphasize that a family's best pathway to healthy coping is the expressing and sharing of the overwhelming emotions of grief. Yet under the emotionally overwhelming conditions of acute grief, families struggle first to reestablish emotional control and the stability of their daily lives. Grief disrupts family stability in the interrelated domains of managing intense emotions, organizing family interactions and patterns of communication, defining effective social roles, and creating an ongoing family narrative of shared meanings. A family's first priority in managing the crisis of grief is reestablishing the stable equilibrium necessary to support ongoing family development. Establishing these new stable family structures requires individual, family systemic, community, and sociocultural resources. The greater a family's resources and supports, the greater the flexibility with which they can reestablish shared family functioning. The greater a family's degree of stress and disruption or discontinuity, the greater its need for establishing constraining strategies for stability, which are designed to limit further disequilibrating change.

Paul's death initiated a period of enormous stress as his family both coped with the emotional loss and tried to reestablish their daily functioning. Looking back on their experience, Nancy could see that she and the children had reorganized their lives and had survived the worst of the emotional upheaval psychologically intact; in overcoming their hardships they had shared a great deal of closeness and satisfaction as a family. But Nancy also knew that they had never forgotten, and in a certain sense never gotten over, the loss of husband and father at such a vital, early point in their family lives. Nancy herself had never remarried. Busy with the often overwhelming demands of teaching, running a complex household, and bringing up her children alone, she seemed never to have found either the time or the energy for dating. Even now, after all the years of successfully coping with her sorrow and rebuilding her own life and the shared family life, she still felt the empty space at the heart of the family and the poignancy of experiencing alone what she and Paul might have shared. Paul was always missing, and missed, at the important milestones of the family. As much as the family had worked to successfully repair the torn fabric of their lives, they were still less than they should have been as a family, less than they would have been with father and husband in their midst.

As our conversation continued Nancy told me that with Mark's graduation from high school and departure for college coming up in a few months the children—now young adults—were beginning to talk with her about their father's life and death. They were asking more questions about their lives together as a family prior to his death and about the agonizing months and years immediately following it. As Nancy began to look back with them, she deeply regretted the difficulty they had all experienced in sharing the enormity of their pain, each struggling in his or her own private way. She now wondered if therapy might have enabled them to more fully share their private experiences of grief with one another.

Resolving the Paradox of Grief and Growth: Balancing Change and Stability

The dual nature of grief, as a crisis of attachment and a crisis of identity for interdependent family members, has important implications for our formulation of optimal therapeutic support for grieving families. We therapists assume that the open sharing of intense, private emotional reactions is a necessary part of normal bereavement for individuals and families. Yet the first priority for a grieving family is reestablishing the stable family conditions that support the family's day-to-day functioning. Moreover, the shared coping with the crisis of family bereavement requires an enormously complex process of mutual awareness and responsiveness. Resonating both consciously and unconsciously to emotional cues from one another, family members responsively adapt to each other's attempts to control overwhelming emotions, reestablish stable patterns of daily living and relating, and reconstruct a sense of self. They become very attuned to the ebb and flow of grief in other family members and try to minimize disconcerting perturbations, hoping to keep their heads above water in what often feel like overwhelming or incapacitating waves of sorrow.

While the family developmental process for managing intense emotions and supporting ongoing development is shared, children and adults also manage grief in distinctive ways that best support their own development. For adults, whose ongoing development is substantially organized by the structures of marriage, parenting, and work, the overwhelming pain and radical discontinuity of bereavement often initiates a period of withdrawal from others and retreat into a private reality within which the enormity of the loss can be gradually acknowledged and from which coherent new life structures can be gradually rebuilt. Children understand death and grief with the cognitive and emotional tools of a particular developmental moment and rely heavily on adults to help them interpret the implications of an overwhelming new reality. For children, the unremitting pace of adult grief is too intense, too much an interference with the necessary work of growing up. Children are more likely to put their grief down and pick it up again, a manner of coping that adults might consider callous if they see the child only during moments of distancing and not during the moments of longing and intense recognition of their loss.

Both adults and children integrate the emotional reality of a death in the family gradually, in ways that are cognitively manageable and that do not totally overwhelm their capacity to cope with the requirements of daily living. The choreography of family members' private grief reactions is seldom synchronous or simultaneous. Nor should it be: The capacity of family members to recognize and respect their differences in grief reactions and coping style is crucial to healthy family bereavement.

Yet sharing one's grief experience, feeling understood and responded to by other family members, and reestablishing a coherent sense of the family's past, present, and future have been found to be important dimensions of a healthy recovery process in the individual. Even when families appear to have coped well with the enormous loss and to have recovered in many ways, as does Nancy's family, members can still feel that their most important life experiences are sealed off from contact with those who would most fully understand the pain and poignancy of the loss. In some families the loss of access to shared grief can substantially compound the losses associated with the death and can contribute to a profound sense of isolation. Especially depriving is a family's loss of shared access to recollections of the deceased, with members refraining from sharing their thoughts and memories out of concern that they might disturb their own emotional stability or that of other family members.

The open emotional exploration and integration of a death and its many implications for every aspect of life is, paradoxically, a necessary developmental luxury. We can risk the potentially destabilizing exploration of our own and our family's anguish only when there is sufficient access to resources that support the safe reestablishment of stable functioning. Such healthy family systems dynamics as strategies for reestablishing equilibrium in the face of overwhelming stress or instituting family communication patterns designed to manage distressing feelings are supportive resources that are mobilized by any family trauma, including a family death. While failures of open communication may in some instances be maladaptive, the control of communication concerning the depths of grief can also be an adaptive support enabling each family member to successfully cope with his or her experience of grief. In fact, both clinical evidence and research suggest that there are many individual and family pathways for coping with grief and that the exploration of distressing feelings is in some instances quite disruptive to the tasks of stable emotional reorganization and functional adaptation (Baker, Sedney, & Gross, 1992; Polak, Egan, Vanderbergh, & Williams, 1975; Silverman & Worden, 1992; Vollman, Ganzert, Picher, & Williams, 1971; Weiss, 1988; Wortman & Silver, 1989).

Sources of Growth-Enhancing Stability

The process of restoring family equilibrium so as to tolerate the massive disruptions and integrate the enormous implications of death and grief requires the creation of new self-organizing structures for the family. The resources for instituting new stable structures for the family include the following:

1. Private individual processes for managing intense emotions and making sense of an overwhelming experience
2. Family system strategies for shared stabilization under circumstances of overwhelming stress
3. Extended family and community supports for managing day-to-day living and interpreting the meaning of the death and loss
4. Cultural rituals interpreting the death and its meanings and prescribing roles for the survivors

All of these dimensions of stabilizing or organizing structure—from the intrapsychic, through the familial and community, to the cultural—contribute to a family's stability during any period of family developmental transition, including the developmental crisis of grief. The greater the realistic stresses accompanying the grief experience, and the fewer the real-life supports, the greater a family's need to rely on growth-constraining psychological structures for stability. From a systemic developmental perspective, we will be most interested in understanding when a family's strategies for stable reorganization have inordinately interfered with its members' access to emotional experience and flexible, creative responsiveness to new situations.

Nancy worried that her family had coped with Paul's death without fully sharing the profound emotional costs and their enduring sense of loss. Yet she herself recognized that Mark's departure for college provided the family with a new developmental opportunity to reconsider their bereavement experience. Mark, only 3 when Paul died, now needed to expand his image of his father as a resource in his evolving image of himself as a man. The ongoing, shared process of development provides families with new opportunities to reexplore their grief experience at later points in the family life cycle, when their adaptation to the death does not feel as new and fragile, and the reexploration of the grief experience in turn allows families to achieve a new integration of their shared emotional adaptation and can serve to expand the emotional resources available for a family's ongoing developmental work.

A SYSTEMIC DEVELOPMENTAL FRAMEWORK
FOR FAMILY BEREAVEMENT

A systemic developmental framework for the understanding of family bereavement is based on the following conclusions:

1. Grief is a family developmental crisis that becomes interwoven with family history and current developmental moment and radically redirects the future course of shared family development.

2. Grief is a crisis of both attachment and identity, disrupting family stability in the interrelated domains of emotions, interactions, social roles, and meanings. Grief mobilizes a family's resources for managing intense emotions, reorganizing daily interactions, and redefining the identity of the complex, collaborative self.

3. A family's first priority in managing the crisis of grief is reestablishing the stable equilibrium necessary to support ongoing family development. Resources for new stable structures include the individual, the family system, the community, and the sociocultural environment.

4. The shared developmental process of establishing growth-enhancing stability while gradually integrating a new sense of the complex, collaborative self is lifelong. The timing of family bereavement will vary with the degree of stress and discontinuity in the circumstances of the death, the balance of stress and support, the nature of the shared developmental history, and the nature of cultural grief practices.

5. The greater the family's degree of stress and the degree of discontinuity, the greater the need for growth-constraining structures (intrapsychic and/or interpersonal) that dissociate overwhelming aspects of the grief experience, reestablish stability, and restrict further disequilibrating change.

6. Over the course of the family life cycle, families continue integrating the reality of the death and its consequences for reorganizing every aspect of the collaborative self. New stages of family development stimulate new realizations of loss but also provide creative new opportunities for growth-enhancing integration of previously fragmented aspects of the grief experience and a new, more inclusive, organization of the complex, collaborative self.

7. Changing family relationships will include transformations of the relationship to the deceased, whose enduring image provides support for the ongoing development of surviving family members. Ideally, the deceased will be reintegrated into the family as a living,

evolving spiritual and psychological presence whose image is brought forward with the family in developmental time and who continues to support the family's development.

8. The goal of family bereavement is to restore the flow of developmental time and resume ongoing family development. Healthy grief reactions involve growth-enhancing strategies for reestablishing stability; problematic grief reactions involve growth-constraining strategies for stability that interfere with ongoing family development.

The systemic developmental model of family bereavement offered in this book is not meant to replace a grief therapist's professional working models and personal style. Rather, it is meant to extend a clinician's awareness of a grieving individual's developmental stage at the time of the death and the impact of the death on the individual's web of life-sustaining relationships. A family developmental model allows us to formulate our interventions as grief counselors and therapists with children, adults, and families so as to expand the family's emotional encounter with their loss while at the same time supporting their growth-enhancing strategies for stability. With a developmental approach that considers the family as a unit of distinct yet inextricably interconnected members, we can help families survive and grow while bearing the burden of death and loss.

PART II

INDIVIDUAL GRIEF IN SYSTEMIC CONTEXT

CHAPTER 3

Grief in Adulthood

ADULT BEREAVEMENT AS A SYSTEMIC
DEVELOPMENTAL PROCESS

If the bereaved adults I have worked with are any indication, Pincus (1974) is right in stating that many of the newly bereaved feel the first blow of grief almost as a death blow, a heartbreak they might in fact not survive. The initial sensations of grief in adulthood are profoundly and simply physical and physiological. The bereaved typically describe a chronic pain like a scraping or rasping in their chest and difficulty breathing and sometimes swallowing, symptoms suggesting the location of heartbreak and the physical stress of holding back torrents of tears and screams of protest. Mourners are vulnerable to disruption of every aspect of their physiological functioning, including disruption of sleep and appetite and even depression of the immune system (Hofer, 1984; Osterweis, Solomon, & Green, 1984).

While the physiological responses of grief and depression have a great deal in common, the physical state of the bereaved cannot be understood simply as equivalent to a condition of profound depression. All of us learn to pattern and regulate our most basic, seemingly private functions, such as emotional fluctuations, thoughts, actions, appetite, and sleep, in responsive relating to others. When these relational patterns of self-regulation are disrupted by death, we have to learn how to reestablish these functions under radically different circumstances. Our own capacity for independent functioning, the supportive resources of others, and, most importantly, a transformed, internalized image of the lost loved one are all essential to the reestablishment of self-regulation. While awareness of the initial blow of grief is cushioned by shock, mourners immediately suffer a radical disruption in their capacity for biological regulation.

Most adults describe an enduring sense of unreality and a thereafter divided consciousness in their initial response to the news of a loved one's death. Part of them has heard the news that their spouse or child has died and begins the slow, arduous process of making sense of it. Part of them refuses to believe, reserves judgment on reality, and hopes the whole episode is a big mistake, someone's idea of a joke, anything but real. In this initial state mourners are unable to break the habits of thought, feeling, and relating by which they construct their sense of self in the world. This initial state has a great deal in common with the shock of a physical injury—the details of the moment are vividly amplified, but the reality of what has happened, including the full sensation of pain, is cushioned by shock.

The blow of death, first and foremost, shatters our view of the world into confusing fragments. The first formidable task is the one of hearing, recognizing, and acknowledging that a disaster has taken place. We feel we cannot live in a world in which our life-sustaining relationships disappear abruptly. When we discover that indeed we can, we have initiated a revolution in the stability of every dimension of our lives, not only in our patterns of relating but also in our patterns of thought and feeling, which themselves depend on our relational world for organization and modulation. The first moments, days, and months immediately after the death of a close family member are taken up with the monumental task of regaining some psychological equilibrium in the face of a shattering blow that has irretrievably changed every dimension of our inner and outer worlds. From my discussions of the initial experience of the news of a death with the recently bereaved, I have concluded that most mourners do not exercise a simple form of denial; rather, they enter a world of unreality characterized by a divided consciousness. The perceptual or emotional defense mechanism the bereaved most often describe comes closest to what we would call *dissociation*: One part of us recognizes the external, lived reality even at the same time that we remove or reject it from working, or ongoing, consciousness.

Very slowly, over many months and often many years, the reality of the death is acknowledged and integrated into ongoing patterns of living, thinking, and feeling. It is always surprising at first to realize how densely "peopled" our habits of mind and of daily living are, how many of our associations lead spontaneously to thoughts of those we love. It is only when these associations become paired with an awareness of painful loss that we appreciate the depth of our interrelatedness. A series of thoughts may begin so innocently and may end unexpectedly with a poignant pang of loss: A recently widowed mother of two young children drives across town to pick up her son at nursery school. She notices in the flow of traffic a car packed for a family vacation, the bicycle racks holding bikes for two adults and two children, the roof rack loaded with suitcases. She is seized with a simultaneous image that begins with what would ordinarily be a pleasurable recollection—she has been on many bicycle trips with the family and knows what it is like to load up the car, remembers the chaos, irritability, and the feeling of reckless relief when the family is finally, whatever they might have forgotten, on their way—but is almost immediately overcome by an associative spasm of pain and grief. She realizes that she cannot lift those suitcases and bicycles to their racks by herself, and that the next time she goes on a family vacation, she and her children will have to go off alone; she is the sole surviving grown-up and parent. The pain of what she and her children have lost washes over her, and she pulls over to the side of the road until she can stop sobbing and continue driving to the nursery school to pick up her son.

It takes many years to achieve the reconstruction of one's adult life and the reorganization of one's adult sense of self, which is shattered by the blow of grief. The mental health field is beginning to realize the long-term nature of the grief and recovery process. Until now the adult bereavement literature in our field has mirrored the commonly held cultural assumption that grief is a time-limited process (of, at most, a year's duration) after which the mourner is ready to go on with his or her life. Indeed, we clinicians ourselves would like to be reassured that grief is a blow from which we can in fact recover; we would like to see those who have suffered the death of a loved one— our relatives, friends, patients, neighbors, coworkers—resume full lives in which they appreciate their surviving relationships and establish new ones.

Our cultural attitude toward bereavement has been reflected in the assumption of many clinicians that a fairly complete recovery should be possible within a circumscribed period of time. This recovery, we further assume, will always include a complete letting go of the relationship with the deceased and the capacity to seek new relationships to replace the lost one. If such a recovery does not occur, clinicians have tended to search for the psychopathology in the adult's early history or in the nature of the relationship with the deceased that is responsible for the prolonged grief reaction. In fact, longitudinal research has been finding that the process of recovery from the death of a close family member is far more prolonged than we would like to acknowledge, that indeed it is in many instances lifelong. Many adults do return to a reasonable level of successful external functioning within 2 or 3 years of a death, especially the death of a spouse (Glick et al., 1974; Koocher, 1986; Lehman, Wortman, & Williams, 1987; Osterweis et al., 1984; Silverman, 1986; Weiss, 1988). The impact of the death of a child on the surviving parents has been found to be more devastating (Koocher, 1986; Rando, 1986; Raphael, 1983; Sanders, 1989; Shanfield and Swain, 1984; Shanfield, Benjamin, & Swain, 1984; Videka-Sherman & Lieberman, 1985).

The research literature on adult grief resolution is plagued by serious methodological problems, especially in the assessment of bereavement symptomatology and life satisfaction; studies may lack adequate control groups or use scales that fail to provide adequate comparison group norms (Osterweis et al., 1984; Stroebe & Stroebe, 1987). Studies reported in the literature on adult recovery differ as to whether they look for formal psychiatric symptomatology (e.g., an increase in depression) or signs of prolonged grief, such as frequent ruminations about the deceased or about the circumstances of the death. After a meticulous review of the bereavement outcome literature for widows and widowers, Stroebe and Stroebe (1987) conclude that the evidence suggests, even accounting for methodological problems, that the widowed are consistently worse off than the married when they are compared for psychiatric disorders, physical illness, or mortality.

The mental health fields are constantly revising their prescriptive understanding of what characterizes the "normal" course of grief and what characterizes its final end point. An illness model would have us look for a return to prior levels of emotional and social functioning within a specified period of time. Yet, as most current observations of bereavement reveal, recovery from grief cannot be taken to mean that we return, unchanged, to the way we were before the loss of a close family member. Weiss (1988) notes that many bereaved people characterize their experience by saying, "You don't get over it, you get used to it." Weiss suggests that traditional notions of recovery do not accurately characterize the deep upheaval precipitated by the loss of a primary attachment figure. However, he finds it useful to assess at what point bereaved people recover their capacity for ordinary functioning in their day-to-day lives and at what point they recover their sense of emotional stability, capacity for pleasure, and energy for living.

In spite of successful external adaptation to their new life circumstances, most adults who have lost a close famiy member describe their lives, their family relationships, and their sense of themselves as inextricably altered. Grieving adults are changed not only by the death but also by the subsequent upheavals in the pattern of their daily lives, their inner emotions, and their relationships with surviving family members. Grieving adults often continue a significant involvement with poignant memories of the deceased—and do so in the face of considerable cultural prohibition. Ongoing family relationships are important sources of support for recovery from adult grief. Yet the demands of family life, especially the now even heavier work of parenting under circumstances of shared grief, can make ongoing family relationships sources of increased stress as well.

Many dimensions of an individual adult's circumstances contribute to the nature of the grief reaction. Factors such as the adult's family history and internalized family-of-origin relationships, history of previous losses, personality organization and coping style, and capacity to make use of existing social supports, as well as the nature of the person's relationship with the deceased and the availability of social supports, do in fact contribute significantly to the depth and duration of the grief experience (Bowlby, 1980; Osterweis et al., 1984; Parkes, 1972; Parkes & Weiss, 1983; Sanders, 1989; Stroebe & Stroebe, 1987). In addition, the actual circumstances of the death, the degree to which the death is experienced as traumatic, and the degree to which the adult can feel realistically (rather than neurotically or defensively) responsible for the occurrence of a fatal accident or the handling of an illness will also prolong the course of adult grief (Bowlby, 1980; Koocher, 1986; Osterweis et al., 1984; Parkes & Weiss, 1983; Raphael, 1983; Sanders, 1989). These dimensions of the grief experience create a continuum along which grief reactions can be found to be more or less severe or prolonged. However, when assessing the grief reaction of any individual or family, we must always keep in mind the extreme upheaval the bereaved are forced to undergo when coping with the loss of a family member. Even the most prolonged and severe grief reactions represent an individual's best efforts to cope with the extraordinary pressures of death and grief.

MODELS OF ADULT BEREAVEMENT

The adult bereavement literature has drawn from three major theoretical approaches: clinical, primarily psychoanalytic, theories emphasizing intrapsychic process (Freud, 1917/1957a; Pollock, 1961; Volkan, 1981); psychosocial theories emphasizing adaptation to crisis or social role transition (Lindemann, 1944; Parkes, 1972; Silverman, 1986); and attachment theory applied to adult grief (Bowlby, 1979, 1980; Raphael, 1983; Weiss, 1988). In the last decade a number of volumes have extensively surveyed the field of adult bereavement (Bowlby, 1980; Osterweis et al., 1984; Parkes, 1972; Rando, 1986; Raphael, 1983; Sanders, 1989; Silverman, 1986; Stroebe & Stroebe, 1987).

A systemic developmental approach to adult bereavement examines the experience of grief and recovery from the perspective of the relationally organized self: How is the adult grief experience a developmental crisis of *both* attachment and identity, functions shaped by the ebb and flow of changing family relationships throughout the course of the family life cycle? Adult development is constructed out of a web of intergenerational relationships evolving together through developmental time. With the death of a close family member, all of these family relationships, including the relationship with the deceased, will be transformed and reconfigured. Changes in our important relationships initiate a crisis of transformation in the collaboratively constructed adult self.

Family relationships will be called upon as supportive resources in the adult developmental process of relational transformation following the death of a family member. Yet the push and pull of new vulnerabilities and demands, the sometimes conflicting or discrepant cycles of grief and need, will make these newly burdened family relationships sources of stress and disappointment as well as support. An adult who loses a marital partner will need to work out a new image of self in marriage that now includes the reality of death and loss. If the adult is a parent, he or she will now be the single parent of children who have lost a parent to death. Grieving children will be struggling with their own sense of loss and will need more from their surviving parent. Adults who lose a child will need to work out a new image of self as parent that now includes both the child who has died and any surviving children. Children who lose a sibling will themselves feel emotionally vulnerable and will need more support from their parents in coping with the loss and making sense of the death. The marital relationship of grieving parents will also be reconfigured as couples collaboratively cope with the heavy new demands, realistic and emotional, associated with a child's accident or illness and death. A systemic developmental perspective on adult bereavement locates the individual adult grief reaction in its family relational context.

In order to make use of the existing adult bereavement literature as part of a systemic developmental theory, we will need to examine the embedded cultural assumptions that shape our clinical theories of grief. Freud's influential writing on grief presents an excellent case study itself, for it shows the mix of accurate observation, cultural belief, and personal distortion based on unique life experience that constitutes any clinical theory. Freud's vivid, in many ways accurate, description of grief is embedded within a much more problematic theoretical framework that has been passed down by generations of psychodynamically informed clinicians as the essential way to think about grief (Frankiel, 1994). The clinical literature on grief is especially vulnerable to cultural bias and personal distortion because clinicians, like most human beings facing the shattering implications of death and grief, want to be reassured that grief is a blow from which one does in fact recover.

The Psychoanalytic Legacy in Adult Bereavement: A Systemic Developmental Critique

The clinical literature on grief begins with Freud's (1917) influential "Mourning and Melancholia," an essay that contrasts normal grief following the actual death of a loved one with pathological melancholia. Melancholia gives the appearance of grief but is stimulated by psychological, rather than real, object loss or disappointment. Freud emphasized that in the normal process of bereavement the goal of recovery is the relinquishment of the mourner's ties to the love object. According to Freud (1917/1957a), we cathect libido, or infuse psychic energy, onto a love object over the course of life, a connection that is "strengthened by a thousand links" (p. 167). When a love object dies, the task of grief is the decathexis or detachment of libido from the original love object so that libido is available for investment in a new object. This process, which Freud called "the work of mourning," is a time- and energy-consuming one because the mourner rebels against the reality of the object loss and is reluctant to abandon the original attachment. The struggle to maintain the attachment will often include a period in which the reality of the death is denied.

Over time, the reality of the death slowly asserts itself; according to Freud (1917), this process of relinquishment requires many small realizations:

> Reality passes its verdict—that the object no longer exists—upon each single one of the memories and hopes through which the libido was attached to the lost object, and the ego, confronted as it were with the decision whether it will share this fate, is persuaded by the sum of its narcissistic satisfactions in being alive to sever its attachment to the nonexistent object. (p. 166)

Freud acknowledged that the process of decathexis is a slow one. However, he asserted that normal grief ends with complete decathexis or detachment from a love object no longer present in reality and therefore no longer offering gratification.

Freud defined melancholia, or pathological grief, whether in response to a death or to some other kind of loss, as a refusal to relinquish the love object. In these cases, often marked by narcissistic or ambivalent attachments, the ego is unable to decathect the love object, which is both loved and hated. The ambivalent ego instead identifies with the love object: "So by taking flight into the ego love escapes annihilation" (Freud, 1917, p. 168). The person experiencing melancholia is then free to attack his or her own ego in an excess of remorse and guilt. This self-criticism serves the dual purpose for the mourner of voicing surreptitious recriminations against the disappointing love object while at the same time refusing to relinquish the object tie, which is now enshrined in the mourner's ego.

Subsequent psychoanalytic formulations of grief continue to incorporate Freud's initial statement that the normal outcome of grief requires the relinquishment of all ties to the object. In fact, very few mourners seem capable of this ideal resolution. To solve this problem, psychoanalytic theorists have turned to Freud's statement that ambivalent attachments are resolved through identification. Since most normal relationships are in part ambivalent, it becomes possible to account for the prevalence of enduring object ties in most mourners by viewing them as a form of identification (Fenichel, 1945). Most grieving adults remain connected to their dead loved ones even when the reality is that the dead person is no longer available to provide relational gratification.

Those of us who have worked extensively with grieving adults can recognize in many of them the applicability of Freud's description of grief as a state often characterized by denial of reality, identification with the lost object, or denial of ambivalence and predominance of guilt. Freud's evocative description of the slow, painful image-by-image process of confrontation with the reality of loss has been echoed by other writers, including the bereaved themselves. A psychoanalytic perspective that acknowledges the complex, unconscious, conflictual nature of our attachments is essential to a complete understanding of our human bonds in life and in death. Nevertheless, Freud's psychoanalytic legacy in the field of adult bereavement is the permanence of two burdensome tendencies: (1) to "pathologize" grief by regarding normal grief in the light of processes more often observed in symptomatic clinical populations and (2) to perpetuate the belief that normal bereavement is concluded with the relinquishment or dissolution of all ties to the lost object. Why, classical psychoanalytic theory asks, would we want to maintain attachments to the dead when they can no longer gratify our needs? The vision of human relatedness and grief perpetuated by this theory, namely, that human beings view each other as interchangeable objects of need gratification, persists in part because this egoistic point of view strikes a resonant chord in our individualistic, self-referential culture.

The Biographical Context of Theory:
Grief in Freud's Life

A review of Freud's writings on grief, both theoretical papers and private letters, suggests that Freud's view was influenced by his own personal losses and was transformed by significant deaths throughout his life. Freud wrote "Mourning and Melancholia" in 1917, a time when thoughts of death were very much with him: He was surrounded by the reality of death in the First World War and feared the deaths of his three enlisted sons, who disappeared from contact for a substantial, and terrifying, period of time. By that time in his life Freud had experienced the death of an infant brother (when Freud was 23 months old), the importance of which he defensively minimized, and the death of his elderly father, which precipitated the life crisis and self-analysis that resulted in his most creative theoretical work. He had not yet experienced the deaths of a daughter and a grandson, which would radically alter his perception of grief in his own life, if not in the official writings of psychoanalytic theory.

At the age of 42, Freud underwent a significant life crisis subsequent to the death of his elderly father in 1894. At the time of his father's death, Freud was in the midst of his ground-breaking self-analysis and was working on the problems of hysteria and the interpretation of dreams. He became preoccupied with thoughts of his own death and was convinced that he would not live past the age of 51 (Gay, 1988). Masson (1984) suggests that the crisis precipitated by the death of his father resulted in Freud's renouncing his seduction theory, which postulated that neurosis is caused by actual sexual abuse. Freud considered himself and two of his four sisters neurotic, and in his correspondence with Wilhelm Fliess prior to his father's death he revealed his assumption that there were incidents of sexual abuse in their own childhood histories. Masson argues that Freud chose to see childhood sexuality as wished-for fantasy rather than abusive reality as a means of assuaging his postbereavement guilt about accusing his own father of sexual perversion. Mitchell (1992) notes that while Freud's ground-breaking studies of hysteria from this phase in his writing were masterfully attuned to issues of repressed sexuality, they were equally notable for overlooking the subjects of death and grief, which were also central themes in the cases upon which the studies of hysteria were based.

Although Freud recognized the considerable upheaval precipitated in himself by his father's death, he felt he had recovered from this loss in the ways he described for the normal course of bereavement in "Mourning and Melancholia." In 1917 he had not yet faced the two significant and crushing losses that would affect the remainder of his adult life: the death at age 27 of Sofie, the second of his three daughters, in the 1920 postwar flu epidemic and the death in 1923 of Heinnele, age 4, Sofie's younger son and Freud's favorite grandson. Both of these deaths were unexpected, occurring outside the normal sequence of life events, and Freud spoke poignantly of the enduring significance of these losses for many years. In a letter of condolence to Binswanger, a psychoanalyst colleague who lost a son to tubercular meningitis in 1926, 3 years after Heinnele's death, Freud stated that he remained inconsolable after the death of his grandson, who had come to represent for him the future of his children and grandchildren. As is characteristic of intense grief reactions of this kind, Freud was unable to gain comfort from the presence of his other grandchildren, including the little boy's older brother, Ernst, who visited his grandparents a few months after his brother's death; in a letter to Samuel Freud in September, 1923, Freud wrote that he "did not find him a consolation to any amount" (Gay, 1988, p. 422).

Six years after Heinnele's death, on the ninth anniversary of his daughter Sofie's death, Freud again wrote to his bereaved friend Binswanger:

> Although we know that after such a loss the acute stage of mourning will subside, we also know we shall remain inconsolable and will never find a substitute. No matter what may fill the gap, if it be filled completely, it nevertheless remains something else. And actually, this is how it should be; it is the only way of perpetuating that love which we do not want to relinquish. (Gay, 1988, p. 386)

Thirteen years after Sofie's death, during his analysis of the poet H.D., Hilda Doolittle, Freud responded to her mention of the last year of World War I by stating that "he had reason to remember the epidemic, as he lost his favorite daugher. 'She is here,' he said, and he showed [the patient] a tiny locket that he wore, fastened to his watch-chain" (Doolittle, 1956, p. 128).

The experience of his brother's death in early childhood remained an unspoken influence that nevertheless inevitably cast a shadow on Freud's early family life and life course. His brother died at the age of 7 months, when Freud, his mother's first born son, was 23 months old. Freud's family had six more children—five daughters and another son. Freud assigned the death of his brother almost no importance in his analysis of his childhood and subsequent development. In a letter to Fliess during his self-analysis, Freud reported his realization that he had greeted the birth of his "one-year-younger brother (who died after a few months) with adverse wishes and genuine childhood jealousy and that his death left the germ of [self-] reproaches in [him]" (Masson, 1985, p. 268).

Freud's experience with the death of a sibling at the vulnerable age of 2 years and the impact of this death on his family undoubtedly influenced many aspects of his subsequent development. Freud minimized the importance of his brother's death, as do his biographers, who tend to emphasize Freud's rivalries with his older half brothers and his same-age nephew as more formative life experiences. Yet many of Freud's adult characteristics—for example, his extraordinary possessiveness of his attachment figures, especially his mother, wife, and youngest daughter, Anna; his intense rivalries with male competitors, which he often explicitly characterized using the imagery of battles to the death; and his obsessive preoccupation with and fear of his own death in young adulthood—were probably influenced by his early loss of a sibling. Freud's early emphasis in his writings on complete recovery from grief was probably, at least in part, defensively motivated by his wish to deny the importance of his brother's death in his own development.

Clearly, Freud revised his understanding of normal bereavement on the basis of his own painful losses in adulthood. He came to recognize that important attachments cannot be relinquished, as he had earlier thought, yet he never revised these early assertions in his formal psychoanalytic writing. The idea that the goal of normal grief is the relinquishment of object ties became entrenched in the psychoanalytic literature, as did many other concepts of Freud's that he himself later came to regard in a more complex, alternative, or multidimensional way. For example, Freud (1923) revised his thinking about identification processes in *The Ego and the Id*, where he states that all object loss in both normal and pathological states is mastered through identification; however, he made this revision in the context of his developing theory of intrapsychic structure and object relationships, rather than in reference to normal bereavement.

Freud's writing on grief, like all of his writing, has remained a touchstone for psychoanalytic theorists, who have insisted on applying the drive theory concept of decathexis and the structural concept of identification in a narrow, inflexible way. The psychoanalytic movement's intellectual climate and character was very much influenced by Freud's intense conflicts over being replaced by the next generation of theorists. Having faced death at an early age and then continuously over the course of his life—with the out-of-life-cycle deaths of peers, children, and grandchildren; with the ravages of World War I; with cancer threatening the last 16 years of his life—Freud sought refuge from his preoccupation with death in his wish for the immortality of his ideas. In a study of the history of the psychoanalytic movement and its educational institutions (Shapiro, 1990), I argue that unresolved grief in Freud's own life gave impetus to his wish to live forever through his intergenerational control of the future of psychoanalysis. Freud gained this immortality—but at great cost to the creative intergenerational vitality of the psychoanalytic movement. No elder can resolve his own conflicts through strict control of the future permitted to his children and grandchildren without creating a stagnant present that merely repeats the past. In the psychoanalytic movement, as in other families, such self-protective control restricts the flexible flow of normal development.

Toward a Systemic Developmental Theory of Adult Bereavement

The Work of Erich Lindemann

The psychoanalytically inspired bereavement literature emerged from the study of clinical populations. Following the Second World War, clinicians began to encounter the many families affected by war casualties and to consider normative reactions to the crisis of death. In one of the first studies of normal grief reactions directly observed in a nonclinical population, Erich Lindemann studied survivors of the Coconut Grove nightclub fire in Boston. He described uncomplicated grief in terms of a series of symptoms that may seem quite extreme from a traditional psychiatric perspective but that are in fact normal following the experience of a death. Lindemann found that normal grief symptomatology includes somatic distress, often pain in the chest and throat; sensory distortions, including auditory and visual hallucinations of the deceased; preoccupation with the image of the deceased; and guilt, hostility, and loss of a person's usual patterns of conduct. Lindemann (1944), like Freud, noticed how disrupted the bereaved's everyday activities become: "The bereaved is surprised to find how large a part of his customary activity was done in some meaningful relationship to the deceased and has now lost its significance" (p. 142).

Unfortunately, Lindemann believed that the normal course of grief, both in its acute symptomatology and in the individual's capacity to invest in aspects of life other than the preoccupation with the deceased, could be resolved in 4 to 6 weeks, especially with psychiatric intervention. In more prolonged grief reactions, Lindemann found, social factors, such as the role of the deceased in maintaining the bereaved's social system, play a more significant role in the nature of the grief reaction than does previous psychological symptomatology. Moreover, a traumatic grief reaction, such as that undergone by the Coconut Grove fire survivors, is in fact a much more prolonged process than 4 to 6 weeks—or even 4 to 6 years. (In 1989, on the 46th anniversary of the 1943 Coconut Grove fire, I heard a Boston radio show in which a now elderly survivor described her still-recurring flashbacks to the fire and her enduring grief at the deaths of her boyfriend and brother.)

Crisis and Coping Theories

Lindemann's work on grief reactions inspired Gerald Caplan's (1964) work in crisis theory. From the perspective of crisis theory, the death of a close family member disrupts the survivor's adaptational equilibrium. In an initial period of disorganization, defensive coping strategies may be exacerbated and underlying personality problems may emerge. The crisis may afford the survivor an opportunity to recognize and transform an existing problematic coping style and create a new adaptation. From this perspective, any life crisis, including the crisis of grief, presents a challenge that can lead to a more adaptive reorganization of the personality. Silverman (1986, 1987) has used crisis theory to describe the experience of widowhood as a developmental transition that requires the reorganization of the widow's social roles and corresponding identity.

More recently, work in the area of adult coping with stressful life events has been applied to the stress of losing a family member (Figley & McCubbin, 1983; Osterweis et al., 1984; Stroebe & Stroebe, 1987). The mitigating or protective effects of social support in reducing the mental health risks for adults in high-stress life circumstances have been documented in both the adult and family stress and coping literature (Belle, 1989; Cohen & Syme, 1985; Dunst & Trivette, 1990; Gottlieb, 1988) and in the adult bereavement literature (Osterweis et al., 1984; Raphael, 1983; Stroebe & Stroebe, 1987; Vachon et al., 1982). Stroebe and Stroebe (1987) argue that the death of a spouse creates a significant deficit in social support for the surviving spouse, since most couples rely heavily on each other for instrumental, emotional, and validational support. The adult stress and coping literature has traditionally not emphasized developmental processes the way the crisis literature does. However, the literature on risk and resilience in developmental psychopathology examines patterns of stress and support that impede or protect child development under high-risk circumstances (Rolf, Masten, Cicchetti, & Nuechterlein, 1990; Rutter & Garmezy, 1983). The view that psychopathology results from the impact of a configuration of stresses and resources on developmental processes creates a bridge between the literature on adult coping with stressful life events and developmental perspectives on adult risk and resilience (Gore, 1994).

Attachment Theory

John Bowlby's (1969, 1973, 1980) work in applying attachment theory to adult grief has also extended the literature on adult bereavement to include relational and developmental perspectives. Bowlby, a British psychoanalyst, observed the separation responses of British children who were temporarily separated from their parents during the bombing of London in the Second World War and generated a theory of attachment in childhood and adulthood that has strongly influenced both theory and research on the nature of grief experiences. Although initially embracing an object relations perspective, Bowlby expanded his theory of attachment to include an ethological perspective on the survival benefits of attachment bonds. Bowlby proposed that human infants are biologically motivated to establish an attachment to a significant caretaker, usually the mother. When this bond is threatened by a separation, the child responds with a series of characteristic behaviors, including crying, protest, and a concerted search for the lost attachment figure. According to Bowlby, this sequence of attachment and separation behaviors, also observed in other mammals, was biologically designed to provide protection to vulnerable infants; the separation protest maximizes the likelihood that an infant will remain close to the primary caretaker and that the caretaker will quickly return if a separation occurs.

Bowlby and his colleagues suggest that adulthood attachment bonds to spouse and children are derived from the same emotional system underlying attachment in children (Bowlby, 1969, 1973, 1979, 1980; Raphael, 1983; Weiss, 1988). They find that the characteristic features of grief in adults resemble many elements of the childhood attachment and separation sequence, including an initial stage of numb disbelief; a stage of searching and pining for the lost person, including restlessness and resentment; a stage of depression and acknowledgment that searching is useless; and a stage of recovery in which the bereaved revise their sense of self and diminish their psychological involvement with the deceased. In order to preserve their capacity for independent action, adults need to maintain an internal image of a secure attachment figure. The frequent finding that widows and widowers preserve a strong sense of the presence of the deceased becomes understandable in terms of the personal stability for new developmental exploration that is provided by a sense of secure attachment.

While positing an instinctual attachment response, Bowlby has also integrated object relations theory and information processing theory to describe internal working models of attachment relationships that help maintain ongoing psychological stability over the course of development. According to Bowlby (1980), under circumstances of emotional stress and disruption of attachment bonds, children and adults will dissociate overwhelming experiences. While this allows them to regain a sense of emotional stability, they lose access to the encapsulated or defended-against painful emotions and associations. Disassociation of the overwhelming experience and related associations creates constricted areas of inner experience and relational adaptations that are not accessible for review and new learning with increasing maturation.

In addition to evoking childhood attachment and separation behaviors, the experiences of grieving adults suggest cognition more characteristic of children, especially in the domain of causal explanation. During the first phase of grief, when adults still hope the death is part of a nightmare from which they might yet wake, the search for a cause of death serves the interest of denial and protest. It is as if they are reasoning that knowing exactly what happened can somehow, magically, enable them to take the moment back and create new circumstances in which the death is averted. Even after the initial acute stages of disorientation, when the death becomes gradually more real, adults often retain concrete, magical, or self-blaming ideas about the cause of the loved one's death. The bereaved grasp for some coherent account of the circumstances of the death, even if the causal explanation they generate is concrete or self-referential. We prefer to live in an orderly universe, even if we must shoulder the painful responsibility for disaster, than in a random one where disaster can strike again at any time (Janoff-Bulman, 1985). Writers in both the grief literature and the trauma literature emphasize that recovery from a stressful or traumatic event requires the creation of a new, coherent account of one's life, an account in which the trauma and its meaning are integrated into a new sense of self (Lifton, 1983; Taylor, 1983). The greater the traumatic stress or violence associated with a death, the greater the likelihood that distorted or dissociated cognitive processes will need to be brought into play as strategies for reestablishing psychological coherence and stability (Herman, 1992; Horowitz, 1990; Lebowitz & Roth, 1992).

Colleagues and collaborators of Bowlby's, including Parkes and Weiss (Glick et al., 1974; Parkes, 1972; Parkes & Weiss, 1983; Weiss, 1988), have integrated his theory of attachment with social role theory in emphasizing the process by which the bereaved create a new iden-

tity or "theory of self." In their extensive study of widows and widowers in England and Boston, this group of researchers has noted that a
grieving adult's initial denial of the reality of death and the gradual process of acknowledgment of it buys time for the main task of adult grief—
the reorganization of identity in adaptation to changing life circumstances. Working from a social role and developmental perspective,
Silverman (1986, 1987) describes widowhood as a developmental crisis in which new roles and previously unexplored aspects of the self
have to be activated and integrated in response to radically changed
life circumstances. She notes that widowhood is an especially radical
developmental transition for women, whose social roles and psychological identity so heavily emphasize the primacy of relationships.

Object Relations Theory

Object relations theory in psychoanalysis views the inner life of the
individual as comprising internalized representations of real relationships with early caretaking figures. In addressing bereavement directly,
object relations theorists emphasize the impact of the loss on these
internalized self and object representations and suggest that the death
of an important person requires a rebalancing of them (Raphael, 1983;
Rubin, 1985; Volkan, 1981). Like psychoanalytic theorists, object relations theorists typically tend to associate the final resolution of grief
with a decathexis of the lost object. Volkan (1981) describes "linking
objects and linking phenomena" that sustain the attachment of the
bereaved to the deceased. However, he considers these to be characteristics of pathological or complicated mourning that are not needed
in healthy or uncomplicated bereavement.

   Rubin (1981, 1985), in contrast, argues from an object relational
perspective that true recovery from bereavement does not require
relinquishment but, rather, the establishment of a new integration of
the internalized relationship with the deceased. He suggests that clinicians need to focus on the patient's capacity for change and evolution in the recollected relationship to the deceased and on the ways
the internalized images of the deceased function toward enhancing
or disrupting self-organization. While this internalized relationship to
the deceased does not take the place of other real relationships, it
continues to exist as an important inner resource for the survivor.

The Interpersonal Object Relational Perspective

Object relations theory, in addition to describing the internalization
of relationships in early childhood, has been extended by interactional

theorists to include the adult relationship process by which spouses enlist each other to collaboratively create a repetition of these historical relational internalizations. Interpersonal object relations approaches have drawn on the work of Dicks (1967), who applied object relations theory to an understanding of marital interaction. According to this interpersonal object relational perspective, a central dimension of grief stems from the loss of the role of the deceased spouse in the interactionally constructed "shared personality." Through mechanisms such as projective identification, marital partners unconsciously agree to divide up functions; for example, one partner can be more emotionally expressive while the other can be more emotionally controlled. After the death of the marital partner, the survivor needs to reclaim and reintegrate these projected aspects of the self into a new, more multidimensional sense of self.

Horowitz, Wilner, Marmar, and Krupnick (1980), drawing on object relations theory and cognitive information processing theory, have likewise proposed that the bereavement process involves the reactivation of latent self-images that, through projective identification, had previously been located in the partner. Pincus (1974), too, studying the impact of spousal bereavement from an interpersonal object relations perspective, found that the grief reaction of adults mourning the death of a spouse was characterized by the reintegration of aspects of the self that had been located in the other through mechanisms of projection, identification, and projective identification. Projective identification, which involves both the projection of defended against aspects of self and their reincorporation through identification with the partner, is an especially useful construct for understanding marital dynamics (Scharff, 1989). She described radical transformations in adults who had adopted one style of personality functioning in their marriage and who revealed a hidden capacity to function much more fully in the absence of the spouse. For example, the loner married to the sociable wife might emerge as much more relationship-seeking than when his wife performed social functions for both of them and the dependent wife who seemed incapable of functioning on her own might launch a successful career or begin to travel extensively. While many widows and widowers are able to reintegrate aspects of the self that had been invested in the dead spouse, others suffer such profound impoverishment of the self after the death that they are unable to survive the loss in a way that enables them to grow in new directions.

The quality of the preexisting marital relationship seems to be an important factor in the bereavement experience of widows and widowers (Parkes & Weiss, 1983; Pincus, 1974; Stroebe & Stroebe, 1983, 1987). If the marital relationship was characterized by conflict, abuse, or dominance, the process of developmental reintegration stimulated by the death of the partner may be much more difficult (Parkes & Weiss, 1983; Shanfield, 1983). Parkes and Weiss (1983) describe conflictual or ambivalent marital relationships as a risk factor for unresolved or pathological grief in widows and widowers.

Gender Roles and Spousal Bereavement. The interpersonal object relations approach recognizes the importance of marital relationship patterns in organizing what appears to be qualities of the individual spouses but are actually implicit arrangements designed to share aspects of the self. While some of these marital arrangements are highly individualized according to a particular couple's personal history, many of these arrangements are also influenced by a society's stereotyped sex role definition. The grief reactions of widows and widowers need to be understood not only in terms of marital dynamics, but also as gender based crises of role functioning and identity.

The predominant evidence on gender effects in bereavement indicates that for every postbereavement dimension—poor physical health, mortality rate, and psychiatric symptomatology—widowers show higher rates of risk than do widows (Stroebe & Stroebe, 1982, 1987). Discussions of this finding suggest that in spite of the centrality of the role of wife in the lives of women, marriage is more advantageous for men than for women. Marriage offers men more satisfaction and support than it offers women and is associated with better health outcomes for men than for women (Bernard, 1972; Stroebe & Stroebe, 1987). Widows seem to lose less realistic support with the loss of marriage and also seem better able to make use of existing networks of support more effectively (Stroebe & Stroebe, 1991). Widowers are more likely to remarry than widows because of the wider age range of potential marital partners. Once remarried, men are once again likely to turn to their new wife as their predominant source of social support—including support for the process of grieving (Glick et al., 1974; Parkes, 1972; Parkes & Weiss, 1983).

Parental Roles and the Death of a Child. Both attachment theory and role developmental theory have been applied in theoretical discussions that try to account for the utter devastation most parents feel after the death of a child (Rando, 1986; Raphael, 1983; Sanders, 1989; Weiss, 1988). Some studies, involving both self-descriptions of grief and objective measures of symptomatology, suggest that mothers suffer more than fathers after the death of a child (Cook, 1984; Lovell, 1983; Rando, 1985, 1986; Shanfield, Benjamin, & Swain, 1984; Shanfield & Swain, 1984). Authors of these studies suggest that factors such as the greater centrality of the parenting role in the lives of women, their greater daily caretaking responsibilities, and their more intimate emotional connection to the child make mothers more vulnerable to bereavement distress. While the interpersonal object relations literature has focused on widows and widowers, the family systems literature in family therapy has focused attention on the fact that children also fill the role of objects of projection, thus absorbing individual adult and family conflict and helping to maintain family stability (Boszormenyi-Nagy & Spark, 1973; Minuchin, 1974; Piercy & Sprenkle, 1986). It has been argued that with the death of a child, especially a child who was central to a system of family projections, the adults in the family lose a major source of the self-organization derived from family interaction (Bowen, 1976; Herz, 1980, 1989).

From the perspective of adult attachment, the death of a child resonates not only to losses associated with the parents' internalized early relationships from the past but, more importantly, to the loss of aspects of the self that the parents invested in the child and that represented their movement into the future (Rando, 1986; Sanders, 1989; Weiss, 1988). From a systemic developmental perspective, the integration of adult grief after the death of a child requires the renegotiation of every aspect of the collaborative self. This developmental process is an extremely long one, especially for mothers whose parenting role was both time consuming and essential to their sense of self. The death of a child also places a strain on the marital relationship, as grieving parents find themselves struggling with overwhelming emotions they feel they cannot share without increasing their sense of disruption or alienation (Cook, 1984; Rando, 1985, 1986; Sanders, 1989; Videka-Sherman & Lieberman, 1985). The literature has been inconsistent in finding a greater incidence of divorce among couples who have experienced the death of a child: Some writers report a higher divorce rate (Herz, 1980; Lehman, Wortman, & Williams, 1987) while others find the divorce rate equal to or lower than that in the general population (Rando, 1986). These writers do agree, however, that the spouses' availability to one another for social and emotional support seems greatly diminished as they each attempt to cope with the death of their child.

RELATIONAL ASPECTS OF GRIEF

In pointing out that development requires the stable internal representation of an attachment figure, attachment and object relations theories have made important contributions to understanding adult bereavement. From these perspectives, adult grief is a crisis in internal as well as external relational conditions that protect the sense of safety necessary for ongoing development. Paradoxically, the death of an important attachment figure challenges us to radically re-create ourselves at a time when the requisite sense of safety that facilitates developmental exploration and creative experimentation with the self has been shattered. Reestablishing stable conditions for ongoing development then becomes a priority in bereavement and requires both intrapsychic and social resources.

Attachment theory, like psychoanalytic and psychosocial approaches, presents adult bereavement as an individual process without exploring the mutual effects of bereavement on the family as a unit. For example, in the attachment literature on the death of a spouse there is extensive discussion of the pair bond in marriage and the impact of its dissolution on widows and widowers. However, when the adult bereavement literature mentions a grieving adult's parenting, it emphasizes the role children play in either aiding or hampering the adult's recovery from grief. Although children in the home assuage feelings of loneliness for the bereaved parent, the demands of child-rearing are likely to interfere with the process of creating a new adult life structure (Glick et al., 1974; Parkes & Weiss, 1983; Sanders, 1989).

In real-life grief experiences, parents and children grieve together. When a parent of young children dies, the bereaved spouse is coping with marital loss as well as the challenging work of becoming a single parent to children who are themselves grieving. When a parent loses a child, he or she is coping not only with his or her own private reaction but also with the grief reactions of a spouse and of surviving children who have lost a sibling. The loss affects each individual uniquely, but the grief reaction of each individual will be shaped by the needs and reactions of the others. In this process of shared grief the parent's reaction will often provide the leadership for what the children will be able to express and integrate. However, bereaved children's emotional reactions and relationships to their grieving parents will also affect the adult's bereavement experience.

For an adult, the death of a close family member, a partner in the creation of the collaborative self, precipitates a life crisis and a radical life review. The adult reassessment of self as marital partner and parent becomes part of ongoing postbereavement relationships, which are reorganized under radically different and highly stressful new life circumstances. With the death of a spouse, the marital relationship is the focus of the inner psychological work, and the surviving parent's relationships with the children assume new burdens of stress in day-to-day living and in managing the intense feelings of loss. With the death of a child, it is the parent–child relationship that is the focus of the inner psychological work, and the marital relationship, as well as the relationship with any other children in the family, assumes new burdens of stress in the reorganization process. Burdened as they are, these family relationships continue to be central to the network of existing supports for the grieving adult. Relationships with members of the extended family will also be important resources for the new psychological structures that the adult will use to rebuild his or her life.

The relationship to the deceased family member will itself remain an important resource for the adult bereavement process. Transitional experiences in the Winnicottian sense (Winnicott, 1971), during which the deceased makes a transition from corporeal external object to internalized object, are a vital part of adult bereavement. Both the British object relations school and self psychology posit that adults need enduring relationships in order to sustain the basic psychological processes of emotional regulation and regulation of self-esteem (Buckley, 1986; Guntrip, 1973; Greenberg, 1991; Greenberg & Kohon, 1986; Kohut, 1971, 1977; Mitchell, 1983; Slavin, 1992). From a systemic developmental perspective, a process of internalization in early childhood establishes a secure inner image of close others and a corresponding sense of a resilient, psychologically accompanied autonomous self. These internalized images of loving attachment figures allow both children and adults to tolerate their loved ones' ordinary comings and goings. When one of the vital members of the collaboratively constructed self has died and will never again be physically present, another step in the process of internalization is required (Rubin, 1985; Valliant, 1985). Working models of the self with others will have to be reintegrated to accommodate realistically to the new characteristics of the relationship to the deceased. The relationship can now only exist in memory and emotion, and the internal definition of the self has to accommodate this new reality.

A systemic developmental perspective on adult bereavement suggests that the end point of successful grief work is not relinquishment of the lost relationship but the creation of a new bond, one that acknowledges the enduring psychological and spiritual reality of someone we have loved and made a part of our selves (Moss & Moss, 1984–1985; Rubin, 1985; Schuchter & Zissok, 1986; Vaillant, 1985). In this culture we have a difficult time granting even to children the need to retain an enduring bond with the dead, so determined are we to promote the reality-oriented "letting go" process. Yet both children and adults require the security and safety provided by the spiritual and emotional presence of their important formative attachment figures.

Grief, from a systemic developmental perspective, is seen as a family life cycle transition that requires the transformation of enduring relational bonds. Grief does not require the relinquishment of the lost love but the reestablishment of a new relationship, still vital and enduring but now internalized.

SUMMARY

Adult grief is part of a family developmental crisis that disrupts adult and family stability in the interrelated domains of emotion, action, and meaning. Grief is a crisis not only of overwhelming emotion but of daily interaction and identity. Adults will have mobilized all the resources at their disposal—intrapsychic, family systemic, community, and cultural—in arriving at strategies for containing the overwhelming emotion, for reorganizing the activities of daily living and family interaction, and for restoring a stable sense of the collaborative self, which now includes the death and its meaning. While grieving adults become preoccupied at first with the pain of all they have lost, they gradually begin to turn to both their external supports and their own psychological resources to reestablish their attachment bond with the deceased, a living, enduring bond in a new place in the configuration of their identity. The restoration of the adult's sense of the flow of time allows movement into a developmental future and casts a new light on the past, as memories of the loved one who has died are now retrieved and reinterpreted in light of the new relational reality (Rubin, 1981, 1985; Vaillant, 1985).

The psychological exploration of changing family relationships after a death requires the passage of time and a supportive environment in order to reestablish a new, coherent sense of the relational self. Grieving parents who have lost a spouse or a child find themselves extremely stressed by the realistic demands of ongoing parenting. The more overwhelming or stressful the real-life circumstances of the death and the scarcer the real-life supports, the more likely an adult will be to utilize growth-constraining intrapsychic and interpersonal strategies as sources of support. These growth-constraining strategies for stabilization may involve intrapsychic processes, such as denial or disassociation, or interpersonal processes, such as restricting the freedom of family communication. While these defenses help adults achieve stability in a state of overwhelming crisis, they restrict full integration of the grief experience. The cost of these growth-constraining strategies may become more evident in subsequent stages of the family life cycle when resonances to the enduring crisis of grief are inevitably reawakened and the capacity for flexible responses to new circumstances is required. Nevertheless, whatever an adult's immediate response to the crisis of grief, new stages of the family life cycle will provide new opportunities for growth-enhancing integration of previously fragmented aspects of the grief experience and for more inclusive reorganization of the complex collaborative self.

CHAPTER 4

A Widow's Story

THE SYSTEMIC DEVELOPMENTAL
EXPERIENCE OF GRIEF IN ADULTHOOD

So far, I have used the theoretical literature to argue that adult grief is best conceptualized as a systemic developmental process. While conceptually useful, this model is also a compelling means of remaining close to the lived experience of bereaved adults, children, and families. The best test of a systemic developmental model of bereavement is its usefulness in helping clinicians understand the family's experience of grief and provide effective support. Gail Kaplan was 36 years old at the time her 36-year-old husband, Stuart, died. The Kaplans were the parents of 6-year-old Alan and 1½-year-old Sam. Gail and I began working together in individual therapy 5 months after Stuart's death, and our work has continued to the present, through the fourth anniversary of his death. Gail is an articulate, psychologically sophisticated, and emotionally courageous woman who has been able to explore and share an extraordinarily vivid depiction of her grief. Her experience illustrates the ways adult grief can be usefully understood as a systemic developmental process (her son Sam's experiences are described later in this book).

THIS IS HOW IT HAPPENED:
A MOMENT FROZEN IN TIME

Nothing at all in Stuart Kaplan's health history or family background had provided any clue to his sudden death of a heart attack. Married for 13 years, the Kaplans had been boyfriend and girlfriend since the age of 19. Having met in elementary school, they had the intimacy of having grown up together. The morning in August when Stuart collapsed in the shower was part of an unusually hot summer; the weekend before had been the hottest of all—a humid 103 degrees. Stuart, as he often did, had spent Saturday working in the yard. He had not let the heat slow him down but, rather, had taken on the strenuous job of digging a new garden bed. The following evening, the night before he died, Gail and Stuart had friends over for a barbecue, and they spent that Sunday evening, with Stuart showing no indication of ill health, planning a trip together. It was only afterward that Gail found herself wondering if Stuart had made himself ill by working so hard in such brutal heat. His decision to work on the garden in spite of the oppressive heat was very much in character, and Gail had long ago settled on a policy of noninterference with his projects.

Stuart's good spirits that Sunday evening were a contrast to his mood of the previous few days. The couple had had a fight earlier in the week, a trivial one, when Stuart prepared a dish of ice cream and told his son Alan that it wasn't fattening. Gail commented that this was in fact not so. She didn't mind that Stuart was eating ice cream; his diet was his own business, and he was only slightly overweight. What she minded was his lying to himself about it and then drawing Alan into the lie. Stuart was indignant and resentful and, as he often did when he was angry, insisted that Gail apologize for her comment or back down. Gail was aware at the time of the fight that for once she was choosing to stand her ground rather than back down to make peace with Stuart. The intensity of Stuart's anger had often led her to make peace to regain their customary easy intimacy. This time, though, she felt his anger was out of proportion to the small event, and she refused to apologize. She was relieved, then, when of his own accord Stuart regained his usual friendliness. Without making too much of it, Gail realized that they had made peace in a new way, and she was pleased about it.

These details, which might easily have gone unnoticed as part of the ordinary texture of their shared life, were dramatically highlighted by Stuart's collapse in the shower a few days later. All the details surrounding Stuart's death, from the profound to the trivial, were vividly remembered as Gail tried to make sense of what had happened to him and to them—the garden bed Stuart was digging, the oppressive summer heat, the barbecue with their friends, the fight over what he said about ice cream, the sound of his dead weight falling in the shower, the paramedics and their equipment, the local hospital emergency room. "What exactly happened?" Gail seemed to me to be asking herself. "Why did it happen? Is it real, or could I be dreaming? Is there anything I can do to take the moment back, make it come out differently?" Gail had been talking to Stuart as he took his shower. When she heard him fall, she called out to him, "Stuart, are you all right?"—as she had done many times before when she heard a sound indicating that some mishap had occurred. She was at first certain that, as usual, he would eventually say, "Don't worry, I'm fine," and she felt annoyed when he seemed so absorbed with the pain of falling that he didn't think to call out to reassure her. Her annoyance lasted for an instant, and when she realized that this was not going to be like any other time, that Stuart was not going to respond, her state of suspended anxiety turned to panic.

Gail called an ambulance and sent 6-year-old Alan to the next-door neighbor's house, asking him to get help and to then wait for her there. Sam, the baby, stayed with her in the house after the paramedics arrived and began to work at reviving Stuart's inert body. As the paramedics made preparations for transporting Stuart by ambulance to the local emergency room, Gail asked them if she should accompany him; they told her that, given his state of unconsciousness, there was really no point to it. She agreed with them at the time, her reluctance to go with Stuart in the ambulance intensified by her worry about leaving Sam without her. Gail was later intermittently haunted by a regret that she hadn't accompanied Stuart, that she hadn't been with him when his spirit left his body, that she had lost a fleeting opportunity to say some kind of good-bye. After reviewing the circumstances of Stuart's death in therapy, Gail concluded that she had in fact been with Stuart immediately after he collapsed, when he, although unconscious, was still fighting for his life, and that by the time the paramedics took him away in the ambulance his spirit was already departing.

Gail's ruminative focus on the moment of Stuart's death and her worry that she had not done everything she might have for him are as inevitable a part of acute grief as is the "denial" of reality. The bereaved, who were going about the business of everyday life in that safe state of routine, like driving a car on automatic pilot, discover abruptly that one ordinary moment was not like any other in its implications. The time of the death gets played back like a film in slow motion, over and over again, as the bereaved try to make sense of and integrate what happened, try to find a different way to say a final good-bye, try to find any loophole in the action that might make it possible to take the moment back. Gail was relatively fortunate in the configuration of circumstances surrounding her husband's death, which gave her almost no opportunity in reality to blame herself. The bereaved often experience an intense wish to find a cause for the death and feel an apparently irrational amplification of their own contribution to it. Embedded within this rumination and self-blame, sometimes implicitly, as with Gail, but often quite explicitly, is the wish to roll back the flow of time and make the final outcome a different one. Just as grieving adults reexperience the attachment protests they made as young children when separated from their loved ones, so too do they resurrect childhood theories of causality in which they would rather blame themselves than feel helpless at the hands of a cruel, indifferent fate that can deliver the shattering blow of a loved one's death.

When I first met Gail, 6 months after Stuart's death, all outside observers—and there were many: her close friends, family, colleagues, constituents of a wide community of people who shared their lives with the Kaplans and themselves deeply mourned Stuart—felt Gail was "doing very well." As a competent, energetic woman with her own consulting business, Gail had increased her hours so as to generate a steadier, more secure income. She continued to spend the majority of her time with her children but had arranged for extra child care from her babysitter to cover her additional working hours. She talked openly with both children about the loss of their father. While she was obviously sad and bereft, she was not taken over by spasms of grief, at least not that anyone could see. She had very capably organized a workable new life within which the family's essential needs for physical and emotional stability could be provided. Everyone who cared about her was relieved that she was handling Stuart's death so well.

Emotionally, however, Gail was precariously suspended in a state of unreality. Like most bereaved people, she had fashioned a state of frozen immobility in response to the need for relief from unremitting pain as well as from the vertigo caused by trying to face a new and unacceptable reality too abruptly. Many grief-stricken people describe this altered state of grief as a nightmare from which one does not wake up, although always waiting and hoping to. Gail and I came to call it the feeling of being frozen in time. At that very early stage in her bereavement her psychological balance depended on her ability to stay very still and live life on a narrow ledge with respect to the flow of time: When she went back in time and remembered the past, she would be flooded by the agonizing grief of loss and by an overpowering sense of missing Stuart. If she went forward in time and thought about the future, she would be again flooded by a sense of loss, this time the poignant loss of a future shared with Stuart. Moving forward in time meant that she would enter a real life within which she would be forced to acknowledge that Stuart was no longer her life companion. For this reason, Gail stayed frozen in time; her life in that first year was characterized by a sense of unreality dominated by a quality of timelessness. Moving from that frozen moment in time required more sorrowful renunciation than she was ready for in the first—and even in the second—year.

When Gail and I first started meeting, she asked me how long she would be feeling so frozen in time, how long it would take for her to rejoin the emotional flow of living. I told her that it was normal to expect that she would continue to experience a sense of unreality and disconnection, punctuated by acute grief, for the first 2 years and that she would probably begin to feel differently during the third year after Stuart's death. She was taken aback with both surprise and relief. While her pediatrician was the first to ask her if she had started dating yet, she knew her friends and family would not be far behind in taking an affirmative answer as a measure of her willingness to go on with life. Like most widows, she was nowhere near ready to sufficiently integrate the reality of her loss to let another person into her life. During the second year of therapy, at a time when she was feeling that the motions she was going through in her life had nothing to do with her private world of grief, Gail said, "I might as well date, I feel so bad." She meant that violation of her integrity could not make her feel any worse, since she already felt so disconnected from herself.

Of course, not all widows have this long a period of emotional and personal reintegration before initiating a new social life, or even before remarrying. Many widowers remarry within the first year of their wife's death. My statement to Gail was based on the evidence, from both clinical work and the research literature, that 2 to 3 years is a common requirement for recovery from the acute phase of bereavement after the death of a spouse. The grief reaction is even more prolonged for those who have lost their spouse to sudden, unanticipated death (Parkes & Weiss, 1983). Most men, and some women, will marry a new partner and then continue to carry through their experience of grief, perhaps asking their new partner to understand or help support them in that process. It can become quite difficult for men who lose a partner when they still have very young children at home to reestablish a sense of shared psychological stability as a family when they are totally dependent on purchased child care. There are many factors, representing both individual emotional qualities and social role realities, that determine when and if widows and widowers choose to seek support from a new partner.

There is no question, though, that when two people have made a life together and this life-sustaining partnership is interrupted by death, the process of psychological reintegration and recovery is a long one, very much longer than our official timetables. Gail was very relieved to hear me affirm that she could not reasonably be expected to move any faster toward recovery, especially when she knew perfectly well that recovery required acknowledging and more fully accepting the ways Stuart was no longer part of her life. In fact, as people continued to talk with her about dating, which they did increasingly once the first anniversary of Stuart's death had passed, Gail remembered with ironic amusement the film *Dona Flor and Her Two Husbands*, based on Jorge Amado's (1968) book. In that film a widow remarries while carrying on an affair with the ghost of her first husband, a plot that well describes Gail's own fantasy of her future household, which would of necessity include Stuart.

Not only did Gail feel frozen in time, but she also felt, and described with a great deal of depth and detail, the sensation of unreality that is so often described by the bereaved. The term that for me best characterizes this experience of unreality is *dissociation*, and I see this experience as related to a sense of disconnection from the flow of time. Ideally, free association is the freely flowing movement of our thoughts through all emotional currents, including those that might be personally or socially "forbidden." Psychoanalytic treatment rests on the analysis of those barriers to the free flow of associational thought and of the defense mechanisms that prevent the forbidden discoveries and connections that might accompany an undeterred exploration of consciousness. Much of what gives our consciousness depth and texture is the often hardly recognized resonance to associations from the past and fantasies about the future. Overwhelming psychological pain, such as the pain of trauma or bereavement, requires the creation of a safe psychic space that will not be disturbed by resonances from the traumatic event. Since so much of our consciousness is organized by the rhythm of our close relationships, the bereaved learn almost immediately that they cannot look anywhere at all, neither outside nor inside themselves, without discovering a connection to the loved one who is now so painfully absent. For a time, it becomes essential not to remain in the ordinary world of the living, where these heartfelt connections to others are as natural as breathing.

The depth and endurance of this initial sense of unreality varies substantially among individuals and is determined by the degree of stress and discontinuity the death represents. The anticipated death of an elderly parent might require little psychological disconnection in order to achieve a process of reintegration; the unexpected death of a child owing to a fatal accident or murder might require massive psychic withdrawal. The experience, like Gail Kaplan's, of a sudden, unanticipated death early in the life cycle has in fact been associated with a prolonged periods of recovery, as would be expected given the high degree of both discontinuity and stress precipitated by such a death. The anthropological literature better recognizes what our own culture denies, namely, that the bereaved exist in a state of "liminality" or transition, suspended between an old, obsolete social structural state and a yet to be established new one, in a nebulous place between the world of the dead and the world of the living.

THE BEGINNING OF THERAPY

Gail, like other grief-stricken people I have talked with, described the quality of this condition of disassociation and immobility or time-lessness as in fact a time when she felt more connected to death than to life. Perhaps more accurately, the bereaved live in a psychological world in which the dead are more alive, more emotionally animated, than the living. The work of grief for Gail, as for others, precipitated a process of life review. Stuart's death forced her to question her life as she had constructed it and to reexamine the assumptions that had worked when Stuart was part of her life but that would no longer work as a way of life for her now. Of necessity, this review required an exploration of the marital relationship and its history, so that Gail could discover who she might be now, without Stuart.

When I first met Gail, not yet 6 months after Stuart's death, she described herself as still "dealing with being left." Like most people who enter therapy, she was describing a profound truth, the full implications of which were far from consciousness but which in a sense would form the core of our therapeutic work. On the surface, it seems obvious that all grief-stricken people struggle with both sorrow and resentment at their loved one's abandonment of them. While my work as a therapist, and my grief work in particular, has taught me never to overlook the obvious, it has also taught me never to reduce private meanings to their simple surface. Gail, in fact, warned me immediately that while she knew she was "supposed" to be angry at Stuart for "abandoning" her, she felt no such thing. "He didn't choose this," she told me. "He would never have wanted to die." The meaning constructed between Gail and Stuart of Gail's "being left" by Stuart would have to be discovered, as an ongoing part of their long-standing relationship, which had now been psychologically interrupted—though not psychologically severed—by his death.

Gail opened our first session by telling me about Stuart as a person, so that I could appreciate the enormity of the loss for her and the family. She described Stuart as an extraordinary man in his emotional depth and relatedness to family, friends, and work colleagues. He was passionately interested in and competent at a wide range of subjects, a lawyer turned university teacher who loved to make things and fix things, not at all the one-dimensional stereotypic professor.

Although not a vigorous athlete, Stuart was a tall, strongly built man, an enthusiastic outdoorsman who led them on hikes and ski trips that were exhilarating though taxing. Gail felt that he could be sweet and loving while still being strong, and she reported that he was very active in caring for the children. However, it was not that Stuart wasn't difficult: Gail was perfectly aware that he could be stubborn, quick to anger, and slow to forgive. She regarded these traits simply as aspects of Stuart's intensity as a personality, and she had learned to live with them. She said she thought that probably everyone who comes to a therapist after the death of a spouse talks about how extraordinary a person the spouse was; it seemed to be the obligatory way to talk about the dead. Stuart was, in fact, extraordinary, she said, as the many people who knew and loved him would confirm.

Gail and Stuart began a relationship when they were both 16; they had gone through their early school years together without taking notice of one another. Once they did, Stuart knew much sooner than Gail that their friendship and bond would become a romantic one. Stuart, the son of Jewish survivors of the Holocaust, was serious, emotionally deep, and passionate about his enthusiasms. Gail recognized and appreciated that Stuart was different from other people their age, attuned to a far wider range of political, historical, and spiritual concerns. But during her high school and college years she had not yet made up her mind to take the relationship seriously. Gail could be imaginative, playful, and lighthearted; she wanted to continue exploring what it was like to be with different kinds of people. Stuart, who made up his mind early that he wanted to spend his life with Gail, persevered in his pursuit of her through the years during which she insisted on dating others.

Although it took Gail longer to recognize the inevitability of their coming together, once she did so, she saw it as very much like the right pathway through life. Her older sister, Shirley, had married a man who was much more in keeping with the family's hopes and aspirations for her—a successful Jewish doctor whose drive for success and sociability fit in easily with the family's style. Stuart was more eccentric, took his Jewish history more seriously, and put material values and professional pursuits secondary to a well-rounded life. Gail's parents had initially protested her adolescent relationship with Stuart, and Stuart never let Gail forget that he had been the loyal suitor and she had been the reluctant one, the "infidel." Once, when Gail asked him, "What would I do if you died?" Stuart responded, "What are you worried about? You'll be with someone else in a minute."

When Gail first came to my office, it was too early to delve deeply into the inevitable compromises and mutual adaptations that of necessity characterize the marital, and any other meaningful, relationship. Gail was involved with a more basic process, namely, fending off her longing for Stuart's physical companionship, which felt so much like an open wound that she could not be tolerate it. After she talked about Stuart as a person and about the terrible loss to her and her children of his unique, special qualities, I was left with the lingering thought that his large, solid, comforting, unwavering presence had been a part of Gail's life for 20 years. I was moved to say, "You must miss him terribly at night. You must keep waiting to feel him come into bed with you and lie next to you. I would imagine, hearing you speak, that that would be the most basic, most visceral kind of missing him, especially now, when you are so much grappling with believing he is really dead." For some widows the recognition of the physical loss comes first and evokes the full sense of the loss most vividly. For Gail, though, those feelings of physical longing appeared to be too dangerous. She looked at me blankly, with a lack of recognition that was too deliberate, and said that she never thought that way and would never give in to such longing: "Stuart is gone, that's all; there's no point in missing him that way." It took another full year for that poignantly physical longing to safely make it to Gail's consciousness.

I was careful not to insist on my interpretation and subsequent observation that Gail seemed to me to be denying the obvious and natural feelings of physically missing her husband. As therapists, we learn always to make our interpretations modestly, in a humble spirit of inviting mutual exploration. First of all, our interpretation could be wrong. Just as importantly, it could be right in a deep emotional or existential sense but wrong in that the person is simply not able at the moment to integrate the insight for his or her own compelling reasons. In Gail's case, my capacity to listen without categorizing her experience became a pivotal prerequisite for embarking on our shared work. I became alerted to Gail's concern from our first phone call: As we negotiated every aspect of our relationship, from practical concerns like scheduling and fees to theoretical orientation, I sensed that Gail was acutely attuned to my capacity for responsive recognition of her own unique experience. I let her know, in every way possible, that I appreciated her need to be responded to as the person she was and that I would not reduce her to the category of patient or widow.

In the evolution of our therapeutic work and in our establishing a relationship that would become a meaningful support in Gail's psychological reintegration and growth, the theme of close relationships as mirrors of the self became a central one. Therapists from a psychoanalytic orientation have used the metaphor of the mirror to describe the work of the therapeutic relationship; the therapist, emphasizing the mirroring function of neutrality, simply reflects the patient's own psychic life. In self psychology and in its more popular therapeutic stepsibling, Rogerian client-centered therapy, the mirroring therapist functions like the parent of infancy, showing, interpreting, and affirming clients' experiences. Few individually oriented theorists and therapists have fully acknowledged the deep relational implications of what every child, and every patient, knows, namely, that therapists–parents can never mirror others with objectivity but only through the prism of their own consciousness, a perspective inevitably distorted by their own emotional responses and corresponding defenses. The mirror is, inevitably, a distorting mirror. Further, the interpersonal process of mutual mirroring is easily distorted by imbalances of power; almost by definition, the more powerful person is the one who gets to define the experience of both, for both. In our culture this socially sanctioned power imbalance rests with parents in relation to children, with men in relation to women, with whites in relation to ethnic minorities, and with therapists in relation to patients.

From her own experiences in her close relationships, Gail was deeply aware of the implications for her personal integrity of the potential skewing in this relational process of mutual mirroring, which would become a crucial theme in our work together. Eventually, over the course of 2½ years of therapy, we would locate her in a three-generational relational process within which she was both shaped by and shaper of important relationships with parents, sister, husband, and children. Without yet concerning ourselves with why, we at first concentrated instead on establishing a therapeutic rhythm in which she spoke and I attentively listened, so that I could offer her my sense of her experience without imposing it and she could make use of it in bringing order to her own experience.

For Gail, the early work in therapy, from 6 months after Stuart's death to the time shortly after the first anniversary of it, was taken over by a panicked anticipation that she was going to have to relive the horror of his death all over again, this time without the cushion of shock. The beginning of this dread began with Gail's anticipation of the unveiling of the grave marker, a ceremony that, according to Jewish custom, is done 10 or 11 months after the death. Gail became concerned, with worries that felt like they could easily become panic, that she would be pulled in too many directions by the compelling needs of other people to observe this early anniversary. She feared she would lose all contact with the rhythm and requirements of her own grief. Both Gail's and Stuart's families, as well as many of their close friends, were planning to travel to Boston for the May unveiling. For them, the unveiling was a ritual of psychic closure, a process of marking the grave and saying good-bye to Stuart as a living person. "It's too soon for me," Gail said. "I couldn't even begin to think about the first-year anniversary until it's safely past us."

We agreed that since the ritual was a meaningful one in the families' Jewish faith and would be an important community and family event, she could participate in it as a means of publicly honoring Stuart's memory without any concessions to the expectation that she was now ready to put the past behind her. We also affirmed the importance of her concentrating on her own needs and the needs of her bereaved children, the people most deeply affected by the severing of their daily ties to Stuart. She would try, whenever possible, not to give in to family requests that she entertain groups of people when she didn't feel capable of it or agree with other people's conclusions about how important it was to go on with her life.

Gail found herself painfully agitated about the unfinished state of the house, which she and Stuart had bought as a handyman's special, relying on Stuart's special talents for fixing it up. She kept anticipating that her father would enter the house and, in an effort to deal with his own pain and his awareness of hers, would anxiously and critically comment on each and every flaw in the admittedly unfinished house. She had no idea how she could bear to do any of the work herself—or even to contract for others to do it. It was clear that the moment of letting a stranger do Stuart's work would be a moment of recognition that he would never come back, and at first Gail wanted no part of it. Also, there were Stuart's preferences to consider; while she felt he would want the work on the house completed, she worried about making aesthetic choices. What if she wanted green counters, for example, when he hated green? He was no longer there to speak up for himself, which in some ways only heightened her sense of responsibility to him. Fixing up the house also meant an expenditure of money at a time when she could easily descend into panic at the thought of having sole financial responsibility for taking care of the children.

As we explored the painful associations and implications intertwined with the decision to do some work on the house, Gail decided that her own comfort and well-being required that she at least fix up her own bedroom and the only bathroom. This she arranged to do and found, to her relief, that she liked the way the work turned out and loved living with a little more of the work around the house completed. Gail had crossed a small but psychologically meaningful milestone in extricating herself from an aspect of her grieving that too much interfered with her ongoing life. She needed to be able to begin to do some things her own way, even in those areas of their shared life on which Stuart would have held strong—and dominant—opinions.

THE FIRST-YEAR ANNIVERSARY:
RESTORING THE FLOW OF TIME

The memorial service turned out to be a meaningful family gathering that Gail felt gave her and the children an important opportunity to remember Stuart with a community of people who also loved and appreciated him. However, after the unveiling of Stuart's grave marker, she found herself anticipating the 8 weeks until the actual anniversary of Stuart's death with a mounting feeling of dread. "I feel," she told me, "like I'm listening to the music from the movie *Jaws*, the ominous music you hear in the background to a peaceful, idyllic swimming scene when you are least suspecting the agony that is about to strike." Every aspect of summer was now weighed down with the portent of tragedy—a tragedy that had already happened but that was once again waiting to happen.

Gail and I talked at great length about the nature of her anniversary reaction. I realized that her mounting sense of dread constituted a traumatic reliving of the reality of Stuart's death, but this time with more awareness and less dissociation. Because the anniversary of Stuart's death brought back associations to the circumstances of his death with such powerful immediacy at the same time that the full reality of his death was still substantially dissociated, Gail had found herself anticipating the anxiety of reliving the event with a terrible sense of dread. It was a source of great relief to her when she realized that her rapidly building panic was generated by her connection of the anniversary with her dissociated feelings. The worst, I reminded her, had already happened. She had already endured and survived Stuart's death. We were both impressed by the relief this realization brought her—not relief from her pain and sorrow, which were intense, but relief from the panic of dissociated retraumatization. Her relief at the realization that since Stuart was already dead, she did not in fact have to suffer the worst feelings again in reality began a deeper process of acknowledgment and integration of the death.

Gail's wish to interrupt the flow of time, her fear of the emotions that would flood her with a renewed flow of time, and her readiness to confront the passing of time were symbolized by an artistic activity she took up precisely at the first-year anniversary of Stuart's death. She felt compelled to create a series of small oblong pins she called "recovery jewelry"; these were composites of various objects assembled on a mirror. Her first piece showed a Spanish fandango dancer suspended over the black hand of death, with the pieces of a broken heart hovering on either side of her. Her favorite piece, which she gave to her sister, included a clock face stopped at the time of Stuart's death, with the number 7 standing for the date of his death, and a jagged-edged broken heart. Gail was amused by our exploration of the death symbolism in these pins, which she had only partially realized as she was making them. In her recognition and acknowledgment of Stuart's death, which became possible for the first time with the one-year anniversary of it, Gail was also declaring that she was ready to restore the flow of time and resume the painful process of grieving and living.

TRANSFORMATIONS OF SELF
AS TRANSFORMATIONS OF RELATEDNESS:
COUPLES' THERAPY WITH THE DEAD

Shortly after the first anniversary of Stuart's death, Gail took a brief vacation to the beach with close friends and their children. One night the three of them hired a babysitter and went out to a club to listen to music. She found herself remembering that she had at one time loved the exploration of new experiences in life and new relationships and entertaining a moment's glimmering realization that she might yet have those pleasures again. Gail's momentary anticipation of pleasure at being alive inaugurated a phase of work on her relationship with Stuart. We began to realize how much she was going to require permission from Stuart to go on with her life. In order to receive this permission, Gail would need to explore in a new way the construction of their attachment, especially the intensity of Stuart's feelings and her guilty response about going on with her life without him.

Gail, it seemed to me at some deep level, responded to the stirring of her own interest in a new life without Stuart as if Stuart needed protection and reassurance of her fidelity, not simply by lovingly remembering him but also by disproving his doubts and showing him that she could remain loyal beyond death. I proposed to Gail that we needed to discover through what interpersonal balance the two of them had achieved a shared psychological stability, and at what cost to each of the fullest exploration of self. Since Stuart was dead, I added, the relationship no longer required that she preserve his psychological stability at her own expense. Gail, so accustomed to the construction of a shared relational reality and to Stuart's unyielding insistence when he believed himself to be right, found almost unimaginable my proposal that she work toward a new understanding of herself that did not give so much priority to Stuart's needs and perceptions. Gail's stirring of interest in constructing a new life exposed a fear that years of marriage had long hidden but that death had resurrected and exposed through her dreams. She found herself returning to issues that had characterized her and Stuart's early relationship, such as the understanding that if she went too far in her exploration of interests beyond their relationship, Stuart could give up on her in anger and go away.

Shortly after her return from the vacation, Gail had two dreams: In the first, she and Stuart were reuniting after a separation. Gail described the air as filled with tension, like the aftermath of a fight: "Stuart did anger well; he got enraged. I didn't do anger as well; I tried to avoid it. He could get mad and not talk. But if he was angry, you couldn't dispel it; it had to be engaged or confronted. His anger required time, but time was not enough. Alan came out like that. In the dream, I was trying not to set him off again. I can still feel the tension in the middle of myself; I would bend over backwards trying to make things better." Later that same night, Gail had a second dream about Stuart and herself, also brief, also speaking to the tensions between them: "We are having a conversation about getting divorced. It felt very real, very serious. I felt awful. I woke up and realized with relief that he was dead."

Gail remembered that in the few days before he died she and Stuart had been in the middle of a fight, but one with a new rhythm leading toward a new outcome. The week before Stuart died they had the fight over ice cream, mentioned earlier in this chapter, which Gail described as a throwback to old fights: "He got furious at me, because I said to him in front of Alan that he couldn't be on a diet and also eat ice cream. I saw how ridiculous his anger was, how out of proportion to the situation. I had learned to fight back. He wanted me to give in so he could feel better; that's what we were both used to. But his anger was passing. One more morning and it would have been totally over." Although the one more morning had never come, Gail now looked back on the fight with Stuart and felt a great deal of clarity about the process between them. "I didn't feel guilty."

At this time in the therapy (8 months into our work and a little over a year after Stuart's death) Stuart vividly entered the therapy room and became a partner in our therapeutic work. Gail typically sat across from me on a long couch, and we both began to turn to the other corner of the couch, the place usually occupied by the second member of a couple. We began a new phase in the exploration of the marital relationship, ushered in by Gail's stirrings toward a new life and the corresponding uneasy dreams. We began to explore the embedded assumptions of the relationship, the assumptions that had made it work psychologically for them both when Stuart was alive but that were an impediment to Gail's rediscovery of her own life direction now that Stuart was dead. At one point in this process Gail turned to

Stuart's place on the couch, then turned to me and said humorously, "I could never get him to agree with me about that when he was alive."

Where in the history and organization of their relationship had Gail's sense of protective responsibility toward Stuart come from? Why did she even now feel compelled to give his perceptions and feelings so much priority in her understanding of herself? We explored the enduring legacies of the three streams of lived experience that contributed to the current relationally organized structure of her consciousness: her growing-up relationships within her family of origin, Stuart's growing-up relationships with his own family, and their history as a couple up to the time of Stuart's death.

Gail's comings and goings had always been a source of tension between her and Stuart, a tension that had been resolved and submerged until it was revived by Stuart's death. In the beginning of their relationship Stuart was much more sure than Gail that they belonged together for life. Initially, Gail regarded Stuart as a friend and had difficulty imagining a romantic attachment to him. From high school through their college years Stuart gracelessly endured her dating others, becoming more and more angry as he began to feel yanked around. Why couldn't she make up her mind? he would ask. What was the fascination for her in being with vapid strangers? They had several confrontations over the course of their college years, when Stuart was pressuring her more and more strongly to make an enduring commitment. One time, while they were both in college, Stuart learned that Gail had dated another man and for the first time he initiated a separation, stating that he had finally had it and couldn't take her vacillation anymore. Gail realized, through this incident, that she couldn't risk losing Stuart. Their confrontation over her "infidelity" deepened their mutual commitment, and 3 years later, after Gail completed business school, they married.

Stuart and Gail had shared so many common values that Gail had felt that most of the decisions made to establish their joint family life could easily have been her own. Yet in some areas of shared decision making, she found Stuart to be so unyielding in his position and so relentless in his attempts to bring her to his way of seeing things that she found it easier in the end to yield her ground. At times when Stuart was angry at her, he could harangue her for what felt to her like the whole night, trying to make her accept his point, while she fell asleep and woke up again. "He would wear me out," she said, "but he would tell you I was exaggerating because I couldn't deal with anger."

Growing up in her own family, Gail had learned from her pliant, good-natured, nurturant mother how to bend and yield to the needs of others. Her father, an anxious, critical, but loving and devoted man, required an enormous amount of sensitively attuned soothing in order to deliver his best, most loving self. Gail had learned from her mother how to let a man's anger run its course, how to avoid initiating a confrontation that would only "set him off" again, making things worse. Eventually, this wish to make things better emotionally for other people became very motivating to Gail herself, more motivating than her own needs. She couldn't bear the tension of someone else's pain or rage and tried to anticipate what would bring the other person emotional relief. Her older sister, Shirley, who was less willing and less able to yield emotionally to others, was always mystified by the intimacy in Gail's relationship with their father. In fact, Gail came to function as a gratifying and soothing mirror to the rest of her family, fashioning close, emotionally substantial relationships with mother, father, and older sister, all hinging on her capacity for responsiveness to the needs of others and awareness of their psychological limits to give to her. She found it more comfortable to satisfy her own dependency needs through this caretaking closeness and was made distinctly uncomfortable by any requirement that she articulate her own needs directly.

It is not that Gail lacked strength of character and clarity about her wants and needs. Quite the contrary: Most people who know her are struck by her strong sense of herself, her unconventional, irreverent sense of humor about her suburban life, her willingness as a business consultant to confront what is difficult but necessary. Gail found that self-assertion was easiest with strangers. The less a relationship mattered, the greater her freedom to be herself no matter what the other person expected of her. The rules were completely different with the people whom she loved and who loved her; Gail felt bound to them by an inextricable mix of love, obligation, and guilt. Paradoxically, the greater our talent for anticipating and responding to the needs of others, the greater our guilt; from here it is only one small step to the conviction that we are responsible for others' pain if we have not succeeded in providing them with relief.

Stuart grew up as the second of two sons born to Jewish parents who survived the Holocaust and met in a displaced persons' camp after the war. His father, a silent, self-absorbed man, had survived through passivity and favorable accidents of fate: He had been drafted into the Russian army, then discharged because he was not a member of the Communist party. Stuart's mother had survived through an act of brazen courage: She hid while the Nazis entered her village, heard them slaughter all the Jews, and then turned herself into the Gestapo as Polish, claiming she had lost her papers. As Gail told me her mother-in-law's story, we were amazed and awed by her bravery and survival.

At the same time, we began to explore the terrible consequences for Stuart's family relationships of the crushing traumas his parents had endured.

Stuart and his older brother, Gary, grew up with the vivid memory of their mother's ordeal, which Stuart visualized as intimately as if he had lived it. Haunted by repetitive, traumatic memories of her experience, Stuart's mother would often sit her sons down and obsessively reminisce about her tortured past, the terror she endured in hiding, and the even more horrible Jewish fate she so narrowly escaped. Both brothers usually felt compelled to listen to his mother to the bitter end of her compulsive monologues, absorbing her pain as a means of trying to ease it. At times, when they couldn't bear listening to her painful stories anymore, they would scream at her to stop.

Gail mused at the enormous difference in emotional style between Stuart and his brother. Stuart had been attentive to and respectful of his mother's experience, had read voraciously about Jewish history and the Holocaust, and had committed his life to commemorating, never forgetting, the horrible injustice done to his family and his people. Gary, while inevitably absorbing the anguish that permeated the atmosphere in their household, tried to absent himself as much as possible, physically and psychologically, from the burden of psychic pain. Their father was too self-absorbed to listen and respond to his wife's pain. Gail respected and appreciated Stuart's responsiveness in the face of his mother's pain at the same time that she realized that he carried the burden of this legacy into his own life, which became a shared burden in their marriage.

In this phase of our therapy, which felt very much like couples' work, I tried to help Gail become aware of the embedded marital assumption that she was applying, although illogically and unfairly, to Stuart's leaving her through death. For the first time, she was able to see past her guilt about her "infidelity" prior to their marriage and her outside interests during it. With my encouragement, Gail began to consider Stuart's possessiveness as a problem of his, a problem for which she did not need to bear full responsibility. We reviewed the dynamics in their families of origin; the assumption they both brought with them that the person who hurts the most deserves priority in being taken care of; and how the anger masking Stuart's or her father's pain didn't change Gail's sense of essential responsibility to yield to their needs but only strengthened her feelings of responsibility and guilt when she couldn't help them feel better.

Our exploration of the nature of the marital relationship, and the psychological burden Gail carried on behalf of Stuart and his family, was accompanied by Gail's sensation of overwhelming grief at losing him. She described her psychological position as one of terrible isolation from other people and depletion from the effort of staying alive herself. "I can't believe," she said, "that this is my life now, this barren nightmare place, and I will wake up to it every morning for the rest of my life. If it weren't for the children, it would feel unendurable, yet the responsibility of taking care of the children is itself a terrible drain. What would happen to them if something happened to me?"

We began to talk about Gail's difficulty considering her own needs, which I identified as a substantial problem in its own right. As a widowed single mother, now coping with enormous financial as well as psychological responsiblity for herself and her children, Gail found herself pushing hard, to the edge of her physical and emotional resources, to be all things to all people. Her parents responded to her obvious exhaustion by pressuring her to move to Florida, where she could live near them and her sister, Shirley. Gail was thrown into intense conflict over this proposal, a response to which I urged her to postpone. It seemed to me much too soon for her to uproot herself and her children from the home they had shared as a family, from the place that most reminded them of Stuart. She was engaged in a community of friends, neighbors, and professional colleagues, which she would have to totally reestablish in Florida, where she felt it would be harder to find people who shared her and Stuart's commitment to spiritual and intellectual, rather than material, values. While her loss of Stuart made her long for the comfort of her own family—and she felt that her children, too, would benefit from the love of their grandparents, uncle, aunt, and cousins—Gail feared she would lose her sense of self and her valued autonomy in attempting such a move. Even though these family bonds were substantial, relocating at this point in the bereavement process would have denied Gail's need to heal in closer proximity to the life she had built with her husband.

It seemed to me that in pressuring her to move to Florida to be near them her family was once again urging a solution on Gail that met their needs far more than her own. I encouraged Gail to consider this dimension of their request, and we explored her vulnerability and confusion about acknowledging her need to be taken care of in her own way. I reminded her of something we had talked about when she first told me about her parents. Her father worked two, at times three, jobs to support the family. When Gail was 5 years old, her mother went back to full-time work, telling Gail that she was doing so because Gail had become "too dependent" and that the independence would be good for her. Although Gail had accepted this explanation, it now seemed clear that her mother had needed to contribute to the family income in order to relieve her husband of his enormous work load and afford him some time at home. This episode became emblematic of Gail's willingness to absorb other people's attributions of her needs or character at her own expense. It also represented the constant confusion in Gail's family over acts that were represented as generosity but were in fact self-serving. Finally, in labeling Gail's normal 5-year-old dependence as excessive, her mother laid the foundation for Gail's sense that her needs were something to keep in close check. Of course, in close relationships, we take care of ourselves when we care for others; when the right hand washes the left, they both come clean. Our focus on the relational structure of her family of origin, represented by the example of her mother's explanation for returning to work, furthered Gail's progress in beginning to untangle her own needs for care from her responsibility to care for others.

I was concerned, though, that Gail was trying to do much more than one person could do alone. I urged her to get herself more household help, preferably a live-in babysitter who would help relieve her of unrelenting responsibility for the children. At the time, I myself wondered just how directive I could afford to be in making this suggestion. After all, she and I talked at length about how vulnerable she was to the suggestions and attributions made by others and how difficult she found it to assert her own needs and preferences in her closest relationships. I did feel, though, that Gail was truly in danger of stretching herself physically and emotionally beyond her capacity to support her own and her children's agonizing, and challenging, emotional integration of Stuart's death. Gail acknowledged that I was only one of many who were insisting that she hire more help. She began the preparations, physical and psychological, to let a new adult into the home.

CHANGING IMAGE OF THE DEAD: MAKING WAY FOR A NEW FORM OF RELATING

Inviting a new adult into the home precipitated an extraordinary crisis in Gail's grief experience, one that served to finally shatter the frozen immobility of time and that dislodged Stuart's spiritual presence in their home in dramatic, unexpected ways. The spare bedroom had been used for storage and contained many of Stuart's belongings. Gail became preoccupied with the details of her new living arrangements: Which of Stuart's things would she keep, and which would she begin to throw away? She became disoriented and overwhelmed by the upheaval of moving Stuart's belongings out of their accustomed places. I encouraged her to get a friend to help and to simply move Stuart's possessions to another part of the house rather than initiate a painful and perhaps premature process of parting with them. Gail recognized that many of Stuart's belongings would be cherished by his children in the years to come, but she also became aware of just how much physical space they took up: What should she do with his collection of math books? Or the enormous model sailboat, handmade, spectacular, and burdensomely fragile? She left it perched precariously in her room, fearing it would eventually come crashing down and remembering how Stuart always anticipated the physical disasters caused by her inadequate sense of spatial relations. The day her Russian immigrant babysitter—a bright, culturally fascinating, but relatively uncommunicative woman who had chosen to separate from her daughter in order to rise in the Communist party hierarchy and gain an American education—moved in, Gail's unease and disorientation again rose to panic. It became impossible for her to decide whether Sonya was in fact a difficult person or whether the process of dislodging Stuart's belongings to make room for her was bringing home, in a new way, the irrevocable loss. She told me that she now felt Stuart was gone forever, felt in a way she had refused to acknowledge before her decision to admit another person into their home. Now it was clear that new people would be needed to do the work that Stuart had at one time lovingly and joyfully done for his family himself.

Gail sensed that introducing a new person into the household had substantially changed Stuart's spiritual presence in their home. In the un-self-conscious intimacy of their own family Stuart had remained a comfortable presence. Now it was as if his ghostly comings and goings were disturbed by this new member of the household, this outsider who had never known him. For the first time, Gail began to speak to me about her changing images of Stuart; vividly present since his death, they were now being dramatically transformed.

Gail, like most people who lose a loved one, felt the presence of the deceased frequently in the year after the death. Knowing that most people would find the idea of these spiritual visitations disturbing, she did not mention them to anyone during the time when Stuart's presence was welcome and comforting. She waited until she entered a period of greater conflict, during which she found Stuart's presence more of a drain, before she talked about it with me. In the initial weeks after Stuart's death she frequently heard him weeping with inconsolable sorrow that he would never hold his children in his arms again. While Gail sometimes saw Stuart in the house, she most often saw him when she went to synagogue. Sometime during the service Stuart would emerge from somewhere left of the pulpit and come down to sit beside her. Initially he looked very sad, but now, a year and a half after his death, he began to look smaller, more neutral. Now when she saw him in the house or the car Gail began to resent his presence. She found herself at one point telling him that he had to go now, that he had to let the children grow up, that they couldn't stay babies anymore.

Gail began to wonder if this sense of Stuart as a presence was a projection of her own needs. Was it she who couldn't let time move on, who couldn't let Sam and Alan grow up because then their father would be that much further away? I suggested to Gail that it wasn't at all essential to find an explanation for her experience of spiritual contact with Stuart but that it did seem important to recognize that at this time in their shared life she needed more freedom than she could gain if Stuart's spirit remained a predominant presence in the household.

Feeling that Stuart was now more spiritually distant, Gail went back to talking about the separation issues we had started on after the first-year anniversary of his death. We resumed our discussion of the way Stuart had handled anger and the ways Gail had responded to his anger, our work punctuated by the continuing flow of her dreams. The symbolism in each dream represented a different angle of entry into their conflicts over intimacy and separation. At one point Gail described these dreams as a first glimmer of the possibility of pleasure in a new life; they reminded her of Monet's paintings, always the same subject but in different lights or at different seasons.

In the middle of March, with the period of daylight lengthening and spring beginning to stir, Gail reports a dream:

"I am in my house, in my bedroom, and Stan, whom I know slightly —he is a friend of friends—has come over and asked me to go to a party with him to be given by the Alaskan embassy. He was asking me as a matter of convenience, as a friend, not as a date; it wouldn't have to mean anything romantic. I went back and forth, I couldn't decide, but I finally said yes. Then I burst into tears, the feeling was so intolerable. I put my head on his arm and felt comforted, but then I couldn't stand that feeling either. I jumped up and left the room. Then the dream shifts: I walk into my bathroom, and there is a washing machine in it—Stan has brought it in there. I start to laugh, because it is the kind of thing Stuart would have done, and I respond as I would have to Stuart, laughing about it and asking how long it is going to be there. Then someone comes to the door, and it feels like an interruption. Stuart's friend Jack comes to the door with a couple—the husband used to work with Stuart—and they don't know Stuart is dead. Jack can't bring himself to tell them, so I tell them. I say to Jack, laughing, 'I've agreed to go out with this guy. He moved a washing machine into my bathroom.' Uncharacteristically, Jack says supportively to me, 'He sounds just like Stuart.' Then I'm getting ready to go, and Stan says, 'The party's at nine, but we have to leave at eight.' Suddenly, I realize I've lost Alan—I didn't know who he had gone home with from school, and I feel panicked, guilty, terrible. I woke up in that state."

There were some obvious reasons why Gail had picked Stan as the object of this dream: While he carried associations to Stuart, which her dream symbolism revealed, he was distinctly someone she was not romantically interested in. Also, it was clear in the dream that she was not important to him either; Gail explained, "Because I wasn't important to him, it made it easier to go out with him. If people feel too much about you, they have more of a claim on you." In the dream Gail made Stan recognizably like Stuart in personality, connecting him with the offbeat humor of a washing machine in the bathroom. Alaska was a place she had always wanted to visit; it represented the possibility of a good and interesting life without Stuart. But with her new-found freedom to go out with someone she did not care deeply about, thus feeling less burdened by his needs, and to go where she and Stuart had never gone, she also accused herself and found herself guilty of forgetting and abandoning her son Alan. In her dream Gail was asking if it is possible to care for herself without forsaking her responsibilities to others. The loss of Alan in the dream seemed to me to be the almost inevitable, unbearable punishment Gail felt would surely follow if she considered her own needs; that is, she would lose those she most loved.

Gail had always found it difficult to leave the children; now she found it almost impossible to do so. The comings and goings of mother and children were fraught with the tension of their shared loss—once we survive the close death of a family member, we know how easily and arbitrarily death can strike again. Sam, so little when his father died, cognitively equated leaving with dying. He was sure that his father had left them to go someplace else—and that he might someday return. When Sam's little playmate moved to another state with his parents, Sam grieved deeply for him, as if he had died and would never return. Gail and I began to explore how she might provide the necessary support for her children, without denying herself the freedom to do things for herself. I pointed out that the children were, in fact, more capable than she realized of carrying her presence with them when they were away from her and that although they needed her there, they also needed her emotionally whole and well, which she could not be for them if she denied herself all rights to a life of her own.

A friend phoned Gail a few weeks later and offered to introduce her to a mutual friend who was interested in going out with her. She found herself interested, confused, and panicked. She had a dream that revealed the same themes in a different light:

> "I dreamed I was in our old apartment, and we had been separated. Stuart came in with his friend Greg, from graduate school, and said, 'I've decided to leave you.' I got very upset and pleaded with him to stay. And then he said, 'Okay, I'll stay. I've changed my mind.' When he said he was leaving, I felt exactly as I did when he said he was ending our relationship—so horrible. Then, when he said he was staying, I was relieved, like everything would be all right."

As Gail and I explored the image of the dream, we noticed how much her guilt in even considering a new relationship with someone else was touching off her old guilt about being the "infidel" from an earlier stage in their relationship. Now, she heard these same reproaches in her children's questions: "Where are you going? When are you coming home?" With typical humor, Gail concluded, "I used to get this from my father, then my husband, and now my children." I commented, "Always someone guarding our virtue."

The final dream in this series, a month later, represented Gail's changing image of Stuart and his spiritual moving on as she too moved on with her own life. Gail described the dream as so vivid a visit to another world that she felt enshrouded by it for days afterward:

> "I was at Cambridge Hospital with two friends I work with now and also with a friend from high school, a woman who was part of our group with Stuart. I'm talking to her, annoyed, while my other two friends are skipping down the hall without me. I didn't feel part of things with them, yet I felt comfortable with that. I knew they weren't going to keep doing the management consulting work I was doing forever, as I needed to because of my need to support the kids. Then I have to leave. I go out of the building. I come to a gateway like the metal detector at an airport, and there is an Indian next to it, a Native American. I try to go through, but he throws little tomahawks toward me—not directly at me, more to scare me, as if I'm going into an Indian burial ground and he wants to keep me out. He is threatening, like he could change his mind and hurt me with them.
>
> Then the dream changes: I realize Stuart has AIDS and wants to go off to deal with his illness by himself, but now I have to find him. I go where he works, and I call his office. He answers the telephone, but his voice is changed; he sounds sick. I tell him I have to see him."

He agrees, and we meet in an elementary school, my school from childhood. Stuart shows up with a skid row alcoholic who is carrying Stuart's belongings, like a man Friday. The man's hands are shaking but he no longer drinks. I tell Stuart, 'I need to see you,' but he won't let me come near him. He says, 'I have AIDS.' He is detached and cold and says, 'I have to go away, and you can't come with me. You can't get AIDS, you have to take care of the kids. You're on your own now. Why do you want to see me?' I tell him, 'We always did everything together. Why can't we do this together too?' But he says, 'No, I have to go. You're on your own now. It's your life.' He is about to leave with this man, and I think to myself, 'Now he's going to go off and die, and I won't even know when.' Then I decide to wake up from the dream, it is so awful."

After reporting this dream that had made Stuart's spiritual presence once again so palpable for both of us, Gail commented to me, "Maybe he'll send me a postcard, and tell me he's dead. I said, "I can tell you that. Stuart is dead." Gail said to me, "I need you to tell me that, every once in a while."

With this dream, Gail's view of death shifted; she no longer saw it as a punishing abandonment but as a spiritual voyage taken by the dead, a voyage in which they cannot be accompanied by the living. Although in the dream Gail feels an enormous sense of loss that she cannot accompany Stuart into the other world, the spirit world, her path is blocked by the Indian gatekeeper and by Stuart himself, who reminds her of her responsibility for their children. The dream blesses her with the burden of staying alive and forbids her to follow Stuart into the world of the dead.

REDISCOVERING ASPECTS OF THE COMPLEX SELF: NEW LIFE AFTER GRIEF

Gail began to explore aspects of herself that she had chosen to put aside when she decided to make her journey in life with Stuart. Self-exploration is an inevitable part of the relational developmental process stimulated by the death of a life partner; in Gail's case this process was evident in her approach to a major life decision. For example, Stuart had always insisted, against Gail's better judgment, that they name his brother and sister-in-law their children's guardians in their wills. Gail had always believed that Stuart's brother was far less related to the world around him than Stuart would ever acknowledge, but she could not overcome her husband's insistence. After Stuart's death it became evident that while his brother, out of his own pain and avoidant characterological style, had become substantially unavailable to her and the children, her sister and brother-in-law had been devoted to and involved with Alan and Sam. After some difficult soul searching, Gail acknowledged that the only thing that stood in the way of changing guardians was the strength of Stuart's attachment to his brother and his skepticism about her family. "He would turn over in his grave if he knew I was going to name my sister guardian rather than his brother," she told me. Yet the evidence of the extended family's grief experience was undeniable: The blow of grieving had preoccupied Stuart's family so completely that they needed far more care from Gail than they could provide to either her or the children. She finally decided to name her sister the children's guardian, saying, "I wish he was here so I could tell him, ' I told you so; your brother is totally unavailable.'"

Gail's reassessment of life on her own terms was also evident in small ways, in the constant flow and texture of her daily life. She went through a great deal of confusion about what style of new clothes to buy; one day she realized she had bought a shirt in a shade of green that she had always loved and that Stuart had always hated. As she did more work on the house, she tried to retrieve what she could recall of Stuart's store of knowledge while at the same time also exercising her own good judgment and aesthetic taste. These experiments with a new sense of self represented an exploration and a resumption of growth in those aspects of her self that had been neglected by choice, by necessity, and by the complex, largely unconscious process of mutual adaptation that takes place in any marriage and creates a shared personality. Now that her husband had moved on in a journey she could not join, Gail gained the freedom to explore the next phase of her life on her own terms. While Stuart would remain an important, enduring presence in her life and in the lives of their children, she did not have to continue taking care of old relational business so as to remain loyal to him.

Gail had a dream: "I was going to India with our friends Bob and Claire, on the trip I had planned with Stuart before he died. They show up at my house, to pick me up, with four suitcases. I'm still packing, because I can only take one, and I need to pack it lightly, because there is only myself to carry it." I asked her, "What do you have to leave out, that other people get to take?" Although it was necessary for her to travel light, because she was without her life's companion, at least, we noted, she was not renouncing the trip; she was finding a way to make it possible to still live out her, and their, shared dreams, even if they are regrettably, undeniably altered.

At that point in the evolution of her grief experience, as the third anniversary of Stuart's death approached, Gail could see the unfolding of a new family life with its own satisfactions and a new sense of self that helped her expand into those areas of living and self-experience that she had constrained as part of the mutual adaptation required by a successful marriage. She was at the same time still struggling with her loss, the enormity of which was sometimes sharpened by very immediate concerns. As the summer wore on in a wave of unrelenting heat, Gail found herself waking in a panic. "It's the air conditioning," she said. "I never turn it on, unless it's brutally hot. As soon as it gets this hot, and I get that sensation again, of terrible heat, of leaving an air-conditioned room and feeling that blast of oppressively hot air, I'm in it again, like it's happening all over again, like no time has elapsed at all. Then I wake up in the morning, and it could be anytime, in any year; it could be that Stuart just died yesterday. The only thing that brings me back to a real sense of time is looking at the children: When I see Alan, a grown-up boy, and Sam, who is so clearly a little boy and no longer a baby, I feel reassured. I know it's 1991, not 1988."

For Gail, as for most bereaved people, especially those who have experienced dissociated trauma and have woven together a series of experiential connections to the death, the triggering of the traumatic memories brings on a dislocation in time and a flood of sensations that directly mimic the original experience. Anniversary reactions are an especially vulnerable time for this kind of remembering, since so many associations with the moment of death are tied in with the rhythm of seasons and with associated rituals or observances, such as holidays and birthdays. Looking into the future was also acutely painful, especially when the children of friends and relatives began to have bar and bat mitzvahs and Gail realized that she would have to experience this milestone alone with her fatherless children; her sense of missing Stuart was simply unbearable at those times. The work of emotional integration in her own life, difficult though it was, in some ways paled in comparison to the challenge of remaining present and responsive while her children suffered their own enormous loss and pain.

Gail sometimes expressed the wish that she and the children could be on a more closely choreographed timetable in the ebb and flow of their grief. It seemed, for example, that she had just made it through the hardest time in the weeks prior to the anniversary of Stuart's death and had begun to feel better when Alan would begin to suffer his own period of acute remembering and deep sadness. At the same time, Gail was alert to any unconscious action on her part that attempted to bring

the children into line with her feelings. She knew from her own experience as she struggled to integrate her grief how constraining the
needs of well-meaning but self-protective family members and friends
could be.

The poignant developmental milestones in their shared family
lives presented Gail with the greatest challenge to her capacity for
emotional integration and expansion. They required recognition of
the passage of time, tolerance of the sorrow and the sense of enduring loss Stuart's death continued to evoke, and the capacity to bear
the bittersweet pleasure of being alive to enjoy their continuing family life when Stuart was not there to enjoy it with them. Yet surviving
her life partner's death, successfully mastering the overwhelming pain,
and meeting the challenge of reinventing herself while continuing to
function and to keep her emotionally vulnerable family afloat have
given Gail new satisfactions and a new sense of personal accomplish-
ment. She can see not only how her family has been diminished by
the crisis of Stuart's death but also how they have triumphed, have
found unexpected sources of strength and capacity for resilience, and
have affirmed their enduring bonds as a family within which Stuart
remains an important member. In looking at her own life, where she
once could see only the ashes of a burned-out landscape, Gail can now
see the green of new growth.

CHAPTER 5

Bereavement
in Childhood

CHILD GRIEF AS A SYSTEMIC
DEVELOPMENTAL PROCESS

When 16-year-old Tim Johnson died in a car accident, each of his surviving siblings—Eric, 15; Greg, 10; and Suzie, 5—responded differently to his death. A stellar academic student and talented writer, Tim had been not only the oldest child of his nuclear family but the first grandson on both sides of the family.

Eric couldn't compete with his older brother, in spite of his own gifts as an artist and craftsman. He skipped school every chance he could and hung out with the wrong crowd in spite of his family's constant criticism and surveillance. After his brother Tim's death, Eric seemed to undergo a personality transformation: He became much more academically motivated and began to hang out with the honor students at the high school, many of whom had been Tim's friends. Eric stated explicitly that his brother's death had catalyzed a crisis in his own sense of self, that he now realized the value of his own life. He seemed sad but was capable of expressing his own enormous sense of loss, and he appeared relatively unburdened by his grief, at least in his immediate adjustment. If anything, his brother's death seemed to benefit Eric's development by catalyzing an expansion of his social and emotional world as he tried to fill in the enormous gap Tim's death left within the family.

Ten-year-old Greg was an intelligent, academically successful boy who seemed by all appearances to be quite unaffected by his brother's death. He had not cried openly at the time of Tim's death, did not speak about him, and did not respond to the few family references to him. However, he was becoming much more difficult to handle at home;

he was argumentative and obstinate and seemed eager to provoke fights rather than contain them. Five-year-old Suzie, energetic and emotionally expressive, was both tomboy and everybody's special girl. She spoke often about her big brother Tim, asked many questions about him, and fought fiercely with Greg over who had the right to inherit Tim's grown-up ten-speed bike.

THEORETICAL ATTEMPTS TO UNDERSTAND BEREAVEMENT IN CHILDHOOD

The Child Bereavement Literature

In evaluating the impact of Tim's death on the three surviving Johnson children, we would be advised by the literature on childhood bereavement to consider each child's cognitive-developmental capacity to understand the death and its circumstances; the immediate emotional reaction to the death; the longer-term adaptation or outcome; and the consequences of these adaptations for the child's full developmental course. For comprehensive discussions of childhood bereavement, see those of Baker, Sedney, and Gross (1992), Bowlby (1980), Furman (1974), Koocher (1986), Raphael (1983), Silverman and Worden (1992), Osterweis, Solomon, and Green (1984), and Vida (1989).

The Influence of Psychoanalytic Thought

The literature on childhood bereavement grew initially out of the psychoanalytic view of adult grief reactions proposed by Freud (described in Chapter 3). Two assumptions from the psychoanalytic understanding of adult grief reactions were applied to childhood grief. First, child analysts emphasized the importance of decathexis or detachment of psychic energy from the love object as the normal outcome of childhood bereavement. Second, they insisted that only when children reach advanced stages of ego development and mobilize appropriate defenses, including identification, can they master the overwhelming affects associated with grief. For many years child psychoanalysts used these concepts to conclude that until adolescence is reached children lack the ego developmental capacity to see grief through to the conclusion of its normal course—the decathexis of the lost object (Fleming & Altschul, 1963; Wolfenstein, 1966). The psychoanalytic literature on childhood bereavement relied primarily for its data on children who were already in psychoanalytic treatment at the time of a parent's death or on retrospective accounts from the analyses of adults who had lost a parent during childhood. The use of treatment cases further reinforced the field's emphasis on psychopathology. On the basis of these distorted clinical observations and theory, psychoanalytic writers argued that children were more likely than adults to rely on pathological defenses, such as denial, splitting of the ego, or idealization of the lost object. They argued that mobilization of these pathological defenses would make the child extremely vulnerable to distortions in development.

Modern Psychodynamic Perspectives

In contrast to classical and ego psychoanalytic perspectives, modern psychodynamic perspectives acknowledge the realistic impact of the child's caretaking environment while also including the child's subjective process in representing the reality of a traumatic event and its implications. These psychoanalytic perspectives continue to contribute to our understanding of bereaved children as well as to our therapeutic work with them. More recent psychoanalytic writings on childhood bereavement have begun to describe the experiences of grieving children from a wider general population as well as from a broader conceptual and theoretical base. Furman's (1974) work, based on children who participated in a psychoanalytically oriented therapeutic school, is one of the major pioneering efforts in documenting childhood grief reactions as they occur. Furman and her colleagues argued that children do, in fact, grieve for their parents and that, with appropriate responses from their surviving parent and other adults, grieving children can be greatly helped to complete their mourning in ways that do not compromise their ongoing development.

Bowlby's Influence

Bowlby (1980), more critical of the traditional psychoanalytic approach to childhood bereavement and the distortions it has generated, has made a strong case for his belief that children are capable of grieving in developmentally appropriate ways when they are not interfered with by the distortions and defenses of adults. He asserts that the more direct the observation of grieving children researchers undertake, the more likely they are to emphasize environmental factors as important determinants of the course of a child's grief. Bowlby especially emphasizes adult defenses as they impact on the child's grief. These defenses are typically manifested in two important way, namely in the adult's tendency to provide the child with distorted information about the nature and circumstances of the death itself and the adult's difficulty in coping with a child's direct questions and emotional expressions of grief. Bowlby goes so far as to say that we know remarkably little about the actual capacity for successful resolution of grieving in children under optimal developmental circumstances, so rarely are supportive environmental conditions met in an ordinary child's life.

Current Beliefs on Child Bereavement

The field of childhood bereavement currently asserts that children can resolve their grief as fully as adults do if they are given accurate factual information appropriate to their age and stage of cognitive functioning; if they are given the freedom to express their many complex feelings about the illness and death of the parent or sibling; if they are included in family rituals such as the funeral; and if their caretakers continue to provide stable attention to their needs in a secure, consistent way (Baker et al., 1992; Bowlby, 1980; Furman, 1974; Sekaer, 1987; Silverman & Worden, 1992).

We cannot evaluate the normalcy of childhood grief in terms of successful adult bereavement. The adult bereavement literature suggests that the response to the death of a close family member is a lifelong developmental process, rather than a finite or completed sequence of stages (Silverman, 1986; Weiss, 1988). Similarly, the child's experience of death and subsequent grief involves a lifelong, evolving exploration of the death and its meaning. Like adults, children establish a relationship with the deceased family member that continues to evolve over time. Unlike adults, however, children are still involved in basic tasks of development; they acquire a more complex understanding of the death and its implications over time. Because so much of a young child's development is yet to be completed, the image of a dead family member, especially a parent, remains a crucial source of support for the child's ongoing development. As a child's cognitive capacities mature, he or she continues to review and transform the internal working model of the deceased parent with new cognitive tools to meet new developmental needs (Baker et al., 1992; Sekaer, 1987; Silverman & Worden, 1992).

THEORIES INFORMING A SYSTEMIC DEVELOPMENTAL APPROACH TO CHILD BEREAVEMENT

The Cognitive-Developmental Influence

Researchers and clinicians who have studied childhood grief reactions have usefully applied a Piagetian cognitive-developmental perspective to illuminate children's understanding of death at different stages of development (Koocher, 1974; Wass & Corr, 1983). Between the ages of 5 and 7, roughly corresponding to the shift from preoperational to operational thought, children attain the understanding that death is irreversible, that it is accompanied by a cessation of all bodily functions, and that it is universal. A cognitive-developmental perspective stresses the importance of the child's cognitive stage in the symbolic representation of experience; in language development; in development of the capacity for systematic, logical thinking; and in understanding causality. The child who has lost a loved one uses these evolving cognitive tools for making sense of the death and integrating the experience of loss and grief as part of ongoing development.

The Psychoanalytic Influence

While psychoanalytic theory has generated problematic assumptions about childhood grief, a psychoanalytic perspective on the child's maturing capacity for emotional coping with overwhelming emotions is important in understanding how a child incorporates the experience of grief into his or her ongoing development. More recent literature on infant and child development has focused on parent–child interaction in providing the foundation for the child's internalized processes of emotional regulation (Sameroff & Emde, 1989) and for the development of secure attachment (Bowlby, 1973, 1979, 1980). The death of a family member will inevitably disrupt the relational developmental processes that become internalized as vital capacities for emotional self-regulation.

Concepts from Developmental Psychopathology

New literature in relational or ecological developmental psychopathology offers an alternative model that examines the child's age-related adaptation to stressful family and social environments. This approach, which assesses the balance of risk and protective factors that determine the quality of the child's adaptation (Anthony & Cohler, 1987; Cicchetti, 1989; Garbarino, 1990; Garbarino, Dubrow, Kostelny, & Pardo, 1992; Rutter & Garmezy, 1983), asserts that the designation of child adaptation processes as symptomatic or pathological is highly subjective and too often dismissive of the struggle all children engage in to make sense of stressful experiences. Writers with this perspective suggest that it is far more useful to assess whether the child's adaptation to stressful life events interferes with the child's ongoing development.

The emerging perspective from the risk and resilience literature in developmental psychopathology integrates ecological or relational approaches to normal development with an understanding of the ways high-stress environments can disrupt the ongoing developmental process. This model makes it possible to examine the developmental impact of childhood bereavement without succumbing to the tendency to pathologize the child's attempts at adaptation. Since adults undergoing the massive stress of bereavement are themselves attempting to adapt to extraordinary circumstances as best they can, our discussion of the ways parents fail to support their children's bereavement is based on a respectful appreciation of their struggle to do the best parenting they can under those circumstances.

Collaborative Construction of the Relational Self

The tension between a child's subjective representation of life events and his or her adaptation to adult needs is a crucial dynamic in the collaborative construction of a relational self in childhood and throughout life. The process of symbolic representation, which is both a private means of making sense of one's experience and a social means of sharing and communicating experience, is under ordinary circumstances mutually negotiated. With mutuality in our close relationships, we can construct socially adaptive selves that also maintain the integrity of our private experience. However, under circumstances of radical discontinuity or stress, such as the death of a family member, a family's capacity for mutuality and for inclusion of the child's perspective is more likely to be compromised.

Bowlby, in ways that follow from his training as an object-relations-informed psychoanalyst, remained extremely sensitive to the fact that children see themselves and make sense of their own experience through internalized models of mutual adaptation in the parent–child relationship. The child's image of self in relationships can be significantly interfered with by the requirements of adapting to a vulnerable parent's self-protective relational demands or views of the child. What Winnicott (1965) called the "true" and "false" self and Masud-Khan (1988) has more accurately renamed "authentic" and "reactive" self addresses this duality in our awareness of our own experience. We are, at the same time, making sense of the world in ways that are uniquely individual and, by using the social and communicational tools of our culture and family, constructing a reality that is socially choreographed.

This dual dimension of consciousness becomes problematic when we are forced to deal with irreconcilable conflict between our own perceptions and those of important others. This normal dialectic in symbolic representation (i.e., between private and social meaning) can lead to pathology when the preservation of our connections to others requires the disavowal of vital aspects of our self. At that point, we are forced to stereotype or dissociate our forbidden, overwhelming, or conflictual perceptions of an event and their associated emotions rather than integrate them. Not only will representations of the overwhelming experience be dissociated, but the associated psychological and relational functions, the tools for understanding a developmental moment, will become entangled with the dissociated event and will become less available for ongoing development. Thus, while the process of adaptation to the parent's reality is initially an interpersonal one, it acquires over the course of development an internalized or intrapsychic component: in a self-perpetuating process that is closed off from new experiences aspects of the self that are associated with personal needs but are in conflict with internalized parental identifications or prohibitions continue to be disavowed.

An Integration of Developmental Theories

These perspectives on child development—the cognitive Piagetian, the psychoanalytic, and the relational–developmental—can be integrated so as to outline the tasks of normal cognitive, emotional, and psychosocial development at a particular stage of child development and the potential impact of a family death on a child's development. The two interrelated domains of *symbolic representation*, or meaning making, and *self-regulation through relational adaptation* are vital to an understanding of the child's creative self-organizing response to any developmental crisis, including the crisis of death and grief. Table 6.1 schematically outlines for each major stage of development the developmental tasks proposed by the following perspectives: the cognitive, or Piagetian; the emotional–defensive, or Freudian; the psychosocial, or Eriksonian; and the relational developmental. While these major theories have focused on separate domains of development, the child's development is in fact an integrated, highly interrelated whole. On the basis of these integrated stages of development, Table 6.1 describes stages in the development of the child's capacity to understand the reality of death and the major tasks of individual and relational development that will be disrupted by the experience of grief. The stages outlined in Table 6.1 (pp. 88–89) can serve to orient grief counselors and family clinicians to the important age-related developmental tasks that determine both the child's tools for understanding death and the potential consequences for the child's ongoing developmental progress. (The developmental dimensions outlined in Table 6.1 will be used to organize the stories of grieving children by stage of development in Chapter 6.)

VULNERABILITIES IN THE
CARETAKING ENVIRONMENT

The optimal conditions for successful childhood bereavement are rarely met in real life for several reasons: First, the caretaking environment is almost inevitably disrupted by the death of an important family member. Disruptions in the predictability and security of day-to-day life place an additional emotional burden on surviving children and parents. The energy absorbed by the need to cope with day-to-day survival interferes with the child's and the family's focus on the loss itself.

Second, discrepancies between child and adult cognitive understanding and emotional coping can lead to confusion communicating about the death and its enduring impact on the family. Children's understanding of death and grief varies with their cognitive stage of development, and adults frequently misunderstand the child's cognitive capacity for grasping the circumstances and implications of the death. Moreover, adults are likely to deliberately give children incomplete information about the circumstances of the death in an effort to protect them from information they might not be able to handle. Adults may also restrict the child's free expression of questions or reminiscences about the dead family member. Often, the motivation to protect the child reflects the adult's own attempts to stabilize and cope with his or her own grief.

Third, cultural practices may limit the representation of the deceased in the ongoing family life cycle and may restrict the access of grieving families to a supportive image of their deceased family member. The dominant culture in the United States is especially reluctant to include the dead as spiritually or psychologically present family members. Our culture emphasizes letting go of the dead and considers a family's focus on a dead member to be disturbingly morbid. Because of these cultural prohibitions, our culture is more likely than others to interfere with the grief of children. With their continually evolving cognitive and emotional capacities, children need to constantly review the circumstances and meaning of the death. This changing review helps children achieve an image of the deceased family member that grows up with them as a supportive resource. An evolving image of the deceased family member helps children meet their ever-changing needs over the course of development.

Parenting by Grieving Adults

The adult bereavement literature has examined the impact of grief on parenting to a limited degree and only with respect to the devastating impact of the death of a child on parental self-esteem. The child bereavement literature has discussed the parent's vital role in providing the right caretaking environment for the grieving child. Unfortunately, that literature has tended either to gloss over discussions of parenting as "good enough" (Furman, 1974) or to document examples of pathological childhood grief reactions that have been greatly exacerbated by such parenting problems as chaotic or discontinuous caretaking, neglectful failures of parental responsiveness to the child's needs, and deliberate parental distortion of the circumstances of the death (Bowlby, 1980).

In order to go further in understanding childhood bereavement, and in helping children and their families, we need a more textured and sympathetic review of the parenting experiences of grieving adults. Parenting, under the best of circumstances, is an extremely challenging demand on the physical, economic, and psychological resources of adults (Belsky & Vondra, 1989). Under the circumstances of bereavement, both the emotional and instrumental resources of parents are taxed to the limit. Grieving parents may find it all they can do to keep their own functioning intact and stable. Grieving children, in turn, will make it their first priority to contribute to the psychological stability of their emotionally overwhelmed grieving parents. Children may help their parents by assuming more direct family and household responsibilities. They are also likely to attempt to help their grieving parents indirectly by constraining their emotional expressions in response to parental messages of what can and cannot be tolerated.

When a parent dies, it is likely that important caretaking functions will need to be redistributed among available adults all of whom are themselves at that point psychologically burdened by their own bereavement. With the death of a mother, a father will need to arrange for alternative caretakers, either within the extended family or through the employment of a child care worker. For many families, distance makes the extended family unavailable, and most family members have other obligations that limit their availability for the full-time caretaking young children require. Few families can afford to replace a young mother's care full-time care of her children with paid child care. Replacing a mother's contribution to the household becomes even more difficult when the mother herself worked outside the home to increase family income, a situation which is becoming increasingly common.

When a father dies, the disruption in the family is more typically a financial one. Additionally, young fathers are more likely now than in previous generations to have been involved in the direct care of their children. A widow is abruptly plunged into the overwhelming experience of single motherhood, dependent on whatever financial arrangements she and her husband made prior to his death. Whether or not she worked prior to the death, a woman often feels compelled to return to work or to increase her work hours after the death of her husband. Concern with financial burdens; an increase of work hours; and the loss of her husband's love, companionship, and support, as well as whatever coparenting he contributed—these factors make it difficult for a widow to attend to her own social and emotional needs, let alone the needs of her grieving children.

The caretaking environment is disrupted in a different but equally important way by the death of a child. On the face of it, it would seem that both parents continue to be available for the caretaking of the surviving children. In fact, most adults are so devastated by the death of a child that they describe themselves as far less available, physically and psychologically, to their surviving children. The death of a sibling is in itself an enormous loss and a difficult emotional experience for the grieving child (Krell & Rabkin, 1979; Raphael, 1983; Pollock, 1986). Compounding the loss for most children is the inaccessibility of their grieving parents, whose slow process of recovery can consume many years of the surviving children's growing-up period.

The terminal illness of a family member provides relatives with valuable opportunities to say good-bye and to more gradually integrate the reality of the loss. However, the conditions created by a chronic illness can create additional stressors for the parent–child relationship. Both the literature on death of an adult and the literature on death of a child suggest that there is an "ideal" length of approximately 6 months between diagnosis of the illness and death (Koocher, 1986; Rando, 1983; Rolland, 1991). The demands of caring for a terminally ill family member with a longer illness are themselves stressors. During the terminal illness of a parent or sibling children often need to be taken care of by adults other than their parents and are often kept uninformed about medical details concerning the illness and death. Rosenheim and Reicher (1985, 1986) found that parents did not accurately perceive their children's involvement in anticipatory grief for a terminally ill parent. These researchers found that children who were informed of a parent's impending death suffered less anxiety than did children who were kept uninformed. In order for parents to provide support for their children's anticipatory grief, parents themselves need to be in a position to cope with their own feelings and to step outside themselves. But, again, a parent's capacity to provide supportive, empathic caretaking is itself compromised by his or her own increased burden of grief and family responsibility.

Given the pragmatic and psychological burdens on bereaved adults, it is not surprising that the ideal or optimal continuity of caretaking is rarely achieved in families. These realities of discontinuity in caretaking are likely to add to the grieving child's emotional vulnerability as he or she adapts to the loss.

Parental Influences on a Child's Bereavement

Most adults tend to misunderstand the process of childhood grief, because they are not aware of the particular characteristics of grief that emerge from the child's cognitive and affective developmental stage. Before the age of 6 or 7, children do not understand the finality of death and will view it as a reversible separation. As Bowlby (1980), Furman (1974), and Koocher (1974, 1986) have demonstrated, however, even preschool children can understand a great deal about death and grief, much more than adults ordinarily give them credit for. Before adolescence, a child's understanding of death and the circumstances that caused it will be concrete and vulnerable to confusion. Koocher (1974, 1986) finds that children who have experienced a death of a parent are immediately concerned with the answer to the following three questions: Did it happen because of something I did or failed to do? Will it happen to me (or to someone else I care about)? Who will take care of me if or when it does happen? Depending on the child's age and stage of development, he or she may be extremely confused or fearful about the circumstances and implications of the death and will need a great deal of support and clarification.

While children's cognitive understanding of logical causality becomes progressively more mature, their understanding of the causality involved in the death of an attachment figure remains vulnerable to distortion throughout life. Rather than feel completely helpless in the face of an overwhelming event, most people, regardless of age and stage of development, choose to feel responsible and blame themselves so as to avoid recognition of the fact that such events can happen randomly, at any time (Janoff-Bulman, 1985; Terr, 1990). For adults, this process of self-blame often involves a reasoning backward from the juxtaposition of events to their causality: "If only I hadn't taken that route"; "If only I had been more careful about keeping an eye on them"; "If only we hadn't had that last fight." For children, the process includes more concrete, self-referential, or magical juxtapositions of self-blame: "Because I asked for that extra cookie"; "Because I was so bad"; "Because I was out playing and having a good time." While adults can apply more mature logical reasoning to counterbalance the deep conviction of self-blame, children are unable to clarify these causal distortions on their own. Whatever the child's age and cognitive stage, his or her sense of self-efficacy at a particular stage of development will become infused with the conviction that certain actions lead to the disaster of death and abandonment.

Parental Distortion of the Death

Adults will in many instances gloss over or deliberately distort details of the circumstances of the death, typically with the hope that they might protect their children from emotionally disturbing facts. These distortions are most often found under circumstances of suicide or extreme trauma. While many parents under such traumatic circumstances may genuinely wish to protect their children from overly painful confrontations with reality, both clinical and research evidence suggests that these adult distortions are often self-protective. When adults convey incomplete or distorted information about the circumstances of a death, they inadvertently compromise the child's capacity to cognitively and emotionally integrate the experience (Bluebond-Langner, 1978; Bowlby, 1980; Cain & Fast, 1966; Furman, 1974). Under circumstances of traumatic bereavement, the family's capacity to tolerate the child's exploration of her or his pain and confusion through insistent questioning will determine whether the child's grief experience can be successfully integrated. An overwhelming traumatic event in the absence of opportunities for exploration and reassurance is more likely to become dissociated information—that is, at the same time both known and inaccessible—at great cost to the child's ongoing cognitive and emotional development.

Establishing a New Equilibrium between Private and Shared Reality

With the shared crisis of family bereavement, children and their parents attempt to reestablish a functional equilibrium that will allow them to integrate the reality of the death and its consequences gradually and manageably. This process of establishing a new equilibrium requires negotiation between the private reality and the shared reality. Because of family power asymmetries, however, the parent's definition of reality will typically take priority over the child's exploration of his or her own reality. Bereavement cases involving death by suicide, such as those described by Cain and Fast (1966), provide the most dramatic examples of the ways in which a child's sense of reality is compromised by the adult's distortion of the death and its circumstances as a means of gaining personal stability.

Most children are happy to make the sacrifice of their own integrity so as to protect a parent's emotional well-being, since the parent's stability is essential to the child's own survival and capacity to proceed with ongoing development. From a systemic developmental perspective, we can say that the process of shared meaning making becomes pathological when a family's attempts to establish a secure base from which to proceed with ongoing shared development has in fact too severely restricted the family's capacity for flexible, adaptive change and has therefore too much interfered with the ongoing development of one or more of its members. Shared meaning making continues in the crisis of grief, where the adaptation made by children, who are still developing in basic areas of cognitive, emotional, and social maturation, to adult and family strategies for stabilization becomes interwoven with and may compromise the work required of them for ongoing development, including the work of making their own private yet relationally negotiated sense of the grief experience itself.

Many dimensions of a family's reorganization and recreation of new stable structures will impact on the child's integration of the grief experience into his or her own ongoing development. Grieving adults may have difficulty supporting the child's emotional expression if they encounter in their children's grieving emotions they are themselves defending against. They might have difficulty encouraging the child's enduring attachment to a deceased parent if unresolved marital conflicts resurface during negotiation of the family's future relationship to the deceased. From an interpersonal object relations or family systems perspective, parents use their children as extensions of their own intrapsychic developmental processes, through projective attribution or projective identification processes that the child absorbs. Grieving families use systemic family structures to help cope with overwhelming feelings of loss and grief and to define the context of permissible responses within which their children's development will unfold.

Cultural Influences on Parenting Bereaved Children

While parenting is essentially an adult and family responsibility, cultures differ a great deal in the supportive context they provide for adults to function as parents. Cultures differ in the caretaking arrangements they establish for developing children: Some emphasize the bond of biological parents to their children while others distribute caretaking over a much wider range of relatives. The work of parenting requires economic resources and a community of other families as sources of emotional and social support, as well as respite care. Stresses in the family's cultural and community context, such as poverty or neighborhood violence, add enormously to the burden of parenting under the best of circumstances (Cicchetti & Carlson, 1989; Egeland, 1990; Garbarino, 1992; Meisels & Shonkoff, 1991; Schorr, 1986). Families who live with the chronic stresses of poverty or neighborhood and family violence and who are, therefore, already struggling to keep their heads above water will be devastated by the loss of a parent. A supportive network of members of the extended family, the church, and other community groups can help grieving parents with caretaking, economic resources, and emotional support. In our increasingly depleted families and communities, these community and extended family supports seem harder and harder to come by.

Cultural beliefs and practices support the expression of certain feelings or coping styles while constraining the expression of others. Cultures also differ in the ease with which they affirm the continuity between the spiritual or ancestral world and the world of the living. Buddhist cultures, which see the individual ego as illusory and which emphasize the enduring spiritual nature of ancestral ties, preserve a reassuring sense of continuity between the living and the dead. Boothby (Personal Communication, 1990) described the experiences of Cambodian children in refugee camps, many of whom had endured and often witnessed the brutal murder of both parents. These traumatized children, alone in the world, felt the enduring spiritual presence of their dead parents, who would visit them in dreams and offer them the guidance and reassurance that helped them survive the camps.

In our technological Western culture, death is seen as the end of life and as the beginning of a process in which attachment bonds are ultimately replaced. In Western culture a child's enduring sense of the presence of the dead parent would be more likely to be considered morbid or pathological. Depending on their own religious beliefs and cultural practices, parents and families vary in how they respond to the child's normal need to achieve an image of the deceased parent that grows with them in developmental time. For many children in our culture, conversations with the deceased parent or sibling remain private and are part of a separate, secret life. Although our culture, compared to cultures that emphasize attachment bonds more strongly, may reap certain benefits in its support for the independence of the isolated self, its emphasis on independence may leave grieving children who are coping with the death of a parent or sibling with attachment longings and fantasies of which they feel ashamed.

SUMMARY

In sum, a systemic developmental perspective on childhood bereavement emphasizes the interweaving of the child's stage of development, family relationships, and culture in determining his or her grief reaction and the impact of death and grief on his or her ongoing development. A systemic developmental perspective on childhood grief considers each child's place in the evolving relationships over the course of the family life cycle. From this perspective, family relationships organize the course of child development and are radically interrupted by the death of a close family member. The death of a family member is a stressful disruption of ongoing family development that forces the reorganization of parent–child relationships in the family system, a reorganization that affects the child's adjustment and continuing growth. The grieving family's capacity to reestablish stable equilibrium without restricting the ongoing development of its members is especially crucial in determining the consequences of the death for its grieving children, who have so much of their development to complete.

Like adults' grief, children's grief is determined substantially by the circumstances of the death, the child's relationship to the family member who died, the amount of disruption in daily living associated with the death, the availability of social support, and the child's temperament or personality style for coping with intense emotions (Bowlby, 1980; Furman, 1974; Raphael, 1983). Unlike adults' grief, children's grief is organized by the cognitive features characteristic of their particular developmental stage (Koocher, 1974, 1986) and by their attuned responsiveness to the expressions of grief their caretakers can tolerate (Baker et al., 1992; Bowlby, 1980; Furman, 1974; Siegel, Mesagno, & Christ, 1990; Weber, 1985). Children are still completing their cognitive, emotional, and social development. For this reason, the child's attempts to absorb the blow of grief and to achieve emotional stabilization in responsive adaptation to other grieving family members become interwoven with the developmental work of a particular stage.

Children's grief is especially vulnerable to distortion by the needs, projections, and instructions of adults. Children perceive the world more concretely and literally than do adults and depend on adults for much of their information about the world around them. In addition, a child's physical and psychological dependence on the parent gives the parent power or priority in defining the child's experiences, even when the parent contradicts the child's direct perceptions (Miller, 1984). The death of a family member generates circumstances in which adults, both protectively and consciously as well as self-protectively and unconsciously, distort the information they give to their children about the nature and circumstances of the death or about their ongoing shared experience of grief.

CHAPTER 6

The Stories
of Grieving Children

WEAVING GRIEF AND COPING
INTO THE DEVELOPMENTAL FABRIC

Our human context is relational, and we weave our life stories out of shared experiences with those we love. Repair of our shattered selves following the death of a loved one depends both on our relationship resources and on the specific tools of a developmental moment. In the previous chapter, I explained how the work of childhood grief is shaped by both the child's cognitive–developmental capacities and the capacities of the adult caretaking environment. In this chapter, I organize the stories of childhood bereavement by age and stage of cognitive, emotional, and relational development, following the stages in Table 6.1. I describe the ways death and grief become woven into the fabric of a child's life. Like grieving adults, grieving children can never be just what they might have been if a parent or sibling had not died. Yet these stories emphasize the remarkable resourcefulness and resilience of children and their families as they create safe havens for continuing their shared growth.

BEREAVEMENT IN INFANCY

Infancy has been a compelling area of study for both clinicians and developmental researchers, who see this time of life as crucial to later development in cognitive, emotional, and social domains. Yet infants are notoriously difficult to study, and clinicians have been especially guilty of projecting all kinds of elaborate theoretical constructs on children of this age. The Freudian view of a disorganized, emotion-

TABLE 6.1. Developmental Stages and Their Implications for Childhood Bereavement

Stage	Designation of stage by developmental theory				Implications for bereavement
	Piagetian (cognitive and symbolic processes)	Freudian (emotions and defense)	Eriksonian (psychosocial issues)	Integrative (relationships and representation)	
Infancy	Sensorimotor	Oral (id/passion)	Trust vs. mistrust (hope)	Emotions patterned through mutually regulating interaction; symbolic representation through action-in-the-body; balance between self-assertion and emotionally attuned environmental adaptation negotiated	Grief experienced through disruptions in caretaking or parental depression; grief represented and remembered in body images or action symbols; potential for deep self-blame because of incomplete understanding of causality
Toddler stage	Representational intelligence (preoperational)	Anal (ego/reality)	Autonomy vs. shame and doubt (will)	Language first used for symbolic processing of emotions; id (passions) now modulated by ego (reality); first individuation accompanies first awareness of dependency; intense conflicts experienced in balancing attachment and self-assertion	Loss experienced directly, with action representations as well as language used to express grief; death understood as a separation; issues of self-blame can become entangled with the beginning of self-assertion
Preschool stage	Concrete operational	Phallic oedipal (superego/conscience)	Initiative vs. guilt (purpose)	More complex capacity for categorization; creative, concrete, magical cognition; dependency issues widened to include exploration of power and gender (man–woman, boy–girl, little–big); internalization of adult prohibitions as private conscience begins	Beginning understanding of finality of death as a concept, although not in relation to close attachment figures, who are viewed as absent and expected to return; concrete language and magical thinking used in understanding of causality; possible interpretation of adult explanations of cause of death in concrete or self-blaming terms

School-age stage	Concrete operational	Latency	Industry vs. inferiority (competence)	New capacity to repress-simplify the complex self through more elaborate categorization and stereotyping of experience (Piaget); better capacity to use the ego's mechanisms of defense (Freud); wish to master grown-up tasks (Erikson); conflicts resolved with adult prohibitions through same-sex identification	Understanding of finality of death, but concrete or confused understandings of cause of death likely; may appear unaffected or uncaring, while maintaining close relationship with the image of the deceased family member and, at times, deliberate illusion that deceased is present; possible sense of shame for being different from conventional, intact families
Adolescence	Formal operations	Genital	Identity vs. diffusion (fidelity)	New capacity for abstract thinking makes possible the re-creation of self in relationship to parents and to wider culture; reworking of previous stages in resolution of identity-attachment processes (individuation); intensification of sexuality, requiring new balance between passion, reality, and conscience	Adult understanding of death and grief, but still vulnerable to fantasies that dead family member might return; possible entanglement of grief and loss with separation processes

89

ally primitive infant focused only on libidinal gratification has given way to a modern view of the socially competent infant. We now understand that infants are highly organized toward the basic developmental tasks of self-regulation through systematic engagement of their social world. During the Piagetian sensorimotor stage, roughly in the first 2 years of life, the child understands the world through the active exploration and coordination of sensory impressions and motor activity. Infants organize and internalize their actions into patterns or structures, which Piaget called *schemas*. These internalized action patterns become the foundation for later intellectual structures.

Complementing Piagetian conceptualizations of infant cognitive development, infant researchers are studying socioemotional regulation through interaction in the mother–infant dyad and are documenting young infants' sophisticated participation in shared action sequences that regulate their affective responses (Bretherton, 1985; Sameroff & Emde, 1989; Stern, 1985; Tronick, 1989). The baby's capacity to engage in highly nuanced, mutually responsive interactions suggests that infants just a few months old are deliberate participants in processes of mutual emotional regulation. These interactions lay the foundation for later, internalized, management of emotions. The success of the child's engagement with the world will depend on the caretaking adults' capacities for responsive care. Erikson's emphasis on the development of trust in this early phase captures the importance of this early mutuality of engagement as a foundation for the capacity to hope in later life.

Most writers do not consider infants capable of mourning in a formal sense, at least not until the cognitive achievement of object constancy, which most typically occurs between 8 and 10 months of age. Yet it is clear from child observation that even very young infants are disrupted in their experience and exploration of the world and in their emotional states and emotional regulation by the absence of a significant member of their caretaking system. Bowlby's work on attachment and Ainsworth's laboratory creation of the "strange situation" to assess an infant's security of attachment generated a substantial research literature evaluating the psychological antecedents and interpersonal consequences of secure versus insecure attachment in children (Ainsworth, Blehar, Waters, & Wall, 1978; Bretherthon & Waters, 1985; Cicchetti, 1989). The attachment literature has not yet focused on infants whose parents die, but it suggests a substantial vulnerability for children separated from the primary caretaker who do not experience stable, continuous caretaking from other adults.

Yet it also seems premature to draw on this literature and predict that young children who lose a parent will have insecure attachment and vulnerable internal working models of self in relationships. While the death of a parent in childhood is associated with some tendency to depression in adulthood, the majority of children who experience this loss do not suffer depression as adults (Bowlby, 1980; Osterweis et al., 1984). The stability of the caretaking environment and the support bereaved children receive in maintaining a relationship with the deceased parent are two crucial factors that enhance their ongoing development.

Preverbal children who lose a parent during infancy arrive at an experience of the death through their internalized representations of the shift in their caretaking environment. The emphasis our culture places on isolated nuclear families increases the bereaved infant's vulnerability to caretaking disruptions. Yet children who lose a parent at a young age can continue, with the support of their surviving parent and other members of the extended family, in a developing relationship to the deceased parent. For infants, the image of the deceased parent exists primarily as received knowledge from others rather than direct memory, and that image can be augmented by photographs, memorabilia, and detailed family stories. Over time, children use their maturing capacity for an inner life in fantasy to request more information directly and to make the image of the dead parent their own. A child's capacity to retain a sustaining sense of comfort from a relationship with a deceased parent will depend on family members' willingness to discuss the parent and share their memories. Too often, parents feel these conversations are morbid; parents who are overcome with their own grief might censor these discussions without appreciating how necessary they are for their child's future developmental course (Baker et al., 1992; Silverman, 1992).

Infants and toddlers symbolically represent experience in body metaphors (Santostefano, 1984–1985). Traumatic experiences are most likely to be encoded in enduring body images and metaphors, as has been shown in the literature on child physical and sexual abuse (Cicchetti, 1989; Terr, 1990). Children who lose a parent during the first 2 years of life attempt to explore and work through preverbal memories of the traumatic separation by means of kinesthetic or sensorimotor images and metaphors. The body-based location of these images makes these children vulnerable to a pervasive, intense self-reproach.

Over the course of intensive psychotherapy Martin, a man in his early thirties, retrieved memories from the age of 16 months, when his father was hurt in a near-fatal car accident, which Martin witnessed. Martin remembered almost nothing of the immediate event, which left his father physically crippled, except for the physical image of running toward his father in his awkward toddler's gait and stumbling before reaching him. Over the course of his life Martin was haunted by vivid dreams in which he struggled to keep his tenuous footing– on a tightrope, on a ladder–while trying to reach his father to save him from certain death. During the course of his therapy 30 years later he discovered the creative web of associations to his father's accident. His enduring dream imagery symbolically connected the toddler's awkward locomotion and magical, self-referential sense of causality with a profound sense of responsibility for saving his father's life on the basis of his capacity to keep from stumbling.

Toddlers often understand much more about a death than they are given credit for by adults. In his attempt to understand his mother's death through the physical representation of the event, Joshua, age 2 when his mother was killed in an airplane crash, began to play a ritualized, repetitive game in which he would jump from the bed to the floor, or the couch to the floor, over and over again.

It is easy for adults to believe that toddlers 1 or 2 years of age are not capable of understanding a death and its circumstances–even in spite of direct evidence to the contrary. When Sandra Sutherland Fox first opened the Family Support Center for grieving families, she stressed, with missionary zeal, the importance of communicating with even young children about the death of a parent. Sandra gave us the following example: After a woman committed suicide by jumping off a bridge, her husband, mother, and children, including an 18-month-old boy, came to the Family Support Center. While the family discussed the death, they assured Sandra that their little boy did not understand that his mother had died, much less the circumstances of her death. As they spoke, Sandra observed the little boy jumping off the couch, over and over again, in the same ritualized way Joshua had. Whatever the 18-month-old had heard and observed, he clearly grasped an image of his mother jumping to her death, which he was repetitively exploring through an action metaphor.

Direct communication with young children does not relieve them of the need to use action images as a means of understanding and working through the death of a family member. Repetitive play is a creative means of coping and mastery, and children rely on both play and fantasy for exploration and integration of events in their lives. The more traumatic the event, the more anxiety the child will need to contain and represent through action imagery. However, direct communication does minimize the young child's sense of isolation and confusion about the death and loss and supports his or her own attempts to cope with the trauma.

The death of a mother or primary caretaker has the greatest potential for developmental disruption in infancy, but the death of a close family member who is not the primary caretaker will also be directly experienced by the child through the caretaking relationship itself. The caretaker's absorption in his or her own grief can lead to massive disruption in his or her capacity for engaging in attuned shared experiences with the child. Research on maternal depression vividly depicts the powerful impact on a baby of a mother who is unable to respond to interactive play (Tronick, 1989). Babies with depressed mothers often step up their interactive pace, trying as hard as they can to evoke a response from their withdrawn mother. They might eventually become withdrawn themselves, giving up on the hope of mutual engagement. Object relations theory suggests that internalization of caretaking interactions with a depressed or withdrawn mother could lead to depression in a child who has not received help mobilizing his or her own engagement with the outside world. Alternatively, interactions between a depressed mother and her young child could lead to the development of what Winnicott called a "false self." Even very young infants who are asked to take too much care of a depressed or overwhelmed parent carefully construct their selves around the task of responding adaptively to the parent's needs and have little opportunity to express their authentic, spontaneous "true self."

While infancy is an extremely vulnerable developmental phase during which to lose a close family member, infants, like all children, are extraordinarily resilient in their capacity to make the best of developmental opportunities. If the child's caretaking environment remains stable and supportive and the parents recognize that the child has also suffered a loss, it becomes possible to minimize the disruptive effects of death and grief. Infants under the age of 8 months cannot understand a parent's direct communication about a death, but they do experience the loss of a family member as a diminution of the relational context within which they form their vital sense of self. Between 12 months and 2 years, children become increasingly capable of understanding a parent's communication about the death of a family member. Young children need to be addressed directly in ways that are appropriate to their understanding of language. As the child becomes more sophisticated in his or her cognitive maturation and use of language, he or she will need to review and explore the death and its circumstances. Children whose families support their maturing exploration of the death and its meaning can continue to integrate the experience of the death and to sustain a living, evolving image of the dead parent.

A Bereaved Infant Becomes a Grieving Boy: Creating a Living Image of the Dead Father

Preverbal children who lose a parent face an especially difficult developmental task; they need to incorporate a sense of their dead parent into their ongoing development without a reservoir of memories and direct experience relating to that parent. The surviving parent's tolerance for sharing a living, evolving image of the dead parent with the child provides a crucial support for the child's ongoing development. Sam Kaplan's father, Stuart—the husband of Gail, whose therapy I discussed in Chapter 4—died when Sam was a year and a half and his older brother, Alan, was 6. Within the tragic circumstances of Stuart's sudden, unanticipated death, we could say that Sam was lucky in that the "holding environment" provided by his mother and brother fully included Stuart as a living, spiritual presence. Gail, who had been working part-time as a business consultant to stay active in her profession, was able to increase her working hours so as to maintain a steady income and sense of financial security. She entered therapy with me and had Alan go into therapy with a colleague, because she knew the family needed help in overcoming this experience without adverse long-term effects on their shared development. In Chapter 4 I described Gail's private reconstruction of her relational self, focusing on her marriage and its history in family-of-origin relationships. Not only was Gail undergoing her private grief, but she was providing the context for Sam and Alan's developmental integration of the loss of their father.

Gail was closely attuned to Sam's evolving, imaginative expressions of his anger, sorrow, and confusion about his father's death. She spoke to him frequently and directly about his father's life and death. Thus, Sam was substantially supported in accomplishing the still overwhelming task of figuring out who he was in relation to his father. Gail had no difficulty invoking Stuart's presence in the natural flow of family conversations or answering Sam's questions about his father, but it was difficult for her to understand and manage expressions of their shared grief when they affected the way she and the children handled separations. Gail had grown up with little tolerance for her own dependency needs and at times misinterpreted the children's vulnerability and need for reassurance during separations, which were direct results of their grief experience.

Because of the confusion following Stuart's collapse, Gail had no awareness of how much Sam was observing as the paramedics worked on his father's lifeless body before taking him to the hospital by ambulance. Afterward, Sam became quite understandably terrified of going to the doctor and of having the doctor touch him in any way. For a period of about a year, Sam's ongoing visits to the doctor required an enormous amount of preparation and sensitivity. Once, when Sam fell while playing and required stitches, he became enraged at the intrusion of the doctors, exhibiting a level of intensity that reflected a traumatized reworking of his father's death. However, by the time Sam was 5, his terror of doctors seemed to have passed.

Like most preverbal children, who understand death as a separation and not as a finite end of life, Sam was convinced that his father was away and that he could come back if he wanted to. Family visits to the cemetery inspired a repetitive search by the boy for small objects, which he would bury and then retrieve over and over again. Sam was acting on his wish to find his father where he seemed to have last been lost, under the earth. At the age of 3, Sam went through a period during which he was overcome with grief and despair at the thought of one of his toys breaking; when he was away from home, he would sometimes cry inconsolably, convinced that one of the toys he had left intact at home had become broken in his absence. In her attempts to comfort Sam, Gail would remind him that even if one of his toys were to break, it could, like most broken things, be fixed; then she would tell him that his father had been marvelously good at fixing things and that he too could learn to fix things. Sam does, as it happens, take after his father in having a talent for making sense of the mechanical world. As he achieved an identification with his much missed father, Sam was able to better master his feelings of fragility and helplessness.

Because of Sam's young age when Stuart died, he had no direct memories of his father. Instead, he had to rely on photographs, memorabilia, and the recollections of others to evoke a living image of his father to warm him and assuage his loneliness. Until he was 5, Sam kept at his bedside a picture of his father holding him. This picture became the focal point around which he organized his evolving understanding of his father and his growing inner image of their relationship. When Sam was around 3, he went through a period during which he proclaimed that he was not going to become a boy but was going to remain a baby. It occurred to Gail that Sam did not know how to remain connected to his father, who had known him only as a baby, as the photograph by Sam's bedside made clear. Gail talked to Sam about how proud his father would have been to see him grow up and do grown-up things, like the kinds of tasks his father loved to do. Sam no longer had to cling to his baby picture as his last remaining bridge to his father; he gradually began to identify with an image of his father as an active man who loved to play sports and to make and fix things.

In our search for objects that might help Sam evoke his father's presence during his growing-up years, Gail remembered that Stuart had taped a speech he made during his son's *bris*, the Jewish circumcision ceremony. In this speech, which Stuart had meant to share with his son later in their lives, the father proudly envisioned his son's growth to manhood and the things he wished for him. While the tape had been meant to record a moment they would share as a family in the future, it became another means through which Sam could infuse his life with a sense of his father actively appreciating his growing-up process.

Gail's greatest area of vulnerability in responding to Sam's grief had been her fear of bringing up her two sons alone without a father's influence. In a home where the parents had emotionally intense, powerful, and often oppositional personalities, both Alan and Sam came by their own strong characters honestly. Sam negotiated the period of toddlerhood with an intense combination of both attached dependence and willful independence. Gail recognized Sam's independence as a quality he shared with both her and Stuart, and she understood how his father's death had heightened his sense of vulnerability and subsequent need to maintain his personal integrity. She didn't fight him to the bitter end—as his father might have done—if he insisted on not wearing his mittens or wanted to pick out his own clothes or refused to eat his food if someone else cut it up for him. She was willing to pick her battles, and then she was a match for him in her own resolve to get her way.

Gail, fearing that Sam might become a mama's boy without his father as an active presence, had a much more difficult time with her son's intensity of attachment and dependence. One night when Sam wanted to sleep in Gail's bed, the two stayed up the entire night fighting because Gail had decided that this was the time and place to draw the line on his emotional dependence. There is no easy solution, as any parent knows, to the struggle over bedtime and the bedtime loneliness that many children suffer. It seemed to me, though, that Gail's decision needed to be made on the basis of her and Sam's psychological need for mutual comfort, as well as their need for privacy. I thought it important that Gail's assessment of the situation not be additionally burdened by the fear that if she gave in to Sam's request, he might never want to grow up to be a man. To a recently bereaved 3-year-old boy a mother's implicit insistence that manhood required the abandonment of all nighttime emotional comfort might itself, I suggested, be a good reason not to want to become a man. Sam was very much the quintessential boy, active and assertive; if anything, he needed to learn how to curb his aggressive side. I suggested to Gail that if we looked at Sam realistically he was exuberantly boyish in his interests. I doubted that the world of girls and women would hold disproportionate appeal for him—as long as it did not become associated with forbidden yet necessary emotional comforts.

Gail's assessment of Sam's desire to sleep in her bed with her was further complicated by the fact that she herself had grown up with an older sister and no brothers. Her father, a loving but anxious, hypercritical man had encouraged Gail and her sisters to be independent, as had their mother, a sweet, devoted, but somewhat absent-minded woman. Gail described her older sister as part mother, part twin; during her growing-up years her sister was her parent figure as well as her constant companion. In our exploration of her paradoxical image of her mother as devoted yet somehow absent, Gail remembered that her mother had gone back to work when she was 5, telling her little daughter that she needed to do so because Gail was too dependent on her and that this move would force her to be more independent. In fact, Gail's father held two or three jobs at that time, and in all likelihood her mother returned to work for economic or personal reasons. Gail retained this attribution of her own great dependence, unexamined, and her conflicts were reawakened in negotiating dependence with her bereaved son. As she uncovered this source of her own fears, it became easier for Gail to tolerate Sam's temporary dependence on her and to negotiate with him a mutually satisfying rhythm of mutual comfort and privacy.

Gail was able to retain for herself and her children a sense of Stuart as a living presence in the household. She did so in spite of feeling personally devastated by the loss and in spite of the encouragement she received from friends, family, and most professionals—almost from the moment of Stuart's death—to "let go and move on." At the time of this writing, close to the fourth anniversary of Stuart's death, his now 5½-year-old son, Sam, has been able to bring an image of his father with him through crucial years of his development. Although Alan, 6 years old at the time of his father's death, had more direct memories of his relationship with his father than Sam did, Gail's willingness to make their father an important ongoing presence in the lives of both children will make a vital difference in mitigating their sense of loss and its impact on their ongoing development.

Once toddlers have acquired and consolidated language skills, during their second and third years, they are in a much better position to communicate with caretakers about the circumstances and nature of a death, and they can begin a process of comprehending death and its causes. In watching Sam Kaplan mature from a preverbal toddler to a linguistically sophisticated 5-year-old, we could observe his maturing use of symbolic representation in the form of language and, eventually, of fantasy. In addition to his increased capacity to use language and fantasy to represent experience, Sam achieved greater maturation in his understanding of physical causality; this cognitive maturation enabled him to review the circumstances of his father's death and permitted a more sophisticated perspective on its causes. Sam's preverbal understanding will probably remain an embedded, unconscious source of vulnerability for him; a future traumatic life event might trigger his fears of basic body integrity, fears that were age-appropriate at the time of his father's death and that were mobilized and accentuated by that trauma..

Even these enduring vulnerabilities, though, can be substantially mitigated as the child matures by direct discussion of the circumstances of the death and its meaning to the child. A traumatic event that is repressed or dissociated as a means of regaining emotional stability seems to enter a developmental time warp. While the rest of development moves forward, images associated with the trauma become encapsulated and isolated. Yet the dissociation of overwhelming experiences can be alleviated even many years later by a supportive relationship in which the reality of the traumatic event and its emotional importance are acknowledged. Any clinician who has sat with an adult enabled by the safety of the therapeutic relationship to recover a dissociated image of childhood trauma will recognize the uncanny sense of suddenly retrieving the conscious memory of a remarkably well-preserved childhood event. Similarly, family therapists have remarked on the immediacy of long-denied grief responses that can emerge intact many years after the death of a loved one. Once the traumatic or forbidden memory is brought out of its encapsulated location and into the open air of full discussion, both children and adults are able to bring to a previously overwhelming experience a more mature capacity for understanding and integration. The more the child's exploration of a death takes place in the context of supportive family relationships, the more effective will be his or her capacity to integrate the death in ways that do not interfere with ongoing development.

BEREAVEMENT AND THE PRESCHOOL CHILD

Having mastered the use of language, preschool children are expressive and responsive participants in family discussions of a member's death. However, they use more concrete and magical thinking than do school-age children or adolescents, as documented by Piaget and other developmental theorists. Piaget considered this stage of child-hood, from age 2 to age 5 to age 7, the stage of *preoperational thought*. Children in this stage have developed a significant capacity for language acquisition and for the symbolic representation of experience in fantasy. However, their thinking remains concrete and is dominated by phenomenistic causality and magical thinking. They use language and imagery to express themselves with a delightful combination of direct-ness and poetry. Creative artists who freely explore their world through the vehicle of their imaginations, children at this age can spook themselves with the power of their own creations. They struggle with all the important questions in life—the nature of birth and death, the dif-ferences between men and women and between boys and girls—although they have not yet acquired, for better and for worse, the adult's stereotyped categories for simplifying complex experience.

Piaget's preoperational stage includes two Freudian stages of development: the anal stage, corresponding to the toilet training years, and the phallic-oedipal stage, from ages 3 to 6 and corresponding to a phase of development marked by exhibitionism, romantic interest in the opposite-sex parent, and rivalry with the same-sex parent. Cog-nitive development in the preoperational years is characterized by an increasingly complex organization of concepts or schemas, which nevertheless remain closely tied to observable reality and do not yet reflect abstract thought. Social and emotional development in the early preschool years is characterized by the infamous struggles with par-ents over the imposition of will. Freud describes these family battles in terms of anality, Erikson in terms of autonomy, and relational theo-rists in terms of individuation or a first awareness of the distinct yet dependent self.

The so-called oedipal stage, in the later preschool years, is char-acterized by the child's struggles with the parents over the humilia-tions of being powerless and dependent, struggles that now involve the child's awareness of gender difference and the consequences of this awareness for self-definition. Preschool-age children try as hard as they can to even the score between themselves and a world of loom-ing, powerful grown-ups who are in a position to tell them what to do every step of the way. They are growing in their awareness of the reality of their lives and of the need to negotiate their desires with the desires of their powerful parents. If it brings them into severe con-flict with their much loved and much needed parents, the preschool child's self-assertion can generate persistent feelings of shame and helpless humiliation. Preschoolers also begin to experience guilt in the form of internalized parental prohibitions, which soon become the child's own standards of conscience.

Children in the preoperational stage of cognitive development typically understand death to be a reversible or impermanent state, like sleep or a separation. They do not understand that the dead cease all bodily functions, that they no longer move or get hungry, lonely, or cold. Most often, preschoolers assume that the person who died chose to go away and could choose to come back. If they are told that the dead person was buried in a coffin, they may imagine that the person is cold or hungry, as they would be in the same situation. If they are told that a dead parent or sibling has gone to heaven, they will assume that heaven is like another city, just "up there" in the sky; to them, heaven is simply a location in which the dead family member could be found and from which he or she could choose to return. Preschool children are also self-referential and concrete in their understanding of death. With their primitive sense of causality, they are likely to attribute the death to factors in proximity to it in space and/or time. If a child fought with a parent immediately prior to the death, he or she will be certain that the death was caused by the fight. The intertwining of their concrete causal thinking and their developmentally appropriate need for self-assertion is likely to lead children of this age to the conclusion that they are responsible for the death.

For many years, the literature on childhood bereavement tended to suggest that children below the age of 7 could not properly understand the concept of death as a finite end to life. However, Bowlby and other child bereavement researchers have pointed out that our culture refrains from discussing death with children. For this reason, preschool children are likely to encounter the concept of death for the first time under the complex, emotionally loaded circumstances of the death of a family member. While even a very young child, these writers point out, is capable of understanding the death of, say, a squirrel or a household pet as a final, irreversible event if the concept of death is explained in concrete terms (often, young children grasp first the idea that lifelessness is equivalent to a total lack of movement), when the child's first experience of death occurs with a much loved parent or sibling, he or she is more likely to think in terms of absence and separation rather than irretrievable loss. In fact, as I mentioned earlier, adults may also think of the death of a loved one as a temporary, reversible separation. For a period of time adults may search for the loved one, imagining that they see or hear the deceased, even though they cognitively understand the physical reality of death.

A preschool child's exploration of death and grief requires a substantial, almost heroic, tolerance on the part of family members of their own emotional pain. It is not surprising to find that adults often wish the child could "get over it" more quickly, in order to avoid a painful confrontation with the child's grief as well as their own. Gail Kaplan found that while her own grief was manageable, the most enduring source of pain for her was the fatherlessness of her children. Because of their acute sensitivity to a parent's needs and their own needs for emotional stability and control, most children are likely to adapt to the adult world's requirement that they "put the past behind them" and "get on" with their lives after the death of a loved parent or sibling.

Yet I am arguing for a culturally counterintuitive position: Children can in fact more substantially continue their own growing-up process if they are supported in sustaining a living image of the deceased parent or sibling. This might be especially true with the death of a parent, given the importance of both parents to the child's ongoing development. In spite of parental and cultural prohibitions, most children who lose a parent in childhood report that they persist, secretly, if need be in holding an image of the dead parent watching over them and accompanying them during difficult times in their lives.

If children are forbidden by the prohibitions of the surviving parent and of other adults, as interpreters of the culture, to turn to the dead parent's image as a source of comfort and developmental support, they become more vulnerable to retaining an image that is frozen in developmental time and characteristic of an earlier stage of development. In addition, associated developmental functions are likely to remain entangled with the frozen imagery associated with the parent's death at a particular developmental moment. Young children, with limited understanding of death and its circumstances and limited knowledge of their dead parent as a multifaceted adult, need the opportunity to add new information to their evolving understanding and growing image of the dead parent. With the support of the surviving parent and other family members, the child can retain the dead parent as a developmental resource, bringing the image forward in developmental time as a living, loving, evolving presence.

A 6-year-old who saw his father shot and murdered by strangers in the living room of their home, was terribly worried when he and his mother, who could not bear to remain in their home, moved in with her sister; the child worried that his father would not know where to find them when he came back to look for them. A five-year-old whose older brother died in a fall during a school field trip, was told that he had gone to heaven, where God and the angels live. Although she had not witnessed her brother's death, the abrupt and confusing nature of the tragedy infused all her fantasies with intense anxiety, and she began to feel frightened at night because she was convinced that her brother was watching her from "up there," perhaps hovering over her in anticipation of snatching her and taking her with him.

And I remember listening to a radio show as a 6-year-old during the Cuban revolution in Havana and hearing about the mutilating torture of an individual graphically described. I was left with the horrifying and confusing image of a man who had been whittled away to a stub and yet was somehow at the same time still able to see, hear, feel pain, and walk away, carrying the horror of his experience with him. I continued to review this terrible, discordant image in my mind until, later in childhood, I finally realized that the man who had been tortured would have been killed and therefore unable to walk away conscious of his pain.

Concrete Thinking and Causality: Does "Sick" Always Mean "Dead"?

Since 2- and 3-year-olds have just begun to make use of language and fantasy, they are especially vulnerable to concrete or magical notions that can lead to surprising distortions of adult communications. When 3-year-old Gretchen's baby brother, Mike, was born with spina bifida, he was not able to come home as planned. Instead, his parents were thrust into an agonizing series of decisions about high-risk neurosurgery that might improve his chances of survival. When her mother explained that Mike was too sick to come home right away, Gretchen was brokenhearted. When Gretchen's brother died 4 weeks later, in spite of the specialized surgical care he received, her parents explained to her that he had been too sick after all and that the doctors had not been able to make him well enough to save his life. Gretchen was deeply grieved, as were her parents and 5-year-old brother, that the baby had not been able to survive. She would often ask her mother where he was and would talk to him during her baths or as she was going to sleep.

Three months after the baby's death, Gretchen caught a slight cold, became extremely agitated, and began to have difficulty sleeping. Her mother realized that the little girl was in a panic because she thought that she was getting sick like Mike and had no way of knowing where the boundary lies between sickness and death. Because Gretchen's mother had explained her pregnancy to her in terms of planting seeds, as they had done together in the garden, she was able to clarify the circumstances of Mike's death in ways the little girl was able to understand. She said to Gretchen, "Do you know how when we plant seeds in the garden, some of them grow up to be plants but not all of them are able to grow? It's like that with babies. Sometimes there is something wrong, from the very beginning, when the baby is not yet a baby but is still a seed, and then that baby doesn't grow like you and your big brother did. You were a healthy seed and a healthy baby and are now a healthy little girl. That's very different from what happened to baby Mike." This clarification of the circumstances of Mike's death, attuned to a 3-year-old's cognitive stage of understanding, enormously relieved Gretchen. Without an age-appropriate clarification, her worries could have become chronic or recurrent, and she might have held on to an unexamined fear that family members could die any time they became sick.

Carrying the Burden of Family Protection: Nobody Gets Mad, Nobody Gets Hurt

David, 5 years old when his mother died in an airplane crash, illustrates how the grief reactions of preschool children are characterized by a complex mixture of factors determined by their cognitive and psychosocial stages of development unfolding in a family context. David was very aware that Roger, his father, and Joshua, his younger brother, were devastated and overwhelmed by the death. By all outward appearances, David made an excellent adjustment to his mother's death. He became absorbed in the care of his younger brother, who had become withdrawn to a frightening, almost autistic, degree and who played a repetitive game of diving off the bed.

As I learned 4 years later, when he entered individual therapy with me at the age of 9, David had in fact created a private and powerful explanation of his mother's death, based on his very literal interpretation of his father's account of the circumstances. From the few initial details available on the airplane accident, it was impossible to ascertain whether or not the passengers had known they were in danger prior to the plane's swift descent. Finding the idea of his wife's conscious fall to her death unbearable, Roger deliberately constructed a more tolerable, but less likely, story, which he then told to everyone, including his children (and, in a way, himself): his wife had hit her head when the airplane's engines malfunctioned in midair and had lost consciousness; thus, she was unaware of the danger and had not suffered the panic and anguish of knowing she was falling to her death.

David, like most children his age, interpreted his father's story literally and concretely: His mother died, not from an airplane crash, but from a blow to the head. David remained unafraid of flying but began to fearfully restrict his activities so that he would never suffer from, or inflict, a blow to the head. But, he wondered, how does one receive a blow to the head if it is not delivered? The explanation David constructed of his mother's death required that he more and more constrict his own expressions of anger, which he feared might lead to blows and perhaps eventually to death. He became an overly good, sensitive, and physically constricted child and devoted himself to the emotional care of his younger brother and his father until his burden of suppressed resentment literally exploded. During a game of touch football, David was blocked by another boy; to his surprise, he totally lost control of his repressed anger, began to strike him, and had to be restrained by the adults.

Over the course of therapy, David and I untangled the web of connections he had constructed between death and anger, the main link being his fantasy that a blow to the head represents the real danger to life. David had made the decision, in the wake of his mother's death, that his potential to act violently had to be suppressed at all costs, thus denying himself a reasonable expression of anger and aggression. In therapy David needed to be coached on how to respond to the children who teased or threatened him and how to express his anger toward his father, stepmother, and brother, all of whom he had been protecting from the violent, explosive danger he imagined his anger to be.

David's response to his mother's death was cognitively constructed out of his preoperational understanding of his father's explanation of the circumstances. At the same time, his age-appropriate self-assertion became entangled with his confused understanding of the circumstances of the death and led to a constriction in his capacity to express his own will and suppression of his capacity for anger. Finally, he was responsively adapting to the implicit message he was receiving, namely, that his family had their hands full with his brother's acute disturbance and could not bear his open anguish as well.

Five-year-old Suzie Johnson, whose 16-year-old brother, Tim (introduced at the beginning of Chapter 5), died in a car accident, was, like most preoperational children, very direct and expressive in her emotional responses to the death. Preschool children will ask questions about the death and make references to the family member who has died. Suzie's position as youngest child enabled her to take less direct responsibility—or perhaps what we can best call a different kind of responsibility—as compared to David. Suzie was not asked to suppress her own feelings of missing her dead brother. If anything, as the family member who by virtue of age, birth order, gender, and temperament was most irrepressible in expressing emotions, she was encouraged to speak of Tim. Suzie spoke for the rest of the family, who had more controlled expressions of grief. In fact, 6 months after Tim's death his deeply depressed father, Steve, initiated a call to me in which he expressed his concern that there was something abnormal with Suzie's insistence on talking about her brother. It was clear that the problem in this family was Steve's insistence that no family member mention Tim to him because the pain he felt was too overwhelming.

BEREAVEMENT AND THE SCHOOL-AGE CHILD

Children in the concrete operational stage of development, roughly age 7 to age 12, are able to understand the concept of death and its finality in more logical and less magical, although still concrete, ways. Children in this elementary-school-age group, which also corresponds to the psychoanalytic period of latency, are typically those who appear to the outside observer to be the least affected by the death of a close family member. Children in these years have acquired the capacity for more mature ego defense mechanisms in response to intense feelings and tend to rely on more stereotyped same-sex identifications as a way of resolving the intense confusion about gender and power of the preschool phase. If preschool children are creative artists whose drawings are expressive and unconventional, school-age children want nothing more than to draw accurate renditions of reality, even if this means confining their artwork to stereotyped and well-mastered cartoon figures.

School-age children tend to be more avoidant of speaking about their grief than either preschoolers or adolescents. Their understanding of causality remains concrete, and although they are especially vulnerable to fears that the death was somehow caused and something they did or thought, there is little likelihood that they will spontaneously voice those fears. Unless they are systematically encouraged to discuss their feelings of distress, confusion, resentment, and guilt, children of this age can appear disconcertingly unconcerned or unaffected by a death. This apparent unconcern masks from others their own internal sense of turmoil, which they struggle to put aside so they can gain for themselves a small island of emotional safety.

School-age children are especially vulnerable to being misunderstood. Their vulnerability differs from that of preschool children, whose cognitive distortion is more obvious. School-age children, with their more sophisticated capacities to repress or avoid overwhelming emotional material, want more than anything to be ordinary, just like other people. They do not want to be suffering the anguish and self-questioning provoked by a family member's death, a terrible burden that marks them as shamefully different and defective. It is not that these children have forgotten their grief; rather, it is as if they believe that if things are not spoken, if they act like everything is all right, life will not be quite so intensely, unremittingly, painfully the way it truly is. Children like 10-year-old Greg Johnson (introduced in Chapter 5), seemingly so indifferent to the death of his 16-year-old brother, Tim, and Nancy's daughter Cara, whom I described in Chapter 2 as believing herself perfectly capable of leaving her mother shortly after her father's death to join friends of the family across the country, are vulnerable to the isolation that can come from being taken too literally at their word. Since so often grown-ups are only too happy to be reassured that everything is all right, school-age children are more often than not reinforced in the avoidant defenses that come relatively naturally to them. An additional effort is needed to reach these children directly, even as one respectfully acknowledges their right to have their grief their own way.

The importance of the cognitive–emotional transition in school-age children and its implications for understanding bereavement processes in childhood were brought home to me by my experiences in working with children during their preschool years and again during their school-age years. These children were often referred for behavior problems in the classroom and at home, and most child therapists would have diagnosed Attention Deficit Disorder. Given my systemic developmental orientation, I was more inclined to look at their symptoms in the light of family processes. In a number of families the grief reactions of members were found to exacerbate already existing family problems. When I first met these children, they were preschoolers who had very real, vivid preoccupations with grief and loss. By the time I saw them again, in the middle of their elementary school years, they had radically shifted in their use of psychological defenses and were trying valiantly to put their existential struggles with grief and death behind them.

The Return of the Repressed: Family Avoidance and a School-Age Symptom

Chris Ogden, age 5 and in kindergarten when I first met him, was referred as a hyperactive, aggressive boy who was driving his mother to the brink of insanity. The middle of three children, Chris indignantly clamored for the parental appreciation he observed his cooperative older sister and adorable baby sister routinely receiving. Chris turned out to be like many of the children I have seen diagnosed with Attention Deficit Disorder. Although he was surely a boy with some unevenness in his neurological functioning, he was also blessed, as well as burdened, with an extraordinary sensitivity to the relational and emotional world and a vivid, artistic imagination.

Chris's emotional sensitivity and active imagination made him the ideal family member for the task of memorializing, through both direct and displaced imagery, his stillborn infant brother's death. Chris was 2 years old at the time of his brother's death, somewhat slow in his language development, and unable to put his fear, confusion, and loss into words. His mother, Sally, felt profoundly bereaved by the baby's death, although rationally she understood her husband's and family's statements that this premature infant with multiple birth defects would have suffered enormously had he lived. At the time of the infant's birth, hospital staff still treated stillbirth as a nonevent, did not permit parents to spend time with the infant, and buried their corpses anonymously. The invisibility of the baby's death left Sally feeling terribly alone with her grief. Sally became pregnant again 6 months after her baby's death, and had a healthy baby girl. The demands of caring for her new baby and her older children helped her put her own grief and confusion aside.

The Ogdens brought Chris in for an evaluation without recognizing the bereavement issues behind their intense emotional reactivity, so that the unearthing of their long-buried grief took place in gradual stages over the course of an initial assessment. Like many child therapy cases dealing with a child's ungovernable behavior problem, the work of assessment and treatment requires sorting out the intergenerational history and current family relationships that accounted for the extreme emotional reactivity Chris and his parents experienced toward one another. Through a combination of play sessions with Chris and sessions with the parents, I learned first about a more recent and also minimized grief reaction.

Chris's paternal grandfather had died the previous year from a heart attack, provoking a life crisis for Chris's father, Bill. Bill no longer spoke of his own father's death and acted as if he had left it behind him. Yet, Chris's first work in play therapy revealed his many fears and questions about his grandfather's death: "Why do some people's hearts stop? Could my father's heart stop too?" he asked me during a play therapy session. Chris drew me a picture of his grandfather with his heart and circulatory system in vivid reds and blues. He used the picture to talk about his love for his grandfather, his sorrow at missing him, and his fear that he might just as suddenly and unexpectedly lose other loved ones. Bill, who had stopped talking about his father's death almost immediately after the event, was mystified that his son carried around this intense preoccupation. Bill, himself, was much more preoccupied by the work demands of inheriting the family bookstore business and suddenly becoming the boss, rather than his father's second in command.

The family grief reaction over the infant's death continued to be a shadow event, fueling Chris's anxiety about helplessness in the face of death. The story of the stillbirth first came up by accident during a parent session, when Chris's parents were talking with me about their conflicts over discipline. As a stay at home mother with three young children, Sally found it easier to deal with her cooperative 10-year-old daughter, Laurie, and her sociable 2-year-old daughter, Donna. Sally found both daughters much easier to care for than her sensitive, physically active, emotionally intense son who seemed to respond only when she overpowered him. Bill felt a special identification with Chris as the only son, and was much more permissive than Sally in his parenting style. Sally's emphasis on control and her overreaction to Chris's misbehavior reminded Bill of his own overcontrolling mother, and he would often, in overt and covert ways, move in to protect Chris from what he viewed as Sally's harshness. Sally then let it be known that at times when Bill stepped in to protect Chris she felt especially resentful of the contrast between his loving understanding of Chris's needs and his total indifference to her and her overwhelming sense of loss. Sally was still enraged at Bill's indifferent reaction to the stillbirth, which at the time of the tragedy and subsequently thereafter was not an emotionally important event to Bill. The distance in the marriage over their very different ways of defining the stillbirth and dealing with their grief continued to be echoed every time Bill bypassed Sally's feelings while sympathizing with Chris.

The uncovering of this marital impasse, with its history in an unresolved grief reaction, enabled Bill and Sally to focus more effectively on collaborating as parents and to avoid making Chris a target for their struggle to communicate with one another. As Sally saw Chris more as an emotionally sensitive, psychologically vulnerable boy—rather than as an example of one more man who wouldn't listen to her needs—she became both more empathic to his emotional needs and more able to set necessary limits without harsh anger. No longer burdened by his role as a pawn in his parents' marriage and by his mother's unhappiness with his father, Chris began to work with concentration and dedication on his own impulse control. Through a combination of brief but intensive individual play therapy, parent sessions, and a school consultation to enhance his kindergarten to first grade transition, Chris's behavior problems at home and at school became much more manageable. After 7 months of therapeutic work, the first phase of therapy ended with Chris's successful transition to the first grade.

While I knew that Bill and Sally had only scratched the surface with regard to the stillbirth and its meaning to their lives and marriage, they were not yet ready as a couple to delve further into this emotionally loaded, potentially destabilizing issue. Similarly, Bill was not ready to emotionally explore the importance of his father's death in his own life at a time when all his energy was being absorbed by the realistic fear that he might not have the business savvy to save his father's life investment, the source of his family's livelihood. The increase in the mutual understanding of each other's emotional needs was just enough to help Bill and Sally respond to Chris more directly. I respected their need to maintain enough emotional stability so that they could go on with the hard work of raising a family under these developmental circumstances at this demanding stage of their lives.

Four years later I saw Chris and his family again. Chris was 10 years old and he had changed from an openly expressive preschooler to a much more private school-aged child whose emotional struggles were less directly accessible in play but not yet readily available through talk. Chris, however, was essentially recognizable; he was, as always, energetic, sensitive, and alternately combative and affectionate. Nevertheless, he was now more emotionally characterized by a wish to look away from the mysteries of life whenever he could possibly do so.

Chris's family came in for a therapeutic "tune-up" because they were having a great deal of difficulty getting along. To Bill and Sally it seemed that the three children were constantly at each other's throats. Laurie, who had tired of being the good daughter and second mother, now fought Chris if he did anything to cross her. I began to work with them all on this new family life cycle transition, which on the surface appeared to be ushered in by Laurie's entry into a more independent phase of adolescent development. Laurie's intense resentment of her central role as a second mother in the family might not have necessarily emerged at this stage of the family life cycle had it not coincided with Bill's postponed depression over the death of his father and its affect on his own sense of manhood. Bill, who had always been a good-natured although absentminded father, became deeply depressed, overwhelmed by a distorted sense of financial insecurity about the successful family business he had inherited from his father. For a period of about a year, he was substantially unavailable as a husband and father; he was uncharacteristically depressed or irritable, and he sometimes exploded with impatient anger at his children. As we explored the background to the family fighting, it emerged that Bill's emotional distress had correspondingly increased to the degree that his children's fighting with each other had intensified.

Her father's unavailability and heightened faultfinding appeared to be too much for Laurie, who, feeling that she was the only one in the family who honored the feelings of others, began to deliver insults at least as good as she had been getting, thus turning family life into a constant melee of explosive bickering. In turn, the family's feuding gave Laurie, in early adolescence, an outlet for the intense insecurity she was feeling about herself (she felt that every single dimension of her looks was seriously flawed). In addition to working with the parents and siblings on better problem-solving strategies and more respectful communication of their grievances, I also supported Laurie's attempts to become her own person without as much rebellious rage and accompanying self-hatred.

While the family sessions reduced conflict and improved the family climate of communication, Chris remained an emotionally vulnerable child and continued to be a lightning rod for family conflict. We agreed to schedule six individual sessions to follow the family work, and an additional two sessions with the parents (one for assessment and one for feedback). In my individual meetings with Chris we talked about his deep conviction that no matter what he did he would always be his parents' least favorite child. With Laurie's fall from grace, the focus of his resentment was his baby sister Donna, who was emerging as a brilliant student, a talented musician, and an amusing, biting mimic who was more verbally adept than her brother. Chris was far more inclined to talk about his emotional experiences than most boys his age, and he and I had already established a history of talking together. There was, nevertheless, a significant shift in the quality of his relating. With vague recognition and amusement, Chris looked at the vivid, expressive pictures he had drawn during his therapy as a preschooler; however, he now preferred to draw orderly geometric shapes and true-to-life pictures typical of school-age children.

Chris's anxiety and sorrow about death and loss, his struggle to control his aggression, and his humiliation at being powerless and at the mercy of more powerful grown-ups came together in the form of an emblematic secret symptom: Chris was afraid that someone was going to kidnap him, that he would become one of the missing children whose pictures are on the back of milk cartons. In a state of vigilant anxiety bordering on panic, Chris began to walk to and from school carrying a large stick which he hid under a bush so he could retrieve it each day. He was incapable of being reassured that he was a large boy for his age, capable of defending himself, and that the chances were excellent that no one could kidnap him if he was alert and refused to enter the car of a stranger. Now 10 years old, Chris showed an age-appropriate lack of enthusiasm for exploring the emotional undercurrents of his unrealistic fear. In defining his therapeutic goals, we settled on a combination of better reality testing and redressing the power imbalance he struggled with in his relationships with grown-ups. Knowing how sensitive Chris had been all his life to the ultimate powerlessness involved in abandonment by death, I tried to bring forward in him a sense of himself as an already powerful boy who was rapidly becoming a powerful young man.

I received Chris's permission to talk about his intense fears with his parents, who had noticed a change in his route to and from school but had no idea he had become so terrified. I worried that Chris's preoccupation with kidnapping could seriously interfere with his development at this time, and encouraged them to talk openly with Chris at home about the many sources of his fear of death. I asked them to speak privately with the two older children about the still-birth, and we reviewed the language that would be appropriate to each one's age and stage of development. The Ogdens followed this course of action, and were surprised at how eagerly Laurie, age 7 when her brother died, and Chris, age 2 at the time, seized the opportunity to make the loss of their brother an open family subject. Laurie, old enough to remember the death and its circumstances, was able to reminisce with her mother about her own worries, which took the form of protecting her mother from family burdens. Chris wondered how the family might have been different for him if his brother had lived. He fantasized that he might have felt less lonely if he had a brother who was an ally in family fights, and who he could play games with.

In our individual meetings, I diplomatically addressed the symbolic meaning of Chris's fear of kidnapping just once, drawing on our shared history of talking about important feelings together. I suggested to Chris that although he knew the probability was low that a kidnapping would happen to him, he had all his life been especially aware of the bad, painful things that could happen to people, leaving them vulnerable to the worst kinds of hurt. I reminded him of his previously experienced and explored losses, like his parents' comings and goings and his grandfather's death. I also commented that his early experience with the death of his baby brother might be part of his enduring sensitivity to the stories of loss and death around him, reported in the newspapers, conveyed among his teachers and classmates, implied in the messages from the bereaved parents on the back of milk cartons. Like most school-age children, Chris squirmed under the intensity of such a direct confrontation with his deepest feelings, although he could acknowledge the importance of these enduring themes in his emotional life.

This phase of the family's work helped to decrease the feeling of burden Laurie and Chris felt for their parents and enabled them to proceed with their own development. However, the Ogdens still felt too personally vulnerable to do more therapeutic work on their own behalf at that time. The further exploration of the stillbirth for this family's shared development had to wait until the next stage of the family life cycle when Laurie's adolescent rebellion had stabilized, Chris was older, and Donna was a successful elementary school student. At that time Sally contacted me because she wanted to explore issues in her own individual development, and felt that her children were independent enough that she could risk the exploration of difficult issues in her own family of origin and in her marriage. I encouraged Sally and Bill to enter couple's therapy with a colleague who worked with both individual and marital issues. I felt sure that their work on improving the quality of their marriage and on unexplored issues in their own lives would help expand their shared developmental possibilities.

Coping with Chronic Illness and Death: Did I Really Grieve My Mother?

The sudden, unexpected death of a parent or sibling delivers a traumatic blow to a family, and the child's ongoing process of development becomes absorbed by the necessity to manage and integrate the overwhelming emotions of self and family. When death occurs after a long period of chronic illness, the bereaved child's ongoing development has already been shaped by the illness and the family's responses to it. The responses that 7-year-old Ann Smith exhibited following the death of her chronically ill mother, Karen, were characteristic of school-age children and, at the same time, indicative of the impact of her mother's illness on her earlier development. Karen had known from early childhood that her cardiac condition made her vulnerable to infection and meant that any physical exertion, including childbearing, would be risky. Each of Karen's two pregnancies had been a hazard for her, although she and her husband, Mike, had agreed from the beginning of their marriage that they wanted to live as normal a family life as possible. Karen's pregnancy with Ann precipitated a heart attack that left her partially paralyzed. Thus, Ann was born into a family whose relationships were already greatly affected by a member's illness.

I saw Ann in therapy when she was 16 years old, 8 years after her mother's death. She remembered her mother lovingly and warmly but mostly as an inert presence with little energy to interact or play with her. Ann recalled her own sense of purpose in being the family's cheerful girl who uncomplainingly accepted her lot in life. In fact, when her mother died, Ann still tried to cheer everyone up, running around the house singing a silly song her older sister, Carol, had taught her, a song Karen herself used to sing when she was relatively well prior to her second pregnancy. Ann's reaction was in contrast to that of Carol, who had known better times with their mother during her earlier childhood and who protested the loss of her family as she had known it. Looking back as an early adolescent on her own school-age reaction to her mother's death, Ann could hardly bear the memory of her "lack of grief" and could not forgive herself for it.

In interpreting her immediate grief reaction with her, I encouraged Ann to try to understand her developmental burden as the youngest child and to recognize the ease with which she might have imagined that she had caused her mother's last debilitating heart attack given the fact that she could not at such a young age have understood that her parents had made their own adult life choices to take enormous medical risks. Ann had never known her mother during her healthy years and had been implicitly asked to make life for the family run smoothly. Moreover, after her mother's death Ann continued to bear the largest part of this burden, as her father remarried within the year and her stepmother, Glenda, was overwhelmed by the task of taking over as the mother in a bereaved family. While Carol was hostile and resentful of Glenda's intrusion and Glenda was critical and demanding of the girls, Ann herself tried valiantly to help Glenda become her much-needed affectionate "mommy."

Once Ann reached early adolescence, her "false self" adaptation to her family's burden of depression began to significantly interfere with both her school work and social functioning. In fact, she herself was substantially depressed. The work of her therapy, in both individual and family sessions, consisted of helping her put down the burden of worry about her bereaved, embattled family. With the help of therapy, and with her family's support, Ann began to concentrate on a more honest exploration of her own needs. She began to grieve her mother on her own behalf and to let her father and stepmother work out their marital problems for themselves without acting as their go-between and mediator.

BEREAVEMENT IN ADOLESCENCE

As the life stage that stands between childhood and adulthood, adolescence is organized by both biological processes of maturation and social processes unique to each culture. Puberty marks the initiation of adult reproductive capacity and is a period of hormonally determined mood instability and radical physical change. Growth spurts enable children for the first time in their lives to approach, equal, and often exceed a parent in height. For most families, the shift in the balance of physical strength catalyzes significant change in parent–child relationships. Because of gender differences in the cultural definition of adulthood, adolescence has substantially different implications for boys and girls. In the cognitive realm, adolescence means the acquisition of formal operations, the Piagetian designation for the period of cognitive development in which teenagers apply a new capacity for abstract reasoning to explore possibilities outside their immediate world.

Adolescence triggers a new stage of self-assertion and connection to others, now broadening to include not only self within family but self within a wider cultural world. Cultures and ethnic subcultures vary substantially in their emphasis on adolescent rebellion from family as part of a coming-of-age ritual. Even in the United States, where adolescent rebellion is considered part of normative development, a substantial majority of adolescents remain close to their families and model themselves after their parents (Ianni, 1989). The Eriksonian process of identity development in adolescence (Erikson, 1968) emphasizes fidelity, or the search for life values that will permit the adolescent to express his or her unique talents in a wider community. An adolescent's opportunities for finding love and work that support the full development of personal abilities and interests will of course vary substantially, depending on the adolescent's position in the hierarchy of social privilege, including gender, race, ethnic subculture, and social class.

Adolescents are capable, from a cognitive standpoint, of understanding death in fully adult terms. The achievement of formal operational thinking, with the accompanying capacity to reason abstractly and from multiple perspectives, enables the adolescent to fully and maturely understand the causes and circumstances of a death. However, bereaved adults are extremely vulnerable to cognitive confusion in understanding the circumstances of a loved one's death. They often attribute self-referential causality to the death of an important person, even if they know better intellectually. Adolescents are in the process of establishing a sense of their own distinct yet family-based identity and negotiating a new balance of separation and connection with family members. When there is a death in the family, adolescents are vulnerable to associating the tragedy with their age-appropriate search for independence. Grieving adolescents may absorb a deep sense of responsibility for their family's survival, which they feel might be compromised if they proceed with age-appropriate separation.

The process of resuming ongoing development in adolescence

after the death of a parent varies, depending on the adolescent's relationship with both the deceased and the surviving parent and on the specific developmental processes interrupted by the death. In early adolescence, when the child is flooded with radical changes in his or her physical, cognitive, social, and emotional development, the death of a parent and the accompanying family disruption can add overwhelmingly to the adolescent's attempts at integration of a complex self. In the case of an actively rebellious teenager embroiled in separation conflicts, the loss of a parent can initiate an enormous burden of guilt in addition to the grief.

When Death Interrupts Family Resolution of Adolescent Conflict

The death of the same-sex parent deprives teenagers of the opportunity to test their evolving sense of their own adult possibilities against the adult they are most like. At the same time, they may be called upon to fill the dead parent's shoes. George Sherman was 19 and a sophomore in college when his 50-year-old father, Bruce, died unexpectedly of a stroke. Bruce Sherman was a critical father and a bitter, frustrated man who had aspired to become an artist but had been pressured by family needs and financial realities to become involved in the family manufacturing business. His conflictual marriage had been deeply affected by his unhappiness, yet he and Alice, now widowed at 46, had also in their own way been very close. After her husband's death Alice collapsed into a deep depression and became inaccessible. Adrift in college and uncertain of any career direction of his own, George found himself taking on more and more responsibility for keeping the family business going. He finally quit school and devoted himself to the business. It was only after his mother died of cancer 30 years later that George felt free to sell the family business, return to school, and complete his studies as a teacher. His own development as a man had been deeply compromised by his father's death and the economic and psychological pressure to become the man of the family and fill his father's shoes. The death of his critical, unhappy father had interrupted George's exploration of a pathway for his own adult life. He dealt with his own confusion and the realistic demands of the family business by taking up his father's unhappy choices. His mother's death afforded him a new opportunity to achieve his own balance of identification with and independence from his father's life.

Depending on the already established trajectory of development within their relationships, adolescents may be brought closer into the family orbit after a member's death. However, an already rebellious adolescent may spin away in intensified acting out. Hilary Walker was 14 when her alcoholic father hung himself in jail after being picked up by police for drunk and disorderly conduct. Earlier in her childhood, she had felt deeply responsible for helping her father with his drinking problem; she had also assumed the role of coparent in helping her mother run their chaotic household. In early adolescence Hilary became an independent, rebellious young woman who openly criticized her father's drinking and her mother's helpless passivity. Her father's death triggered profound rage at her family and an enormous increase in Hilary's angry impulsivity and delinquency. She began to drink heavily herself, initiated fights both in school and on the streets, and was caught stealing. Although she had always resented her mother's passivity, after her father's death Hilary's animosity toward her mother escalated to such a degree that she was forced to leave home and live in a halfway house. In Hilary's case, an already established process of childhood overresponsibility and adolescent rebellion against this burden of responsibility was intensified by her father's death. Determined not to become helpless and passive like her mother, Hilary then identified more closely with her father; at the same time, she resented the impact of his alcoholism on the family. With his death, she shot herself out of the family like a rocket, fueled by her rage at her father's senseless death and by her fear of being sucked back into her earlier developmental position of coparenting her family.

Rebellious adolescents are embattled in the temporary warfare they see as essential to becoming their own person. For these adolescents, the death of a parent interrupts the working through of a conflictual stance, a process that, when successful, leads to the re-creation of connections at a later stage of young adulthood. This moment of normal family developmental conflict, now frozen in developmental time, can create a barrier to the adolescent's ongoing exploration of his or her relationship with the dead parent and retention of the parent as a developmental resource. When Meredith Levine's father died of a heart attack, she was 16 years old and engaged in a pitched battle for her adolescent rights. She saw her father as substantially controlling her mother who was housewife. Her struggles with her father over dating privileges, curfews, and dress codes contained not only her own drives for independence but her need to symbolically address the issue of her father's dominance over her mother. After her husband's death, Meredith's mother experienced a deep depression; at the same time, she urged Meredith to go on with her own life as independently as possible.

Only later, in couples' therapy as a woman in her forties, did Meredith realize the extent to which she had erected barriers against receiving comfort from a man. The legacy of her parent's marriage, its exploration interrupted by her father's death, had endured in her marriage as a barrier to the intimacy she could permit herself with her husband. Meredith's exploration during the course of couples' therapy of her relationship with her parents prior to her father's death and of her parents' marriage in the more mature light of her own adult understanding enabled her to seek and gain comfort from a reestablished connection to her father.

Adolescent Grief and Identity Development: A Living Parental Image as a Developmental Resource

The grief reaction of most adolescents is very much complicated by the grief reaction of other family members. With the death of a parent, adolescents can also lose the support of the surviving parent, whose grief makes it impossible for him or her to function as a developmental resource. Adolescents under these circumstances are forced to bring themselves up at the same time that they struggle to salvage an enduring image of their family as a developmental resource. Peter Russell was 15 when his mother died from a very rapidly progressing breast cancer (the time from her diagnosis to her death was barely 3 months). At the time of her death, Peter described himself as a "mama's boy," a description supported by an enduring image he held of his mother standing at the back door of the house calling out to him while he was playing, always within earshot, with his friends. At the time of his mother's death, Peter's brother, 5 years his senior, had already left home and was living on his own. Their father immediately moved out of their home and into the home of a woman with whom he was already involved. He left Peter alone in the house to take responsibility for his own care and the care of the household. Peter somehow muddled through high school, totally overwhelmed by both his grief at his mother's death and his resentment at his father's abandonment.

Peter ran into academic problems when he was a 19-year-old college freshman. His college academic counselor evaluated him and discovered the overwhelming nature of his bereavement experience, which was still fresh and which was significantly interfering with his cognitive organization and capacity to concentrate. Peter gratefully accepted this interpretation of his academic difficulties and initiated a very successful short-term treatment (with a colleague whom I supervised) during the end of his first college year. Peter was living with his mother's brother and wife while attending school. For the first time in the 5 years since his mother's death he was living in a stable care-taking environment, where an adult was willing to take appropriate responsibility for him. As it turned out, his uncle and aunt's solicitude was a mixed blessing, since they were struggling with their own grief and resentment at Peter's father. Thus, in exploring his grief experi-ence, Peter had to figure out how to separate their emotional reac-tions from his own.

Peter made an extraordinary statement at the beginning of his therapy about what he saw as his current dilemma in life: He saw him-self as all alone in the world and needing to create for himself the images of adulthood toward which he could strive. One important function of the therapy became the retrieval and exploration of his images of his mother and father, that is, of the memories he could salvage of the important adults in his life and bring with him through the growing-up process. Peter, like many bereaved children, felt his mother's presence and engaged in private internal conversations with her. His reluctance to talk about his mother with his uncle and aunt, however, had led them to tell him repeatedly that he had not mourned his mother. His therapist made him realize that everything he said showed just how much he did, in fact, grieve for and miss his mother, even though he chose to keep this grief to himself. The therapist's recognition of his intense inner experience caused Peter to feel al-most immediately a palpable sense of emotional relief and relaxation of the inner tension that had been generated by his terrible sense of isolation and feeling of guardedness at being misunderstood.

The therapist's recognition of Peter's grief and her respect for his own good reasons to keep his feelings private freed him to explore his relationship with his mother more fully. He began to seek out conversations about his mother with his uncle and aunt, his father, and especially his older brother, whom he most trusted to talk to him about their mother without imposing his own needs and feelings onto Peter. Their mother emerged as a complex, multidimensional woman rather than the housebound homemaker who called to Peter from the kitchen doorway. In the year prior to her death she had confided to Peter that she was having an affair. Peter had dismissed his mother's confession as a fantasy based on her attempt to relieve the ordinari-ness of her life with material borrowed from the soap operas she fol-lowed. However, after talking to his brother and thinking over the quality of his parents' marriage, he began to believe that his mother had, in fact, told him the truth about her affair. Peter's ability to see his mother as someone with a life more complex than the one she appeared to be living with her husband and children began to give him more room for a more complex image of himself as her son growing into manhood.

The therapeutic listening of Peter's young female therapist, halfway in age between a peer and a mother, affirmed in him his sense of himself as a young man growing away from his family and into more independent interests. This new image of himself and his evolving image of his mother as a complicated and worldly woman loosened the binding ties of his younger image of himself as a mama's boy limited by the length of his mother's apron strings. No longer frozen in developmental time, Peter was able to find new ways to relate to his mother that would support his growing up and would enable her image to grow up with him. By including, but not yielding to, other people's images of his mother, Peter was able to bring his sense of her as a person into his current life. The question with which he began therapy—"How can I become an adult all on my own?"—was reworded to include the support he felt he was receiving from his new inner image of his mother. Peter ended the therapy with a much fuller and more expansive inner life than when he began, having been enriched by the exploration of his grief and by a shift into a new level of development within which he still felt accompanied by his mother. Less encumbered by a burden of grief, Peter moved into the college dormitory, resumed age-appropriate relationships, and attended to his studies.

CONCLUSION: CHILD GRIEF IN A FAMILY DEVELOPMENTAL CONTEXT

Although Peter Russell and 2-year-old Sam Kaplan were at totally different stages of life when they lost a parent, they were both faced with the same developmental dilemma: How do you tolerate moving forward in time when this movement brings you into a world in which your loved one no longer exists? Adults struggle with the same sense of preferring to be frozen in time rather than bear the painful remembering of the past or the empty loneliness of the future. For children, the consequence of freezing time to minimize the sense of loss is that it also freezes developmental time. Yet Peter's and Sam's therapeutic work shows that the child's accompanying image of the parent can be explored and enriched by new information and by the continuing development of the child's capacity for more complex understanding; in short, a child's image of a deceased loved one can be brought forward by the child in developmental time. This process of develop-

mental integration dislodges the tangled knot of symbolically connected developmental functions that were dissociated along with the
grief experience itself. Energy is no longer expended in protecting
an unexamined area of overwhelming pain and is freed up for further
growth.

While children and adults essentially share the same emotions of
grief, in sorrowfully pining and yearning for the lost person, children
are less likely to show acute grief in the initial phase and more likely
to pace the process of grief over a much longer period of time. Adults
are often mystified by a bereaved child's capacity to shift gears and
go from a state of deep sorrow to a state of apparent forgetfulness.
"How," ask adults, "can these children grieve and at the same time
pursue play activities with such apparently full involvement? They
must not be grieving in the same way we do, for we cannot put down
the burden of grief even for a moment." In fact, children do not forget their grief; neither do they constantly keep it in the front of their
minds as do adults. Adults often want to believe that children do not
remember a dead parent or sibling and that they more quickly get over
their grief than do adults, but evidence from the child bereavement
literature suggests that this is wishful thinking and not developmental reality.

As children grow older and gain a greater capacity to cognitively
and emotionally understand the death of a loved one, they continue
to process the death and arrive at new understandings of it. One
mother described the process as a developmental spiral: Her son,
whose father died when he was 3, kept returning to the same place,
to the same questions, about his father's life and death, but he did so
each time with a greater sophistication and depth of understanding,
which characterized his new stages of cognitive and emotional development. Anniversary reactions, which at one time were considered
pathological, can now be seen from a systemic developmental perspective as important and integral parts of the grieving process for
both adults and children. Anniversary reactions evoke a reexperienc-
ing of the grief reaction at a new level of maturity and understanding
(Fox, 1984; Plotnik, 1985). For children especially, anniversary reactions become important opportunities to rework the meaning of a
death in the light of more mature cognitive and emotional functioning. The internalized image of the parent is brought forward in time
by the developing child, who needs to create an image of the parent
that is capable of supportively responding to his or her new developmental dilemmas.

While the outcome literature on childhood bereavement is inconsistent in its assessment of the long-term developmental effects of a

death in the family on a child's adult functioning, it does seem that school-age children who lose a parent or sibling are especially vulnerable to reacting with depression and with lowered self-esteem for a period of some months, if not longer. Children are very likely to equate death with abandonment and to feel that if a parent died it was because the parent didn't love them. The bereaved child's depression, heightening of self-blame, and lowering of self-esteem occur at a point in the developmental process when the child is establishing a sense of self and working on crucial areas of competency and relationships with peers. Given the crucial developmental consolidations taking place in childhood, even a minor depression of a year's duration is likely to interfere with the child's normal development. Given the even greater potential for disruption of the caretaking environment and of surviving family relationships after the death of a family member, it seems highly probable that children will adapt to the death but will be burdened by thoughts and feelings that will interfere with optimal ongoing development.

While children can be helped to resolve their grief experiences through the active support of their parents, it is often the case that bereaved parents, struggling as they are with their own grief reactions, are themselves too emotionally vulnerable and psychologically overextended to offer their children the support, clarification, and constancy in caretaking they need. Parents who lack supportive resources to help them integrate their own grief experience are likely to be much less available to their children than they were prior to the death. Provision by grieving parents of a supportive caretaking environment for their children is an ideal outcome; the reality is that grieving parents who lack other supports are more likely to need their *child's* instrumental and emotional cooperation in preserving their own and their family's stability. The process of mutual adaptation in relationships toward the restoration of stability after a death in the family is a necessary part of family development and is not in itself pathological. However, the process of mutual adaptation can become problematic if the parent is relying too heavily on the child's support in ways that interfere with necessary aspects of the child's ongoing development. The interdependent bereavement reactions of grieving children and their grieving parents become inextricably woven into the mutual adaptation process that shapes their shared movement as a family system through subsequent stages of the family life cycle.

Children are extraordinarily creative in their grief reactions as they achieve an understanding of the death that stabilizes their own inner turmoil and harmonizes with their family requirements. The stories of grieving children illustrate the importance of understanding the many dimensions out of which each individual child and each family constructs a grief experience. With sympathetic understanding for the child's and family's original dilemma, it becomes possible to support the child's continuing creative work of incorporating death, loss, and sorrow into an evolving life story. While the sorrow of death and loss is never finished, neither do we ever exhaust our sources of energy and of new images of renewal in our storehouse of memory. Children preserve their important relationships with dead family members in memory and spirit. These evolving relationships can be revisited and restored as sources of comfort and havens of safety throughout life.

PART III

GRIEVING FAMILIES AND THEIR SHARED DEVELOPMENT

CHAPTER 7

Family Systems Theory and Models of Family Bereavement

FAMILY SYSTEMS THEORY: BASIC CONCEPTS

The field of family therapy has studied family bereavement only relatively recently. The field's historical neglect of individual psychology as a contributing resource in our understanding of families has been especially limiting to an understanding of family bereavement. In their introduction to a recent edited volume of family systems papers on family bereavement, Walsh and McGoldrick (1991) describe what they see as the barriers in the field of family therapy to a systemic analysis of family bereavement:

> The neglect of loss in family therapy was furthered by the split that occurred in the development of the field regarding the relative importance of the individual vs. the family system, of "content" vs. "process," and of history vs. the here-and-now, for the understanding and treatment of family dysfunction (Madanes and Haley, 1977). With the paradigmatic shift to a systems orientation, focus on the individual, on content issues, and on past influences was regarded by many as unsystemic, associated with more reductionistic traditional models of psychotherapy (Fisch, Weakland, and Siegel, 1982). . . . Loss was dismissed as "merely" a content issue, involving intrapersonal feelings and reactions to events, particulary in the past; accordingly, it was relegated to the domain of psychoanalysis. More recently, constructivist theorists further devalued the significance of life events (presumably including death) by arguing that reality can never be known, that all experience is subjectively coconstructed, and, therefore, that any attempt to "discover" the factual occurrences is misguided and irrelevant to changing current views (see Hoffman, 1990). (p. 6)

Walsh and McGoldrick's critique does not include the schools of family therapy, such as their own intergenerational approach, that have remained focused on family life cycle events, including family deaths, as they influence subsequent generations.

The study of family development has been more actively pursued by family systems thinkers than has the area of family bereavement. However, family therapists have been more comfortable turning to concepts from family sociology, such as the family life cycle, as the conceptual basis for a systemic approach to family development (Carter, 1989; Falicov, 1988; Carter & McGoldrick, 1989; Walsh & McGoldrick, 1991). Writers in the field of family therapy have become increasingly interested in the interface of individual and systemic processes (Sugarman, 1986; Wachtel & Wachtel, 1986). The integration of social, ecological, and relational views of human development with concepts from family systems theory can further our understanding of family bereavement from a systemic developmental perspective.

The conceptual frameworks of family systems theory contribute a crucial missing dimension to an understanding of both child and adult bereavement experiences as they interact within the family. According to family systems theorists, families are governed by the same rules that govern the organization of other biological systems (Bateson, 1972, 1979, 1992; Hoffman, 1981; Piercy & Sprenkle, 1986). First and most important, the family is seen as an organized whole, its constituent members interdependent. Most simply, the whole is greater than the sum of its parts. From a systemic point of view, the family is composed not only of individuals but also of relationships between individuals that themselves define the structure or organization of the family as a unit. Further, biological systems are viewed as circular rather than linear in their causality: The action of any one member or constituent part of a system affects all others, which in turn change and affect the functioning of all others yet again in an ever-changing spiral. In a family system the same triggering event in a sequence can lead to different outcomes. Yet an outcome is caused not by a particular triggering event but, rather, by the interplay of responses that are governed by the structure of family relationships.

The processes of adaptation and self-regulation in family systems are seen as including both *stabilizing mechanisms* for the maintenance of continuity, or *homeostasis*, and *transformational mechanisms* for the integration of new information and adaptation to changing circumstances, or *morphogenesis* (Hoffman, 1981; Keeney, 1983; Keeney & Thomas, 1986). In their early work with extremely disturbed families, family therapists and theorists primarily emphasized homeostatic mechanisms, which maintained the stability of the family under changing circumstances. Disturbed families often experience change as overwhelming and tend to use especially rigid mechanisms to maintain a sense of enduring emotional stability. More recent writings in family therapy emphasize the balance of change and continuity; that is, families need to be able to adapt to changing circumstances while maintaining a sense of cohesiveness and stability.

In addition to the balance of change and continuity, family systems theorists and therapists have identified the balance of connection and self-assertion that characterizes family relationships. In their early work many family theorists and therapists described a continuum of differentiation of self from family, with extreme overinvolvement or "enmeshment" at one end and extreme isolation or "disengagement" at the other. In highly enmeshed or emotionally reactive families the self-assertion of any individual member is experienced as a threat to the family's shared self-definition and is strictly controlled. Differences of perception or opinion are considered dangerous to family stability, as they might lead to too great a separation between members. More recent family therapy writings emphasize the balance of self-assertion and connection achieved through an exploration and acceptance of family members' differences in feelings and perceptions. A family that achieves an inclusive balance of self-with-others recognizes both similarities and differences and permits family members to feel fully included in a differentiated and authentic, rather than "pseudomutual." family cohesiveness.

Family systems theorists have historically focused on patterns of communication in families as they organize emotional responsiveness and reflect shared family patterns of adaptation. Any one individual's symptom is seen as an expressive act resulting from a shared family process, an act that conveys the meaningful way in which a family has arrived at a stable self-organizing structure. Family interactions consist of a constant flow of nonverbal as well as verbal exchanges through which members communicate to one another tolerable ideas and emotions, that is, those that will not threaten family cohesiveness or stability. Most schools of family therapy, whatever their theoretical orientation, concentrate their efforts on restructuring those patterns of family communication that affect the organization of family experience and family symptomatology.

From a family systemic point of view, individual symptoms are understood and treated in terms of their function in the current organization of the family system. Symptoms located in an individual may serve the function of maintaining homeostasis for a family. They may also represent an individual's attempt to "meta-communicate" that all is not as it should be in the family; in this way they represent an attempt to change. Interventions that address the problematic interactional or communicational patterns, rather than the particular individual in pain, are considered a more powerful and effective means of addressing individual problems.

In recent years the field of family therapy has been increasingly fragmenting into separate theoretical schools, which emphasize somewhat distinct, although overlapping, perspectives on family functioning. Concepts from structural, strategic and systemic–epistemological, and intergenerational schools of family therapy can make significant contributions to a systemic developmental understanding of family bereavement. Each of these approaches begins with the shared systemic perspective that the family is a group of interacting, interdependent individuals. The intergenerational approach emphasizes the ways family history is mapped onto here-and-now relationships, especially for families under stress (Boszormenyi-Nagy & Krasner, 1986; Bowen, 1978; Framo, 1982; Kerr & Bowen, 1988; Stierlin, 1977). The structural approach tends to focus on formal patterns of organization that characterize well-functioning families but are missing in disturbed families; these normal family structures include hierarchical organization, clear boundaries between family subsystems, such as parental or sibling subsystems, clarity about how family roles are organized and performed, and flexible communication between subsystems (Minuchin, 1974; Minuchin & Fishman, 1987). The strategic/systemic–approach emphasizes the family's construction of a shared reality and views symptoms as communications of the family's best, if problematic, attempt at adaptation and stable organization (Haley, 1974; Madanes & Haley, 1977; Selvini Palazzoli, Boscolo, Cecchin, & Prata, 1978). Each of these schools can contribute to an assessment of the developmental transformations precipitated by a death in the family.

BEREAVEMENT IN THE
FAMILY SYSTEMS LITERATURE
Intergenerational Family Therapy

Most of the bereavement literature in the field of family therapy has been generated by the intergenerational family therapists, who focus on patterns of emotional relatedness established in families of origin and imposed onto current family situations. The more stress experienced by the family over the course of the intergenerational family life cycle, the more rigid or inflexible will be the preservation of past images or patterns of relationship at the expense of direct emotional engagement in current relationships. Family patterns that arise out of the need to manage an overwhelming loss, such as the death of a family member, become a central focus of intergenerational family therapy. Family therapists who construct a family genogram (McGoldrick & Gerson, 1985) are immediately provided with a historical account of the intergenerational flow of the family life cycle, an account in which the interweaving of births and deaths over the course of a family's life suggests the potential impact of family deaths on family development.

Delayed Grief and Operational Mourning

Intergenerational family therapists have written about the continuing impact of delayed grief observed in their patients, as well as about grief reactions immediately after a death. Family therapists often note the significant number of symptomatic families who over the course of treatment discover that it was an unrecognized grief reaction that triggered a family disruption. In some families unfinished mourning remains a current problem even though the death occurred many years ago. In one of the earliest contributions to the family systems bereavement literature, Paul and his colleagues (Paul, 1974; Paul & Grosser, 1965, reprinted in McGoldrick & Walsh, 1991; Paul & Paul, 1989) observed that disturbed families of psychiatrically hospitalized adults could not tolerate the object loss of normal separation and individuation. Paul proposed that these family failures of individuation were generated by difficulties with mourning in the parental generation over deaths sometimes occurring as many as 50 years earlier and usually before the birth of the identified patient. The parents denied the emotional significance of the actual loss in their lives at the same time that they maintained unchanged feelings about and images of the lost person, which they imposed on current family relationships.

Paul and his colleagues found that one possible repercussion of incomplete mourning that affects current family functioning is the parent's projection of aspects of the lost person onto the child. These parents also try to limit the child's growing independence as a way of limiting further losses and disappointments. This parental attitude creates a condition of rigid or pathological equilibrium that restricts the growth of all family members. Paul suggested that these rigid defenses were at their most extreme in families with schizophrenic members. Walsh (1978) also found that a significant number of the parents of hospitalized schizophrenics had suffered the death of a parent immediately preceding the birth of the child.

Paul and his colleagues found that when these families share a belated mourning experience in the context of therapy, they often experience significant improvement. They introduced the concept of "operational mourning" to describe the "corrective mourning experience" they offered these families in family therapy: The therapist stimulates the grief work through concrete discussion of the events of the death and the associated feelings, thus providing the family with a powerful emotional experience that allows for mutual empathy through the expression of shared feelings of loss and pain. Once the emotional anguish of grief is out in the open, the family can be helped to explore their anxiety about loss and abandonment, including the system of projections designed to provide connection with the lost family member. According to Paul, operational mourning creates a temporary disorganization and disequilibrium for the family but is followed by a reorganization that permits freer emotional expression and greater individuation of family members.

Intergenerational family therapists apply Paul's concept of operational mourning by encouraging a full emotional remembering and recounting of the details of the death, an emotional expansion of the grief experience, from each family member. With the support of the therapeutic relationship, families are often able to reopen the suppressed but still vivid subject of a family death, to explore the shared emotional implications of the event, and thus to better integrate the experience and separate past from present. Other family therapists have applied the concept of operational mourning by prescribing rituals outside the therapy room that enhance the family's grieving. Williamson (1978) reported the greater individuation that results when patients are encouraged to visit the grave of a dead parent and more fully experience their grief.

Grief and Differentiation of Self

Theoretical discussions by Bowen (1976) and Herz (1980) of family grief reactions immediately after a death address both intergenerational and structural dimensions of a family's grief experience. Bowen's clinical obervations concerning family grief reactions are rooted in his theory of the differentiation of self from family of origin, which emphasizes that anxiety and stress increase a family's fusion, mutual emotional reactivity to one another's states, and reliance on overly rigid family structures, such as triangles, for emotional stability. Bowen (1976; reprinted in Walsh & McGoldrick, 1991) notes that most people, including dying patients and many physicians, have a tendency to deny death or to experience intense anxiety when discussing terminal illness and death. He proposes that under circumstances of intense anxiety family relationships unconsciously shift from an open to a closed communication system to protect the self against the anxiety that would be generated by an open discussion of the anxiety-provoking situation.

Bowen further discusses the disruption of family equilibrium that occurs at the time of a death. He proposes that when a family member is added or lost, the family has to establish a new equilibrium based on the new circumstances and changes in relationships. The family's level of emotional integration and the severity of the change determine how long it takes the family to achieve this new equilibrium. Bowen notes that while the death of a family member is always a severe disruption, the family's previous adaptation, level of differentiation, and system of communication are crucial elements of a family's grief reaction. He adds that simply helping a family express feelings at the time of a crisis does not necessarily increase the family's level of emotional integration.

Bowen has observed the presence of an "emotional shock wave," or series of additional disruptive family life events that often follows a death or life-threatening illness. These disruptive events can be any human problem, including the more frequent occurrence of relatively mild illnesses, the first occurrence of a more severe illness, the appearance of emotional symptoms, and a greater frequency of failures in functioning or of accidents. For undifferentiated families the emotional shock wave is likely to be more severe. Most families deny the connection between the death or life-threatening illness and these later family disturbances and thus continue to deny the emotional importance of the loss.

Bowen argues that in addition to the family's level of differentiation the importance of the individual to the family system also determines the occurrence of an emotional shock wave. The death of either parent in a family of young children, the death of a grandparent who is considered the head of the clan, the death of a child important in family equilibrium—all are likely to be followed by an emotional shock wave. Bowen distinguishes between grief, which is a characteristic of individual family members, and the emotional shock wave, which is a characteristic of family structure and organization. For example, he suggests that there will be prolonged mourning but no emotional shock wave after the death of a dysfunctional family member or after a suicide, unless the member who died fulfilled an essential functional role in the family.

Bowen states that it is important in conducting family therapy at the time of a death for the therapist to know the total family configuration, the functional position of the dying or recently deceased person in the family, and the overall family adaptation. Further, the therapist needs to use direct descriptive words rather than euphemisms, because direct language enhances open communication. Bowen finds that the funeral is a vital opportunity for the family to share fully in the emotional experience and acceptance of a death. He speculates that funerals were probably more effective when people died at home, with their families present, thus bringing family members into direct contact with the harsh facts of death and with each other at a highly emotional time. Present-day funeral customs—such as the use of euphemisms, refusal to look at the dead body, refusal to include children in a funeral, private funerals segregated from the larger community, the use of ritual to the exclusion of intimate or personalized acknowledgment of the dead person—further avoid the shared emotionality of death. Bowen frequently coaches families about the best use of the funeral in enhancing family emotional adjustment.

Herz (1980, 1989) uses Bowen's family theory and draws on her own work as a family therapist and nurse who has worked extensively with dying patients and their families. Following Bowen, Herz agrees that both level of differentiation and level of stress are dimensions of a family's capacity for open communication. With sufficiently high stress levels, such as after a long and difficult terminal illness, even highly differentiated families are likely to restrict the openness of their communication or to develop some dysfunction. She suggests that this restriction of open communication about death is exacerbated in our technological and death-phobic society, which has developed "death specialists"—medical staff, morticians, and funeral directors—who separate communities and families from the realities of death. Herz finds that the degree of disruption to a family system caused by a death will be determined by the timing of the death in the life cycle, the nature of the death, the openness of the family system, and the family position of the dead family member.

Herz argues that not all deaths have equal importance to the family system. The emotional significance of a family member depends both on his or her functional role in the family and on the family's degree of emotional dependence on the individual. The more the family depends either functionally or emotionally on the family member, the greater the disruption it suffers after the death. Herz suggests that the death of an elderly family member is the least disruptive to the family because the elderly are seen as having lived a full life and have fewer caretaking responsibilities for other family members. In contrast, the death of a parent of young children is the most disruptive because it leaves a gap in the functioning of the family and may interrupt its ongoing development. The death of a child is also severely disruptive, according to Herz, because of the importance of children in the family projection process. The more emotionally incomplete the parents, Herz suggests, the greater the projection onto the child, the more extreme the fusion between parent and child, and the more severe the degree of family disruption at the death of the child.

Whatever the level of family fusion, any family death interrupts the ongoing tasks of that particular phase of the life cycle. The nature of the death, such as whether it was sudden or anticipated, will also influence the family's reaction. A sudden death does not permit anticipatory mourning, and preparations such as a will or other financial arrangements may be incomplete. An anticipated death due to illness permits anticipatory mourning but means that the family has had to bear the stress that accompanies prolonged illness.

Herz notes that of the four major factors affecting a family grief reaction, three cannot be changed by the therapist: the timing of the death, its nature, and the position of the person in the family system. The family therapist can only intervene in expanding the openness of the family system. For this Herz recommends the following interventions: using open and factual terminology and information; establishing at least one open relationship in the family system as a facilitator of more open communication within the family; helping the family balance the focus on death with a focus on hope for life and living; checking on the progress of relationships and issues, especially in areas where symptoms show up as an indication of stress; and utilizing the family's own rituals, customs, and styles. She adds that it is important for the family therapist to remain differentiated, that is, emotionally calm and nonreactive, in the face of the family system's intense emotional stress and reactivity.

Like Bowen and Paul, Herz finds that most families do not seek help with their grief reaction but, rather, come for therapy because of later symptoms in the family, that is, aspects of the emotional shock wave. After the symptom is addressed and the family's attention is redirected to the grief reaction, the focus of family therapy becomes the resolution of the past relationship. In these families seeking treatment for a delayed grief reaction Herz finds that dead family members are typically either idealized or vilified; they are not seen as people with both strengths and weaknesses. Often, the dead family member either is not mentioned or is spoken of as if he or she were still alive. Unresolved issues with the dead family member typically cannot be openly discussed, and the facts surrounding the death are often confused. Herz urges families to review the events surrounding the death, to review family relationships with the deceased in a full way, to make frequent references to the dead family member, and to reestablish connections with other important people in the extended family or community network who knew the deceased.

The Shared Tasks of Family Bereavement

Walsh and McGoldrick (1991) discuss family grief reactions from a systemic theoretical framework that includes intergenerational and family life cycle perspectives. They describe two major family adaptational tasks in response to the death of a family member: (1) a shared acknowledgment of the reality of the death and a shared experience of the loss and (2) a reorganization of the family system to enable reinvestment in other relationships and life pursuits. Families who have suffered the death of a family member are especially vulnerable to isolation, and these writers, like most others in the field, stress the importance of open communication of feelings between family members, taking into account that family members may be out of phase with each other's grief. They also note that many families make precipitous moves, such as remarriage or relocation, in an attempt to restore emotional and functional equilibrium but fail to address the underlying grief.

Walsh and McGoldrick also identify a number of factors that can adversely affect family mourning processes, including the type of death, the prior functioning of the family and social network, the life cycle timing of the loss, and the sociocultural context. Losses that involve sudden or lingering death, ambiguous loss, such as disappearance, or violence are likely to be more stressful for family members and to precipitate more disturbance. Disengagement or enmeshment in the family's previous level of functioning; a lack of flexibility in the family system; blocked communication or secrecy concerning death; a family belief system invoking blame, shame, or guilt surrounding the death; lack of kin and of social or economic resources—all are risk factors for a more complex or distressed family grief reaction. If the deceased performed an important function in the family or had a conflicted or estranged relationship with other family members, the family grief reaction will be adversely affected. Multiple losses or other family stressors concurrent with the death; a multigenerational legacy of unresolved loss; a sociopolitical and historical context fostering denial, stigma, or catastrophic fears—all are important warning signals for a therapist working with a bereaved family.

Other Family Systems Concepts Used in Understanding Bereavement

Grief and Disruptions of Homeostasis

Jordan (1990), like Walsh and McGoldrick, integrates systemic and developmental approaches in understanding family bereavement as a disruption of family homeostasis. Using Stierlin's (1977) and Combrinck-Graham's (1985) work on centripetal and centrifugal forces over the course of the family life cycle, Jordan argues that families at a particular phase of the family life cycle are characterized by an emphasis on either centripetal forces, or a turning inward, or centrifugal forces, or a turning outward. He proposes that a family bereavement experience is best understood as a crisis of attachment in which the natural oscillation between centripetal and centrifugal forces in the family's development is interrupted by an increase in a family's centripetal or fusionary forces. Jordan observes that in order to proceed with optimal family development, families require a balance between change and stability.

In a theoretical paper based on structural family therapy, Bowlby-West (1983) states that the death of a family member creates a structural void that requires homeostatic adjustment. She presents a list of common homeostatic adjustments in the family, including displacement of feelings through triangulation or scapegoating; increase in enmeshment, especially in becoming mutually overinvolved and fearful of separations; creation of family secrets related to the death; idealization of the deceased; infantilization, parentification, and role reversals; and attempts to replace the deceased. According to Bowlby-West, these homeostatic adjustments will be especially needed if family members are having difficulty communicating their emotions about the death or if emotions are repressed or misunderstood. The family therapist can facilitate open communication and can encourage the family to seek support from a wider social network, including the religious community.

Child Symptoms and Their Family Function

A number of published case studies in the family systems literature have discussed grief reactions. These discussions tend to emphasize the role of the "identified patient," usually a child, in expressing unacknowledged grief reactions for the family as a unit (Hare-Mustin, 1979; Rosenthal, 1980). Selvini-Palazzoli et al. (1974) treated a disturbed 2-year-old girl, who had not been told of the death of her infant brother, by prescribing a symbolic burial in which she and her parents participated. Yates and Bannard (1988) describe three nonpsychotic children, ages 9 to 14, who experienced hallucinations of the deceased family member. They argue that the children's symptom served two important family functions: (1) It expressed the family's, especially the mother's, incomplete mourning and (2) it served to bring the child in closer contact to a mother made emotionally unavailable because of her own intense grief. Their discussion includes a developmental as well as a family systemic perspective on the child's hallucination of the deceased inasmuch as the "symptom choice" is viewed as a reflection both of an unmet developmental need and of the systemic problems in the family that have left the need unmet. According to Yates and Bannard, these three children were using hallucinations to grieve the loss of the unavailable mother, vicariously do her grieving for her, and flag the problem in the mother–child subsystem for the family as a unit.

Structural Change in Grieving Families

Family-systems-oriented bereavement therapists also emphasize the structural changes in the family system as the result of a family member's death. These structural changes have two dimensions: impaired functioning in family roles, caused by loss of the family member or by the survivors' incapacitating grief, and the loss of a stabilizing member maintaining family equilibrium, or homeostasis. Rosen (1989), in a discussion of family systems therapy with cases of what he called "interminable grief" after the loss of a child, describes a frequently occurring structure for reestablishing family homeostasis in which one of the parents forms a subsystem with the deceased child and becomes isolated from the rest of the family. In his work with these families, Rosen tends to do individual grief work with the isolated grieving parent in preparation for reintegration of the family as a unit.

Gelcer (1983) reports on two cases of family therapy after the death of a parent and the remarriage of the surviving parent. In both cases the dead parent was described as a ghost whose presence shifted the structural balance in existing family triangles. Unresolved mourning in both these families interfered with the acceptance of the loss and the recognition of the new family configuration. In these families the stepparent was thrust into the position of parent in an attempt to deny the loss and counterbalance the ghostly presence of the dead parent. Family therapy in both cases emphasized open discussion of bereavement issues, encouraged rituals to commemorate the family death, and supported the emergence of a more appropriate role for the new parent in contributing to the family system. Gelcer warns that many of these families involving remarriage after the death of a spouse enter therapy because of current family dysfunction, and are often at first reluctant to discuss past grief and trauma. These families are especially concerned that exploration of the bereavement history will disrupt the fragile new family relationship. Only through the process of therapy do these bereaved families realize the degree to which an enduring relationship with the deceased is interfering with the commencement of their shared new life.

Terminal Illness and Family Bereavement

A number of family systems theorists and therapists have discussed their work with families who have a chronically or terminally ill family member. Reiss (1981), on the basis of his research into family epistemology, describes the ways in which families with a chronically ill member construct shared meanings for understanding the illness, meanings that can enhance or impede what he calls "processes of recognition and growth through experience" (p. 192). Reiss contrasted families who grew and changed from the illness experience with families who instead became preoccupied with connecting the illness event to past experiences or beliefs. Reiss suggests that families differ in the fit between their family organization and the demands of chronic or terminal illness. He suggests that ordinary middle-class families, with their complex goal-oriented structure, may do well in coping with the initial crisis of diagnosis and treatment but often cannot cope with the demands of terminal illness. These families are likely to turn over a chronically ill family member to the medical system for care, because of the massive disruption to their ongoing functioning precipitated by the chronic illness. In contrast, poor or so-called "disorganized" families may not do as well in the initial treatment phase but do better during the chronic care phase, because they have greater access to extended family members and put less emphasis on goal achievement, factors that often allow them to care for a chronically ill family member within the home.

Rolland (1987, 1991) describes a family systems–illness model, a systemic conceptual framework for helping families cope with anticipatory loss. Rolland sees anticipatory grief as determined by the type of illness, the phases of the illness, and the intersection of the "illness life cycle" with other aspects of family organization and family development. He makes the crucial point that illnesses vary in terms of onset (acute or gradual); course (progressive, constant, or relapsing); outcome (shortened life span or no effect on longevity; gradual deterioration or possible sudden death); and incapacitation (ranging from none to severe). These psychosocial characteristics of the illness itself, as well as the phase of the illness process, intersect with family characteristics, especially phase of the family life cycle, to determine the family's adaptation and response.

Grief and Coconstruction of New Family Narratives

Walker (1991) describes her team's work at the New York, Ackerman Institute with families who have a family member dying of AIDS. Based on a systemic perspective that emphasizes the family's shared construction of meaning, Walker's work is especially important for its exploration of the meaning of AIDS in the larger culture and its impact on the family's mutual adaptation and meaning-making process. Given that the AIDS epidemic is currently most associated with lifestyles the culture considers both deliberately chosen and morally reprehensible (homosexuality, substance abuse, and heterosexual activity outside of marriage), families experience a great deal of social pressure to expel the dying family member or to define his or her death as a punishment for transgressions. Walker and her team describe the importance of creating a new family narrative that moves from a narrative of shame to a narrative of pride and allows the full positive integration of the dying family member and his or her illness. The most intensive work of Walker's team with families tends to occur prior to the death of the family member with AIDS, although the team engages as many families as possible in follow-up subsequent to the death. Walker's discussion of case material reflects both theoretical sophistication and clinical sensitivity in examining the enormous pressures on these families as they struggle with the physical stresses and emotional demands presented by AIDS.

SUMMARY: FAMILY THERAPY APPROACHES TO BEREAVEMENT

The family therapy literature on bereavement emphasizes the interpersonal, interactional nature of grief. The death of a family member disrupts the family equilibrium, and new family mechanisms for stable organization need to be established. The quality of the family's organization and interaction prior to the death of one of its members is crucial in understanding the family's grief reaction after the death. According to family therapy writings on bereavement, the test of successful bereavement is the family's reestablishment of equilibrium and resumption of functioning.

Implicit in this literature, as in the bereavement literature, is the assumption that severe grief reactions represent some family dysfunction, such as a high degree of fusion, enmeshment, or rigidity. Since Bowen, Herz, and others equate severity of grief reaction with degree of importance of the deceased's family functions, they conclude that a severe reaction to the death of a child, who has no caretaking responsibilities, must mean that the child had an important function as the receiving object of significant family projections. Unfortunately, this assumption by family systems theorists leads to the attribution of a great deal of psychopathology to families who have lost a child and have not recovered in accordance with a preestablished timetable proposed by the therapist, just as psychoanalytic theory condemned the prolonged grief reaction as an indication of a pathologically ambivalent relationship. In fact, work with families who have lost a child suggests that the death of a child provokes a crisis of long duration for most families. The death of a child in a "healthy"—that is, emotionally open, mutually attached, and functionally successful—family can be a profound, enduring blow precisely because of the loss of the good relationships the child had with family members and the destruction of the family's dreams of their shared future.

As an alternative to applying these pathologizing perspectives from both family systems theory and psychoanalysis, it is possible to assume that the relationship that existed between survivor and deceased, whether the relationship was between parent and child or between spouses, involved deep human interrelatedness coconstructed by processes that characterize normal family relational and developmental processes. A survivor's reaction to the death of a family member is a profound, shattering developmental crisis of both attachment and identity that is precipitated by the loss of an important constituent of the collaborative self.

Research findings increasingly support the clinical observation that while most children, adults, and families go on living and growing after a family death, many families make substantial compromises that affect the ongoing development of their members (Osterweis et al., 1984). While a family's previous level of adaptation or enmeshment will influence the severity of its bereavement reaction, which is itself a potential opportunity for growth and more successful adaptation, the death of a family member is nevertheless a developmental burden for all families.

In understanding family bereavement, it becomes important to examine closely the aspects of family life that are disrupted by a death and the mechanisms that families rely on in reestablishing the stable self-organizing structures that support their ongoing family development. The circumstances of the death—that is, how it occurred, the extent of violence at the moment of death, the degree of disruption in ongoing family functions—constitute a more powerful organizer of family bereavement than do characteristics of prior family functioning. The degree of discontinuity, the degree of accompanying stress, and the availability of supportive resources to help reestablish the flow of daily life are important determinants of a family's capacity to re-create stable family structures that support and enhance, rather than constrict and limit, family growth. The pool of resources a grieving family draws from includes their previous learning from earlier stages of the family life cycle and the strength, warmth and flexibility of their surviving relationships with one another. The test of a family's recovery from the death of a family member becomes whether or not the establishment of new stable family structures enhances or constrains the ongoing development of its members and of the family as a unit.

The integration of a wider range of concepts from the family systems field greatly enhances the usefulness of a family systemic model in understanding family bereavement. Family therapists have long fought against the pathologizing of ordinary family processes. They have traditionally emphasized the creative ingenuity of symptoms as problem-solving strategies that create the necessary stability for family change. In bringing together a wider range of systemic developmental theories to our work with family bereavement, we can expand our own resource base for supporting a grieving family's best developmental outcome.

CHAPTER 8

Family Development and Adaptation to the Crisis of Grief

The out-of-life-cycle death of a family member, whatever its circumstances, will have to be integrated into an ongoing process of family development. At the same time, a death in the family radically shifts that ongoing developmental process and makes overwhelming new demands on it. A systemic approach to family development can help evaluate the interweaving of the current normative stage of the family life cycle with the transition precipitated by the death itself (Falicov, 1988; Walsh & McGoldrick, 1991). In this chapter I apply a model of family development (Shapiro, 1988) that examines the shared process of individuation in response to family life cycle transitions as a means of understanding the systemic developmental impact of family bereavement. Table 8.1 provides an overview of this family developmental model.

RELOCATING "PATHOLOGICAL GRIEF" IN ITS NORMAL DEVELOPMENTAL CONTEXT

Under the shattering blow of grief, family members immediately reach for the most basic human strategies that will enable them to survive the agony of the moment and to restore a sense of stability to their world. With this temporary stability, family members can gradually begin the radical transformation of every aspect of their lives precipitated by the death. Child and adult bereavement theorists and therapists refer to denial of the reality of the death as a basic human strategy for survival immediately after a death (Bowlby, 1980; Parkes, 1972;

TABLE 8.1. Model of Family Development

1. Human development is systemically organized through collaborative choreography in multiple interlocking systems that include individuals, families, communities, and cultures.

2. Family life cycle transitions are opportunities to observe family developmental transformation of the collaborative self through mutual adaptation to shared family change.
 A. The collaborative self is renegotiated and re-created through processes of mutual adaptation, over the course of the family life cycle. Family life cycle transitions include changes in family structure (e.g., birth and death of members, school entry, retirement, divorce), as well as changes initiated by individual development (e.g., puberty). When any family member changes, all family members must reorganize the collaborative self.
 B. The reorganization of the collaborative self can be called individuation, defined as an interpersonal, dialectical life span process in which both the establishment of a distinctive, autonomous self and the establishment of relatedness or connection are dynamically or dialectically balanced. The balance of self-assertion and connection will be renegotiated and reestablished throughout the family life cycle.

3. The circumstances of family development determine whether or not the process of individuation, collaboratively negotiated during family transitions, is characterized by an optimal integration of complex, contradictory perspectives, a normative stereotyping of conflict and complexity, or a symptomatic fragmentation and dissociation of overwhelmingly painful or conflictual contradictory realities.
 A. Optimal family development requires the balance of continuity, or stability, and discontinuity, or change, so that families can integrate change in a manageable way. Under circumstances of overwhelming change, a family and its members will act interpersonally as well as intrapsychically to reduce the rate of change. The more radical or traumatic the circumstances of transition, the more extreme the measures the family will use, including radical denial of change, to establish a necessary sense of stability.
 B. A family's capacity to integrate changes into an ongoing, coherently experienced family life will depend on the balance of stresses and supports at the time of a transition. Under sufficient stress and lacking adequate supports, a family is more likely to fragment or dissociate in the face of change and to rely on severe intrapsychic and/or interpersonal symptomatology to control the rate of change.
 C. A symptomatic adaptation to overwhelming stress or discontinuity is one in which the sacrifices of the complex self necessary to maintain stability of personal coherence and of mutual adaptation interfere with the flexible responsiveness to new situations necessary for ongoing development. Symptoms continue to represent an individual's and family's best attempt at stabilization and integrative adaptation to changing developmental circumstances.

4. Although the collaborative self is created through mutual adaptation between all family members, power asymmetries make it possible for

(continued)

TABLE 8.1. (*continued*)

the more powerful family member's projective attributions of others to take priority in the collaborative creation of the self. Healthy relationships are characterized by mutuality and flexibility in relational adaptation. Disturbed relationships will be characterized by exploitation and dominance and the use of authoritarian definitions of the realities of others for the purpose of stable self-regulation and rigid control of differences.

   5. Human relational development takes place within, and is further organized by, the sociocultural context within which family relationships are embedded.
      A. In the dialectical organization of the complex, collaborative self, cultural roles and values offer alternative models for ways of being as well as coherent values and beliefs with which we make the simultaneously shared and uniquely personal meanings that help organize a personally coherent and relationally harmonious sense of self.
      B. In culturally constructing the process of individuation over the course of the family life cycle, every culture creates its own configurations, which take into account age, gender, and social role, in the balance of self-assertion and connection for its members.
      C. Culturally determined power asymmetries, such as racism or sexism, give members of the dominant group the power to define the less powerful person's reality so as to regulate and enhance the dominant group's sense of self at the expense of less powerful others. Under conditions of social injustice, a culture accepts the dominant group's negative attributions of the less powerful group. As in family abuses of power, cultural abuses of power interfere with the integration of a coherent complex self and enhancement of all members through flexible collaboration and mutual adaptation.

Parkes & Weiss, 1983). Family theorists and therapists refer to comparable mechanisms of family interaction and communication that permit, through shared denial and avoidance, a family's immediate emotional survival and psychological restabilization after a death (Herz, 1980, 1989; Walsh & McGoldrick, 1991). How do these mechanisms of psychological survival under extreme stress, both intrapsychic and interpersonal, enhance, rather than constrain, further individual and family development? While both individual and family-oriented grief therapists have tended to emphasize factors in individual and family history that predict normal versus pathological bereavement, the actual circumstances of the death, including the degree of violence and disruption that accompany the death, and the supportive resources available to the family will be major determinants of the family grief reaction.

   Rather than rely on mental health models that emphasize psychopathology, a family developmental approach to family bereavement can make better use of models from both child and adult development that look at successful or maladaptive coping to stressful life circumstances. In the newly emerging areas of developmental psychopathology (Cichetti & Carlson, 1989; Rolf et al., 1990; Rutter & Garmezy, 1983; Sameroff & Emde, 1989), ecological development (Bronfenbrenner, 1979; Garbarino, 1990; Garbarino et al., 1992), and risk and resilience (Anthony & Cohler, 1987; Rolf et al., 1990), clinicians are joining with developmentalists to examine the normal developmental context of childhood symptomatology. Rather than begin with the study of childhood psychopathology, developmental psychopathologists begin with an assessment of normal development and of the environmental circumstances to which the child adapts and that either support or impede normal developmental progress. Developmental psychopathologists (Rolf et al., 1990; Rutter & Garmezy, 1983; Sameroff & Emde, 1989) acknowledge that the boundary between normal and disturbed development in children is often fluid and constantly changing as developmental tasks change. These writers conclude that we can best assess a symptom's seriousness by evaluating its interference with the child's ongoing developmental process.

Risk and resilience models of child development and developmental psychopathology emphasize the dimensions of a child's developmental context that either support or impede successful coping with stressful life events such as severe parental psychopathology or abuse. An extensive literature on adult and family coping with life stress suggests that social support is a key dimension in successful adaptation to stressful life circumstances, including the stress of family bereavement (Figley & McCubbin, 1983; Osterweis et al., 1984). The more stress and discontinuity in the circumstances of a death and the more restricted the available supports, the greater the likelihood that the family will be forced to rely on growth-constraining psychological structures as the only available resources for personal and family stability.

In the chapters on adult and child bereavement I emphasize the fact that a characteristic dimension of the grief experience, especially if it is overwhelmingly stressful or traumatic, is a sensation of being frozen in time at the moment of the death. This interruption in the flow of time gives individuals and families the opportunity to more gradually explore and integrate past memories, present reality, and future possibilities and to thus repair the torn fabric of family developmental time. The developmental moment at which a family endures the traumatic blow of death, which interrupts ongoing developmental tasks, determines the developmental resources a family can bring to bear in coping with the crisis so as to support their ongoing development. Fundamentally, successful resolution of grief requires the restoration of movement in the flow of developmental time.

In supporting a family's capacity to integrate the death and restore the flow of developmental time, we need to consider the following five dimensions of a family's developmental motion:

1. The movement of each individual, adult or child, through his or her unique life cycle
2. The interaction of these individual life cycles at this moment of family history
3. The developmental motion of this interacting family organization over the course of the family life cycle
4. The interweaving of intergenerational family life cycles, the young parent in a family of procreation being at the same time an offspring in a maturing family of origin
5. The movement of a family through the course of historical time in its given sociocultural location

At all times in the course of family development there are interrelationships between individual, systemic, intergenerational, sociocultural, and historical lines of development. Each of these interconnected domains of development, which ecological theorists call "nested structures" (Bronfenbrenner, 1979; Garbarino et al., 1992), generates an adaptational context with stresses and supports for the dialectical renegotiation and reintegration of the complex, collaborative self. The private psychological processes of each individual and the nuclear family's here-and-now interactions, its shared history as a developing unit, its extended family history and current relationships, its social role organization, and its cultural traditions and meanings—all are supportive resources for the tasks of family reorganization and bereavement after the death of a family member. Grieving families need strategies for managing intense emotion, reestablishing disrupted family functions, reorganizing family interactions, and re-creating a collaborative family identity that locates the death and its meaning in the ongoing flow of the family's shared intergenerational development.

The process of reestablishing a stable, growth-promoting sense of the collaborative self after the death of a family member requires the reexamination of both patterns of relating and of underlying relational assumptions developed over the course of a shared family life cycle as sources of stability and support for ongoing family development. These underlying relational structures and accompanying meanings are cast in a new light by the circumstances of the death itself, by the new challenges to the self that are presented by the overwhelming emotions of grief, by the demands of coping with new life circumstances, and by the need to construct a new relational world, external and internal. The capacity for flexible responsiveness to the overwhelming blow of grief may already be compromised in families who have already experienced overwhelming stress during previous stages of their family life cycle in the current or in previous generations. For some families, a good-enough adaptation to previous family life cycle transitions may have involved strategies for stabilization that leave the family vulnerable during the far more stressful developmental demands of shared adaptation to the death of a family member.

A family developmental perspective gives us a powerful means of understanding the "relational phenomenology" of grief, that is, the subjective process of examining life structures previously taken for granted and the accompanying sense of self catalyzed by the loss of a self-sustaining relationship. A systemic developmental perspective also makes it possible to assess the ways we as therapists might better support the developmental integration process, even under circumstances of extreme developmental distress. An understanding of the stresses and supports that contribute to the capacity for growth-promoting, as compared to growth-constraining, adaptation after a family death will give us a theoretical basis for intervention strategies designed to enhance the ongoing process of family development. An intervention approach that emerges from an understanding of optimal family development and of the barriers that impede a healthy developmental process will allow use of the family's developmental motion as leverage in supporting more effective family developmental solutions to the crisis of death and grief.

PRINCIPLES OF FAMILY DEVELOPMENT

Family development can best be understood as a whole life cycle process in which aspects of the developmental progress of children and parents, normative, optimal, and symptomatic, are inextricably intertwined. A comprehensive theory of family development under the high-stress circumstances of family bereavement needs to address the conditions under which development proceeds in normative, optimal, and symptomatic forms. What circumstances permit the optimal flow of family development for all its individuals and for the family unit over the course of its shared life cycle? What circumstances constrain or restrict the process of change and generate symptomatic individual or family responses in which the flow of change is defensively controlled? As clinicians working with bereaved families we are especially interested in the family developmental processes that help grieving families cope with overwhelming experience and in the impact of these stabilizing mechanisms on the ongoing process of shared development.

Integrating the Complex Self

The integration of a complex sense of self and others over the course of the family life cycle requires a high tolerance for contradiction and difference. Dialectical (Riegel, 1976) and organismic developmental (Werner, 1948) theories both propose that development moves forward through confrontation with discordant or apparently contradictory information that is explored, integrated, and organized into meaningful, coherent patterns. Family life cycle transitions are opportunities to re-create the collaborative self through mutual adaptation during periods of shared family change.

Healthy human development requires a balance between connection and self-assertion, a harmonious adaptation within relationships that is negotiated to permit and include the distinctiveness of its individuals. As suggested by Werner's (1948) organismic developmental theory, the view of self within relationships becomes increasingly more articulated and organized with maturation and with the integration of new information from new situations. Riegel's (1976) dialectical developmental theory further suggests, in agreement with clinical theories of individuation, that the impetus for growth is provided by discordant information that has to be organized into meaningful patterns. Systems theory adds the important perspective that these individual transformations take place in mutual exchange within the family system; that is, change in self requires change in others, and change in others requires change in self.

Under ideal family developmental circumstances various routes for family change—the individual developmental progress of family members, family life cycle changes of structure, changes of life circumstances—generate opportunities for a shared process of mutual adaptation. Under these optimal family developmental circumstances, which I will call *integrative*, the family generates and acknowledges multiple perspectives on developmental experience, both between family members and within a complex self. When family members encounter conflict, contradiction, or difference—within the self, between the self and other family members, or between the self or family and the culture—these can be explored and included in the shared thinking of the family.

A number of clinical and developmental fields show remarkable agreement about the characteristics of the aforementioned ideal, or integrative, developmental process. Symptomatic, or pathological, family development involves opposite processes: intolerance of multiple perspectives, denial of differences, and attempts to control or restrict the process of change. When social supports and family resources are unavailable or are simply no match for catastrophic life circumstances, a family and its individuals are more likely to resort to psychological structures, intrapsychic and interactional, as the means for reestablishing a sense of stability.

From an integrative developmental perspective, change precipitated by changing family circumstances will be explored, negotiated, and integrated into new ways of relating. In the process of negotiating family developmental change, family members acknowledge and include the distinctiveness or difference presented by each family member while preserving the mutuality necessary for maintaining family bonds. When individual family members' feelings or needs come into conflict, these conflicts will themselves be the impetus for change through this process of empathic recognition and negotiation of a mutually acknowledging adaptation.

This idealized view of family development has a great deal in common with Werner's (1948) view of development as a process of differentiation, articulation of parts, and hierarchical integration into a coherent whole, as well as with Riegel's (1976) dialectical developmental perspective on the integration of contradiction or conflict in development. The definition of ideal developmental process as integrative also correlates with, and includes, perspectives on the optimal development of relatedness proposed by object relations theorists (Bollas, 1987; Buckley, 1986; Winnicott, 1965, 1971, 1975), on intersubjectivity, as proposed by self psychologists (Stolorow & Lachmann, 1980), and theories of gender proposed by feminist psychoanalysts (Benjamin, 1988; Goldner, 1989). More traditional drive or ego psychoanalytic perspectives typically focus on defenses against intrapsychic conflict and would view exploration and integration of conflicting aspects of the self as characteristic of healthy intrapsychic functioning. Loevinger's (1976) theory of ego development, which integrates cognitive and psychoanalytic perspectives, also emphasizes a process of mutuality and negotiation between the needs of the self and the needs of close others, as does Selman's (1980, 1990) theory of social development.

Defense and Constriction of the Complex Self

From an intrapsychic perspective, aspects of the complex self that are defended against, rather than included, do a great deal more than impoverish the personality; conflictual aspects of the self are retained and find indirect expression through compelling yet problematic symbolic representations of unconscious associations. Grieving children make sense of overwhelming experience with the tools of the developmental moment, weaving together a web of associations and meanings that represent their best capacity at the time to face and master the event. Aspects of experience that are overwhelming are repressed or dissociated, gathering with them aspects of the child's development that were intertwined with the stressful event and with the child's attempts to cope. The trade-off seems worthwhile at the time of the original event, for the child gains stability and reduces conflict with important others; however, this is accomplished at the expense of full development of the child's capacities, which denies the child the possibility of optimal functioning. Adult models of intrapsychic coping with traumatic stress similarly emphasize the dissociation of overwhelming experience but view the style of coping as determined by an already established characterological style (Horowitz, 1986).

While family systems perspectives on normal family processes focus on the interpersonal rather than the intrapsychic, they would agree that the capacity to acknowledge, include, and integrate differences in family members' points of view characterizes ideal family relatedness. Research on the normal family (Walsh, 1982) suggests that optimal family functioning requires flexibility and adaptability to change, whether the change is generated by individual differentiation (Beavers, 1977, 1982; Olson, 1988; Olson et al., 1983) or by a stressful life event, including a family death (Crosby & Jose, 1983; Walsh & McGoldrick, 1991). Family communication disorders can be understood as family responses that systematically suppress differences or obscure acknowledgment of them, because the emergence of differences would require disequilibrating growth in self-awareness. Interpersonal tactics for avoidance of overwhelming shared feelings create associated areas of family feeling and functioning that have to be controlled and restrained so as to protect the safe encapsulation of the original distress. At their extreme, these strategies for family stability may radically interfere with the family's exploration of new developmental opportunities. Emotionally constricted families may come to associate all family separations and differences with overwhelming disintegration and danger (Boszormenyi-Nagy & Spark, 1973; Bowen, 1978; Minuchin, 1974).

Families (through the use of interpersonal defense) and individuals (through the use of intrapsychic defense) relegate overwhelming experiences to the never-to-be-opened storage closet of history. Because these encapsulating defenses restrict access to the original disturbing experience, the individual or family never has the opportunity to learn that originally overwhelming feelings might be more manageable under new developmental circumstances. On the other hand, if family and individual adaptation are sufficiently flexible, new stages of the family life cycle that resonate to the original event can provide individuals and families with new developmental opportunities for integrating dissociated or forbidden feelings and memories and associated aspects of the collaborative self. Flexible responsiveness to new developmental opportunities, in spite of the emotional pain or disorientation they might also evoke, restores lost developmental functions and resumes the flow of developmental time in an area of family functioning that had been lost to developmental time.

In sum, there is substantial agreement in these diverse clinical literatures on the nature of human relational health. Nevertheless, family development seldom takes place under these theoretical optimal circumstances in which family members fully share in a collaborative process of integration and self-transformation. The "news of difference," as Bateson (1979) calls it, that is, the information that a change in the family is taking place, a change that requires complementary change in all family members, is not always welcomed. While Werner's (1948) organismic theory and Riegel's (1976) dialectical theory are useful starting points for understanding the cognitive processes that organize and catalyze change in our understanding of the world, neither theory addresses the emotional processes to which cognitive understanding is inextricably linked and that sometimes compel the need for psychological defense against the process of developmental exploration.

The emotional responses associated with new learning are often intense and themselves require organization and stabilization in the exploratory developmental process. However, our cognitive-developmental theories have not customarily addressed the process of emotional development, let alone the continuum between normal and pathological mastery of emotions (Schultz, 1990). And although clinical theories have addressed the process of pathological emotional development, they are typically removed from an understanding of normal cognitive and emotional development.

Models from developmental psychopathology examine the continuum between normal and symptomatic development as mediated by developmental context. Cicchetti (1989) describes normal development from this perspective as an integrative process of organization in response to increasing maturation and changing environmental circumstances. Under circumstances of high environmental stress, such as childhood physical abuse, normally integrated developmental functions—such as the efficacious exploration of the environment, the development of self-awareness and self-esteem, and the development of secure attachment—may become disrupted and fragmented. Yet not all children exposed to high-risk developmental circumstances, such as severe parental psychopathology, physical and sexual abuse, or poverty and urban violence, develop symptomatology. Researchers in the area of developmental psychopathology have been especially interested in the protective factors that characterize so-called invulnerable or resilient children (Anthony & Cohler, 1987; Werner, 1990). Systemic ecological developmental models and risk-resilience perspectives on childhood psychopathology increasingly recognize the importance of contextual stresses that burden the child's capacity for successful adaptation and of contextual supports that foster that capacity even under circumstances of high developmental risk.

The ecological and risk–resilience models of developmental psychopathology are consistent with family systemic views of family adaptation, which see family symptomatology as the family's best adaptation to stressful family life cycle circumstances. From a systemic developmental perspective, we can say that the process of communication, mutual adaptation, and shared meaning-making becomes symptomatic when a family's collaboratively constructed attempts to establish a secure base from which to proceed with shared ongoing development has in fact too severely restricted its capacity for flexible adaptive change, has too much interfered with the ongoing development of one or more of its members. Nevertheless, symptoms remain creative expressions that organize and communicate symbolic representation of experience. Symptoms connote a complex web of private meanings and at the same time convey aspects of the self that cause the family discomfort, and are therefore forbidden by it, but are nevertheless in some way essential to the individual's and family's ongoing development.

Integration and fragmentation represent extremes in our human capacity to make sense of new experiences. Most of our human experiences in fact take place in a more ordinary middle ground, in which we organize an understanding of our critical life events and relationships using workable, if abbreviated, schemas or images for encoding complex experiences. As we develop in cognitive capacity, we create categories of increasing sophistication for new experience; however, these categories, or schemas, become more conventional or culturally stereotyped and less infused with the complex personal and emotional meanings of early childhood. In his book *Metamorphosis*, Schachtel (1958) argues that our adult talent for categorizing and stereotyping experience prevents us from living more fully and directly and deprives us of a vital source of immediacy and creativity. Yet without some categorization and corresponding censoring of experience, we would be very quickly overwhelmed by the cognitive, emotional, and relational complexity of the world around us.

In most cultures it falls only to a few unusually creative individuals—the artists and revolutionaries of their times—to transcend cultural givens in the construction of a sense of self. Erikson, in his discussion of Luther and Gandhi, describes the arduous personal process and unique combination of historical moment and personal character that make it possible for a rare individual to transcend his or her times. Erikson also describes the normative process of identity construction in adolescence, in which the individual looks for a socially sanctioned means of making a unique contribution to the community while affirming his or her connection to its values. Ideally, the Eriksonian self connects to the wider society through the medium of identification while remaining infused with personal meanings uniquely its own.

In the cultural structuring of experience, we rely on the tools of a culture, that is, its rituals and customs and language, to forge an identity that is both publicly affirmed and privately meaningful. Yet individuals vary in the creative freedom or compulsive conventionality they use in the creation of a complex self. In his book *The Duality of Human Experience* (1966), philosopher and psychologist David Bakan describes the human tendency to structure complex experience through polarization or stereotyped duality, especially under circumstances that feel too complex for a fuller integration. This process of polarization is especially well illustrated by gender stereotyping, in which males and females are seen as having separate, nonoverlapping, characteristics. Individuals also differ in the extent to which their socioeconomic level grants them the freedom to create themselves along the most expansive lines of their personal creativity and ideals. Adolescents of middle and upper classes, who have the financial backing for their identity explorations and a secure knowledge of some comfortable place in the working world, have a wider range of options than do adolescents of working-class or poor backgrounds, whose future possibilities are more restricted. The restrictions that accompany social class may well be compounded by restrictions associated with racism and other forms of social prejudice, which limit still more the pathway by which an adolescent transforms talent and possibility into a future life and sense of self.

A family's capacity to integrate changes into an ongoing, coherently experienced family life will depend on the balance of stresses and supports at the time of a transition. When it is under sufficient stress and lacks adequate supports, a family is more likely to fragment or dissociate in the face of change and to rely on severe intrapsychic and/or interpersonal symptomatology to control the rate of change. Over the course of our lives we sacrifice our greatest human complexity in exchange for the stability we require to feel like complete individuals. Our ordinary life circumstances often require that we develop along the lines of the possible and conventional rather than the ideal. Under conditions of extreme or traumatic stress, such as those generated by the death of a family member, we find ourselves dissociating aspects of self-experience that we cannot integrate, thereby gaining a sense of stability and personal coherence, a developmentally necessary illusion of wholeness. Grieving families are faced with a painful developmental paradox: They are forced to radically re-create themselves as a family under family life cycle circumstances that, because of stress and discontinuity, are least hospitable to the open exploration of difference and the reintegration of a complex, mutually negotiated collaborative self.

STRATEGIES FOR MANAGING DEVELOPMENTAL STRESS: CONTROLLING THE RATE OF DISCONTINUITY AND CHANGE

Why is exploration of difference and integration of complex, contradictory perspectives so difficult to achieve under circumstances of radical family transition, such as bereavement? Systemic theories of development argue that family development is characterized by a constant organization and reorganization of spontaneously occurring fluctuations, some of which lead to radical reorganization of family structure (Hoffman, 1981, 1990; Keeney, 1983; Keeney & Thomas, 1986). Because development, in the Wernerian sense, can be viewed as a constant process of organization, one can postulate that a new organizational configuration in a family can lead to a revolution of understanding, even if the catalyst is a relatively minor event. Families, like individuals, are dynamically organized and maintain growth-promoting coherence and stability through self-organizing structures of patterned interaction. Receiving the "news of difference" from family change can catalyze a radical reorganization and transformation of the patterns of organization out of which the collaborative self is formed.

The capacity for transformation of the collaborative self requires a basic stability in the sense of self and a degree of change that can be managed and integrated. Under circumstances of radical instability or discontinuity, such as those that characterize family bereavement, individuals structure their perceptions of self and others so as to create a manageable rate of change. Ordinarily, families manage a balance of continuous and discontinuous change so as to maintain a sense of stability in the face of change. When change is radically discontinuous, families find mechanisms to restrict the information heralding change. Nowhere in the clinical literature is the relationship between overwhelming, discontinuous change and restriction of information clearer than in the traumatic stress literature, which documents the radical use of disassociation and psychic numbing as mechanisms for regaining psychological stability after an overwhelming event (Herman, 1992).

Our psychological processes for managing overwhelming emotion and controlling the flow of change so as to maintain continuity of organization in the face of discontinuous life events emerge from two major, and interrelated, sources: family interactional structures and cognitive–symbolic representational structures. Patterns of socioemotional regulation, from the infant–caretaker system through family interactions in the ongoing family life cycle, create what systemic developmentalists call internalized relational structures and family systems theorists call family structure. Infant researchers have documented the infant's extraordinary social skills and readiness to participate in a highly choreographed sequence of interactions in which both the mother's and the infant's moods are stabilized and regulated. Beebe and Lachmann (1988), Stern (1985), and Tronick (1989) have documented, in their written work and films, the baby's sophisticated capacity to shape social interaction. Babies are remarkably resourceful in evoking needed social responsiveness from a depressed caretaker or terminating overstimulating exchanges. Over the course of the family life cycle, couples and their children generate patterns of interaction and communication that organize their responses to constantly evolving family circumstances. The second source of organizational structure in the process of development is provided by patterns of cognitive organization and symbolic representation of new, complex, or contradictory information, as described, for example, by Riegel (1976) and Werner (1948). The development of cognitive structure, the capacity to make meaningful sense of self and other, has neuromaturational, family relational, and sociocultural dimensions.

Family communication and the mutually adaptive negotiation of shared meanings in families provide the connection between these two interdependent pathways—the cognitve and the interactional—to the stabilization of structure.

Assimilation and Accommodation in Family Context

I have applied Piaget's concepts of assimilation and accommodation to the process of family development as a bridge between cognitive and family interactional pathways to stabilizing structures during transitions (Shapiro, 1988). According to Piaget (1954), progression from the stages of sensorimotor development in infancy to the fully developed capacity for abstract reasoning involves the processes of *assimilation* and *accommodation*. In assimilation, the child perceives information and fits it in with an already existing "schema," or concept. That is, the information is matched to and made to fit an already explored and familiar category of action or thought. In accommodation, the child encounters new information that does not fit any such existing category of thought, one of which must then be modified to create a new schema.

The recognition and integration of new information causes a change in the child's existing cognitive organization. For example, in early infancy, the child developes the schema "things to be sucked" and applies that schema to a diverse range of objects encountered in the environment. With cognitive and motoric development, the child encounters objects that do not readily fit the schema for sucking, objects that are best conceptualized as "things to be banged on the floor." According to Piaget, children selectively ignore objects that are too novel or complex for them to integrate into an existing schema. Rather, children are most curious about objects that are at the same time somewhat familiar and somewhat novel, in this way gravitating toward opportunities to expand their cognitive development.

Although Piaget did not intend the concepts of assimilation and accommodation to be applied beyond an understanding of childhood cognition, they provide a useful model for understanding family reactions to change, especially the creation of stable family structure during periods of family transition. Because the definition of the self is an interpersonal one, changes in any member of the family require reorganization of the self for all family members. The constantly changing adults and children in a family relentlessly present to each other new information, new ways of understanding the self or of being with others, that requires responses from others. Family members can respond to the new information with an "accommodating" change, by creating new schema for self-with-other, or with an "assimilating" change, by making it fit already existing categories of thought.

There are two important differences between the process of cognitive learning as described by Piaget and the process of interpersonal learning experienced in family development. First, interpersonal learning has an emotional component and often requires the integration of both intense emotions and new information. Second, our relationships do not permit us full control over what new learning we take on. While our exploration of the physical world proceeds with a great deal of control over the information we choose to encounter, the interpersonal world presents fewer such opportunities. When new information is provided by the differentiating process of one family member, the others are forced to respond, either with accommodating changes in self or with assimilating attempts to prevent change in the other. Under conditions of interpersonal change, assimilation can involve an individual's distorted perception that no change has occurred, and/or an interpersonal attempt to actively prevent the change.

As in optimal cognitive development, in which there is a balance of assimilation and accommodation, optimal interpersonal development involves a negotiation of the process of mutual change. With too much assimilation in response to family change, an individual has too rigidly denied the news of difference; with too much accommodation as the response, an individual has too fluidly denied his or her own needs for stability and continuity. This discussion of assimilation and accommodation in relationships parallels Buber's (1970) discussion of the "I/it" versus the "I/Thou" relationship, in which an "I/Thou" position involves a full recognition of another person's subjectivity and "I/it" involves an objectification of the other along the lines of our own categories of thought. Buber argues that "I/Thou" relatedness is an ideal, that none of us could tolerate the instability and spiritual challenge of being constantly emotionally open to the full experience of others, and that "I/it" stereotyping of others makes it possible to achieve moments of "I/Thou" relating.

Power Asymmetries and Control of Family Change

Although the self is created through mutual adaptation between all family members, power asymmetries, for example, between parent and child or between male and female, make it possible for the more powerful family member's projective attributions of others to take priority in the collaborative creation of the self. The role of dominance in relational development has been substantially unexplored in the mainstream psychological and developmental literatures. Inspired by

Ferenczi's (1932/1955) work on the reality of abusive parenting and by Marxist thought on the psychological consequences of class exploitation (Fromm, 1961, 1970; Held, 1980; Jay, 1973), the work of the neo-Freudians, especially the work of Sullivan (1953) on parental exploitation of the child, of Horney (1967) on feminine development in the light of male dominance (Westkott, 1988), and of Fromm (1970) on human alienation in an exploitative market economy, presents the most articulate psychoanalytic discussion on the internalization of unjust social conditions.

The role of dominance in human development is returning as a topic of psychological study through the work of critical postmodern cultural studies of race, class, and gender (Aranowitz, 1990; Benjamin, 1988; Dinnerstein, 1978; Hare-Mustin, 1988; Nobles, 1978; Pinder-hughes, 1989; Stanley, 1990; Tyler, Brome, & Williams, 1991). In these studies of power asymmetries and the perpetuation of social injustice, the psychologically important new definition of power imbalance emphasizes the capacity of the powerful or dominant group to define the self of the dominated other. In recognizing the role of power in relational development, we are acknowledging that the partners in a human interaction do not have equal power to define self and other along lines that will create maximum stability for the self. Rather, the less privileged, more vulnerable, members of a society—children, women, the poor, the racially and ethnically different—struggle against broad sociocultural as well as intimate interactional power asymmetries that enhance the self definition of the dominant culture group or partner at their expense. Using Buber's terms, dominant partners remain the "I" or subject of their own experience while objectifying others and denying them the power to define their own subjective view. From a perspective of social justice, then, liberation or empowerment does not require the capacity to dominate or control others but, rather, the capacity to reclaim the power to define the self (Aranowitz, 1990; Benjamin, 1988; Freire, 1970,1985; Miller, 1986).

In adding a social justice perspective to our understanding of family development, we acknowledge the unequal power family members have in controlling the process of mutual adaptation. The uneven distribution of power between parents and children can be handled within a family in ways that are more or less exploitative and that depend to some extent on the sociocultural attitude toward authoritarian dominance in parenting. The role of cultural ideology in the construction of the self, especially ideology that promotes unjust power asymmetries with respect to sex, race, and income, is currently being addressed in a wide range of social science literatures (Garbarino et al., 1992; Levin, 1987; Miller, 1986; Nobles, 1978). From two quite different disciplines, family therapist Boszormenyi-Nagy and radical educator Paolo Freire both propose that recognition of social injustice—what Freire (1970) calls "conscientization"—is an important first step toward healing the psychic wounds created by socially sanctioned dominance and exploitation.

SUMMARY

What circumstances in the course of family development make the difference between a flexible, responsive capacity for mutually adapting change in self and a rigid disavowal of change? Optimal family development requires a balance of stability and change so that families can integrate change in a manageable way. Under circumstances of overwhelming change, a family and its members act interpersonally as well as intrapsychically in ways that attempt to reduce the rate of change. The more radical or traumatic the circumstances of transition, the more extreme the measures a family will use—including radical denial of change—to establish a sense of stability. Under stressful family developmental circumstances parents are more likely to exploit their greater power to dominate the process of adaptation; they do so by giving their own needs for stability greater priority in generating self-protective meanings and rules for family functioning.

The death of a loved one inevitably results in a more limited relational life for family members than they would have had if the loved one had remained alive. In balancing the radical discontinuity of grief with strategies for creating stable new structures of shared adaptation, individuals and families inevitably constrict aspects of self and relational patterns. Later stages of the shared family life cycle, however, can provide grieving families with new opportunities for relational exploration and for more inclusive integration of the complex self. The process of coping with death and loss over the course of life offers us the opportunity to stretch and grow in new ways: to deepen ourselves and our understanding of what it means to be alive, to renew our commitment to appreciating our lives, to cherish our enduring relational bonds.

CHAPTER 9

Helping Bereaved Families

ENHANCING STRATEGIES
FOR STABLE REORGANIZATION

A GRIEVING FAMILY'S FIRST PRIORITY:
ESTABLISHING EMOTIONAL EQUILIBRIUM

The psychological structure of any single individual is derived from collaboratively created patterns of relationship. Shared structures provide the family with the continuity and stability required to negotiate the instability and change generated by ongoing family development. The importance of these relational patterns in preserving growth-promoting stability is perhaps most evident at times of abrupt family transition, when coping requires the radical reorganization of the family at a time of severe challenge to its functioning. An assessment of the transformations in family structure that contribute to the radical disorganization and reorganization of family equilibrium is crucial to an understanding of family bereavement. With the death of a family member, the family structure, derived from patterns of family interaction, is radically disrupted. Since stable family relationships are the source of family equilibrium, or homeostasis, the death of a family member presents the bereaved family with the challenge of managing overwhelmingly intense emotions at a time when the patterns of family interaction that provide structural stability are radically disrupted. The existing mechanisms for maintaining the bereaved family's stability are thrown into significant disarray precisely at a time when members have the greatest need to draw on these equilibrating relational structures.

The reestablishment of a stable new family structure and of functional family equilibrium immediately becomes the highest priority for families who have suffered the death of a member. In the face of overwhelming emotional despair, families immediately struggle to cope, that is, to continue to manage ongoing family functions. For families of young children, there is an urgent need to reestablish family stability so that responsible caretaking can continue. While a certain equilibrium is achieved early in the family's grieving process, this stability is often achieved at a price, namely, in restricting family flexibility or emotional expressiveness.

Emotional Avoidance as a Stabilizing Strategy

The consequences of establishing a necessary but restrictive emotional equilibrium in the early stages of family grief are apparent in the case of the Johnson family (mentioned in Chapters 5 and 6), whose 16-year-old son, Tim, died suddenly in an automobile accident. The Johnson children are described briefly in Chapter 6 as examples of how age, temperament, and family relationship processes all contribute to the grief reactions of children and the father, Steve, is described at length in Chapter 10 as an example of the impact of a child's death on adult development. Steve and Denise Johnson came with Eric, age 15; Greg, age 10; and Suzie, age 5, for family support and therapy less than 24 hours after the death of their son. The parents, wanting to cope with this terrible tragedy as well as possible as a family, came in for six family sessions immediately after the death, sessions in which the children and parents openly shared their experience of loss and grief. After these sessions the family felt well enough to go on a planned summer vacation and to suspend family meetings.

When school began in the fall and Suzie entered kindergarten, Steve called to report that Suzie was clearly having trouble with Tim's death because she insisted on talking about her dead brother constantly. In a family meeting it became clear that Steve himself was struggling against a flood of emotions about losing his son and wanted to avoid all mention or reminders of him. Family members had removed all photographs of Tim from Steve's sight and, as Denise put it, were "walking on eggshells" to help keep Steve emotionally stable. Although the rest of the family had cooperated by avoiding discussions of Tim's death so as to spare Steve's feelings, Suzie was, both by her ebullient nature and her young age, unstoppable. In a family and a couples' session the problem was redefined as Steve's avoidance of his inevitable, necessary grief. The collaborative protection by Denise and the children of what they experienced as Steve's emotional fragility greatly limited their opportunities to share their grief as a family. Without intervention the family might have pursued their pattern of avoidance still further, which would have made Suzie comment more and more on the family's missing grief. Eventually, Suzie's normal grief reaction might have become truly symptomatic, with her grief becoming a vehicle for the symbolic communication of a vitally important yet avoided family subject. Once Suzie was no longer in the position of having her normal grief defined as the problem, the family confronted Steve's psychological isolation and thereby exposed deep problems in his adult development and in the development of the marital relationship. The family's prior collaborative developmental adaptation had successfully brought them through earlier stages of the family life cycle, although it involved a strong emphasis on the couple's collaboration as parents and neglected other areas of their adult and marital development. Only the extraordinary stresses generated by the crisis of grief exposed the vulnerabilities in the family's seemingly effective structural organization and family life cycle adaptations.

Family Triangles as Stabilizing Structures

From a structural point of view, the family system is hierarchically organized into subsystems that function with flexible but distinct roles (Bowen, 1978; Minuchin, 1974; Minuchin & Fishman, 1981). The death of a family member disrupts the family's organization and requires new relational patterns to fulfill absent social role functions and restore missing emotional functions. From a structural family therapy perspective, family triangles are normative patterns of organization in which unstable dyads use a third party through which to communicate, contain, and stabilize otherwise unmanageable feelings. While all families are essentially triangular in their organization, they differ in the flexibility of function and openness of communication permitted by these relationships. In families stressed by the overwhelming emotions in response to a death of a member, an existing family triangle that functioned in an open or flexible way prior to the death may become more emotionally reactive and defensively rigid as a means of maintaining emotional equilibrium or stability.

Conceiving a Replacement Child

Bill and Sally Shaw, whose 15-month-old daughter, Mary, was killed in an accident, were devastated by the loss of their baby. The Shaws generated new structural stability in their lives by intensifying already existing family triangles with their older children—Laurie, age 7, and Josh, age 4—and by having another baby. From a structural family developmental standpoint, the birth of their new baby boy re-created

the lost family structure, restored the triadic relationship, and rein-
stated the couple's abruptly lost parental function of caring for a baby.
While the clinical literature warns of the developmental danger to
"replacement babies," that is, offspring who are meant to make up
for a family's loss after the death of a child, parents who lose a child
while still in their childbearing years are not necessarily making a
pathological decision in choosing to bear another child. If the family
is unable to include the death and their grief as indelible realities in
their ongoing family development and tries to behave as if the death
never happened, the memory of the dead child may come to symbolize unintegrated overwhelming emotions and may become a constraining presence in family relationships. Unintegrated grief responses to
the dead child will be all the more oppressive to a child born after the
death, whose contact with his or her dead sibling will be entirely
mediated by other family members. The Shaws were very clear that
their newborn son, Danny, was simply his own person. It probably
helped that their new baby was a boy and that he, a feisty, demanding (but delightful) child, was temperamentally different from Mary.
It was quite impossible for the family to confuse Danny with the sweet-
tempered, compliant Mary, who continued to be psychologically
present as a member of the family.

More problematic for the family's ongoing development was an
intensification of Bill and Sally's needs that made them more demanding in their expectations of Laurie and Josh. The death in the family
deepened Laurie's role as the child who absorbed both parents' anxieties. After Mary's death, the Shaws believed that it was possible to
maintain the safety of the family only by avoiding separation—in the
psychological as well as the physical sense. Laurie became more and
more of a problem for her parents, in part because she, like other first-
born children, was forcing her parents to the growing edge of their
own developmental experience. Additionally, she was the focus of a
family triangle for temperamental reasons: She had always been a creative, artistic child who marched to the tune of her own drummer,
aware of the big picture but inattentive to details. Her temperamental mismatch with her relatively exacting parents had always required
a great deal of mutual tolerance. With Mary's death, Laurie and her
parents went through a phase, corresponding to Laurie's elementary
school years, in which they recognized and resonated to each other's
emotional fragility. Laurie herself did everything she possibly could
to reflect her parents' image of a good, devoted daughter. She excelled
in school as well as in sports, music, and dance, following a rigorous,
regimented schedule that included lessons in these activities. She had
many close friends, whom her parents knew well and of whom they

approved. Josh, himself fearful and perfectionistic, found it easy to respond to his parents' needs for compliance. Danny, an active, intensely self-assertive baby, so thoroughly disregarded his parents' controlling overprotection that they described themselves as giving up on controls and following his lead.

It would be hard, at this phase of their family life cycle, to call the Shaw family's structural reorganization rigid. Yet their deeply inflexible dependence on this shared adaptation, especially on Laurie's capacity to remain the "good girl," and their interference with Laurie's ongoing development became evident when their daughter entered adolescence. Their assumption that safety could only be ensured by proximity became explicit only when it was challenged by ongoing family development. Laurie's age-appropriate separation needs were intensified by the family's imposition of close controls over separation as a means of generating a shared psychological equilibrium. Once Laurie initiated moves toward greater separation and independence, and began to reject her previous position of emotionally protecting her parents, she exposed a relatively inflexible yet equilibrating family triangle. Laurie's initially age-appropriate requests for independence and her rebellious response to her parents' control of her life became intolerable to Bill and Sally who intensified their attempts to protect and control her. Laurie, in turn, shifted the family confrontation into high gear by abruptly abandoning her many activities, sneaking around with her friends, making a colossal mess throughout the house, and staging angry confrontations about her right to do whatever she pleased. Parents and adolescent then entered a cycle of escalating mutual hostility, one at first all too typical of many families during a child's adolescence; however, the intensity of the intergenerational confrontation in this case was fueled by this family's inflexible structural adaptation to the emotional challenge presented by the death of their baby daughter, an adaptation that had nevertheless been effective until then. The Shaws required the intensive support of family therapy and the experience of struggling unsuccessfully to make Laurie the "identified patient" before they found a new stable relational structure for managing the demands of her adolescence.

The Shaw family's experience of grief will be discussed again in Chapter 10, with a greater focus on the adults as parents and the consequences of their own developmental struggles and its impact on Laurie's adolescent development. The brief vignettes of the Shaw and Johnson families show how early attempts at achieving emotional stability after the death of a family member only tell a small part of the story that evolves over the course of the family life cycle. Many therapists have the experience of working with a family, as I did with Chris

Ogden and his family described in Chapter 6, where unrecognized grief reactions emerge over the course of clinical work. We often wonder whether a family might have handled their grief experience differently and more optimally had they received some help at an earlier time after the death of a family member. The Johnson and Shaw families illustrate how the story of grief is an evolving story, one which has to flow from the family's need to balance overwhelming change with strategies for stability. Often, the best we can do is support a family's need for stability while keeping the door as open as possible to future opportunities for growth and change.

TRIANGULATION OF THE DEAD

In families where there was a family disturbance prior to the death of a member, the disruption of a central family triangle adds substantially to the subsequent psychological work generated by the family grief reaction. The Abbot family included Ed and Alice and their four adolescent children; the youngest, 13-year-old Bobby, was recognized by the entire family as the parental favorite. He was described by his family as a charming, lively boy with a sunny disposition who could always be counted on to cheer his parents up. His parents needed a considerable amount of cheering up: They had been in and out of marital counseling, and Ed had suffered serious business setbacks. Bobby was seen by his family as instrumental in keeping his parents' marriage together. For his more reserved older siblings, too, Bobby was the emotional center of the family. He was the one who could freely express his loving feelings as well as his need for love, an important emotional function he fulfilled for his siblings as well as his parents.

When Bobby was killed by a hit-and-run driver as he and a group of friends crossed a busy street, the family's first response was to mobilize themselves into a well-organized, well-publicized yearlong search for the driver of the automobile, which the boys accompanying Bobby had been able to identify. Any accidental death, especially one that is the result of another person's irresponsible behavior, ends up being compared by family members to a cold-blooded murder and evokes its own distinctive grief reactions and emotions, which are often dominated by murderous rage and an urgent need for justice, if not vengeance. Bobby's parents responded to his death in ways that were characteristic of their marital and gender roles: Ed became obsessed with the search for the distinctive red Thunderbird that had struck down his son. Given the speed at which the car had been traveling and its erratic path, the family was quite reasonably convinced that the driver had been intoxicated and was now doing everything possible to avoid discovery. The family's plight was treated sympathetically by the media, which cooperated in printing every available detail about the car and driver. Ed spent close to 2 years actively searching for the hit-and-run driver and searched every automobile body shop in the city for a red Thunderbird that had been brought in for repainting. By the 2-year anniversary of his son's death, Ed was finally convinced that his search for the driver, and therefore for justice, was futile. Ed's search for his son's killer is an appropriate and understandable response to a violent, senseless death. However, as Ed himself acknowledged, continuing the search prevented him from coming to terms with the reality of Bobby's death; in fact, during the search Bobby became, in a sense, even more of a presence in his life.

Bobby was also the predominant focus, the full emotional center of life, for his mother. While her husband concentrated on the search for the killer, Alice constructed a shrine in honor of Bobby that dominated their bedroom. On top of their dresser she kept several photographs of Bobby along with commemorative candles that were lit day and night. Ed and the children complained that their home felt like a mausoleum and that Alice was living more in the realm of the dead than of the living. Alice herself agreed with this; in fact, she acknowledged that she visited the cemetery daily, as this was the only way she felt able to maintain the spiritual contact with her son that had become compellingly necessary for her. Alice had often considered suicide: She frequently imagined crashing her car into an embankment as a way of ending her own misery and being spiritually reunited with Bobby. The only consideration that stood in the way of her own selfish desire for suicide was her concern for her family, especially the children, whom she could not bear to subject to another violent death and agonizing grief. This concern kept her alive through the period of her deepest mourning.

The unity of this emotionally fragile family had been maintained by Bobby's active intervention. His death greatly exacerbated the family's burden of emotional and psychological problems that his central systemic position had kept in abeyance. Both Ed and Alice, each in a unique way, intensified their use of Bobby as a structurally triangulated family member, one who was now all the more needed to help them cope with the unbearable grief evoked by their loss and its agonizing circumstances. Alice's bereavement reaction of maintaining spiritual contact with Bobby both in a household shrine and at the cemetery emphasized her feelings of overwhelming sorrow and loss. Ed, in contrast, concentrated on his feelings of rage and the search for justice. In fact, one of their original marital problems was rigid gender specialization. Now they related to each other only through their intense involvement with Bobby.

Ed and Alice entered couples' therapy for their marital problems at the time of the second anniversary of their son's death, when it was clear to them both that the driver responsible for their son's death would never be found. With the suspension of the search, Ed lost his all-consuming mission of angry revenge, which had warded off his agonizing feelings of pain and loss in recognizing the finality of Bobby's death. At this developmental moment in their grief experience, Ed began to face his own feelings of sorrow and to ask Alice to emerge from her own deep isolation. Alice found it terrifying to consider that her grief reaction might be having a negative impact on the rest of the family, since her spiritual contact with Bobby was so compelling a source of comfort to her. She was uncertain of her readiness to give him up in order to relate more fully to her husband and surviving children. In a therapy session attended by the whole family, the children poignantly described their own despair in losing not only a beloved brother but also the member upon whom the stability of the family depended. Although each adolescent had tried to support the parents and maintain family cohesiveness, each felt unable to provide what Bobby had provided. Three years after Bobby's death, and after a year of couple's therapy, the family began the slow process of remembering him in a way that no longer involved seeing him as the emotional center of the family.

Discussion

The process of commemorating the dead and the nature of the memorial is as much determined by cultural custom and spiritual belief as by psychological realities. In contrast to other cultures, which acknowledge the importance of a spiritual continuity with the dead, our culture is profoundly lacking in spiritual beliefs that promote a reassuring, developmentally constructive sense of ancestral continuity. Our mourners are left with a sense of shame about their need for the spiritual presence of their dead loved ones, since our culture regards such attachments as morbid and promotes "letting go" and "moving on" to a new life with new relationships. Even more destructively, it condemns as psychological disturbance mourners' own privately constructed means for maintaining this contact, the need for which is typical of mourners across cultures.

While the enduring presence of the deceased in the household is a necessary part of healthy grief and recovery, the family focus on the deceased can be so extreme that it dominates the psychological life of the family and sacrifices the ongoing development of surviving family relationships. In these instances of obsessive focus on the deceased it becomes important to understand the role of the deceased in the original psychological stability of the family as well as the stabilizing functions of his or her new role in an even more powerfully triangulated family structure. We worked with several families in Boston's Family Support Center who maintained a dead child's bedroom intact even when it meant significantly crowding for the rest of the family. For these families, as for the Abbots, the death of the family member was so disruptive that the new structures they generated for regaining stability severely limited their capacity for ongoing developmental change. In responding to such rigid structures, however, it is important to respectfully acknowledge the cultural, family systemic, and private psychological conditions that make the enshrinement of the dead psychologically necessary for the family.

As with most symptoms, a family's triangulation of the dead represents a family's best solution to a psychological dilemma. Thus, it can best be addressed through a respectful acknowledgment of the needs that are being met through the symptomatic solution. The presence of a shrine to the dead in a household, especially one in which the development of surviving children seems to be sacrificed to the worship of a ghost, can evoke in a well-meaning family therapist the desire to "restructure" the obviously pathological symptomatology of morbid grief. Yet systemically informed grief therapy recognizes that the restructuring of family relational patterns needs to take place in a way that fully recognizes and includes the family's emotional perspective. This process of respectful joining may be especially difficult for therapists in cases of such extreme family adaptation to grief, especially since our cultural emphasis on "letting go" makes these perpetual memorializations seem simply disturbed. Families who have coped with overwhelming loss and grief by keeping the dead family member as an idealized (but immobilizing) family ghost may need an enormous amount of sympathetic support in order to achieve a new memorial arrangement. Hopefully, the new means of memorializing the dead will sustain a meaningful contact with the loved one while permitting more freedom of developmental movement within surviving family relationships. We cannot afford to view the symbolic representation of a deceased loved one as an unequivocally pathological means of creating coherence and stability in the face of unbearable pain. Like every attempt to make one whole life out of the shattered fragments left behind by the blow of grief, the enshrinement or triangulation of a dead family member has to be evaluated in a cultural and family developmental context for the ways in which it supports family stability even as it constrains freedom of developmental movement.

THE GRIEVING CHILD'S INCREASED BURDEN OF FAMILY RESPONSIBILITY

Families who have suffered a grief experience often find that they turn to a child for emotional comfort and perhaps for replacement of the hopes once invested in the deceased. The Johnson family focused on Eric because of his willingness to move into the position of good, responsible son left vacant by his older brother's death. This left in the position of family scapegoat 10-year-old Greg, who was more withdrawn (in fact, more like his father, Steve) and whose complex grief reaction was characterized by avoidance and by behavior problems as a means of expressing his pain. The Johnsons' daughter, Suzie, the only family member who felt free to make frequent references to her brother, also took on a new role in the family as a result of her brother's death: As the youngest child and only girl, she carried the family's emotional expressiveness. The new roles assumed by the children can also be viewed as roles delegated by the parents, with each child being assigned a particular psychological position as a means of helping to restore emotional stability for the family.

Boszormenyi-Nagy's concept of parentification (Boszormenyi-Nagy & Spark, 1973; Boszormenyi-Nagy & Krasner, 1986) is useful in analyzing family grief reactions, more obviously with the death of a parent but also with the death of a child. When a parent dies, there is a natural need to redistribute family responsibilities among alternate caretakers. While these new responsibilities would ideally fall to other adults, there is often more work and fewer resources than a family can arrange. Even if the functional work of parenting is redistributed, some of the emotional and psychological work of the family, including gratification of the need for family intimacy, often falls to the children. Any single-parent family inevitably requires more from its children. The important thing to consider in assessing the child's new responsibilities and the potential for parentification is the extent to which the child remains free from the assumption of full adult responsibility, whether functional or emotional.

Rafael Gomez was shot in the living room of his own home, while his wife Ana and 7-year-old son, Carlos, were tied up in an adjoining bedroom. Rafael had owned a small-appliance repair business in their working class neighborhood and had been known to his family as a scrupulously honest man. His widow, Ana, in a state of confusion and terror, fled her home after the murder and moved in with her older sister in their already crowded apartment. The Gomez family's grief reaction will also be discussed in Chapter 13 to illustrate traumatic grief reactions due to violent circumstances. Ana and Carlos slept together in a fold-out couch in the living room, both plagued by incessant nightmares in which they relived every detail of the murder. Carlos was just past an oedipal-stage attachment to his mother and had been deeply attached to both his parents. He was terrified not only by the violent circumstances of his father's death but by his own proximity and helplessness during the murder. Carlos was also disturbed by the shattering impact of the trauma on his mother, who entered a profound depression punctuated by panicked fearfulness. He refused to be separated from his mother, saying frequently that he would now be the man of the house, "el hombre de la casa", and that she did not have to be afraid because he would protect her. The sight of this traumatized little boy who was struggling with his own totally overwhelming emotions after his father's violent murder drawing himself up to his full height and insisting on becoming his father's heir in the protection of his mother was enough to break my heart.

It would be grossly unfair to view Carlos's attempt to protect his mother as pathological, especially at this early phase of their traumatic grief reaction, so fully dominated was it by terror that it did not yet allow much space for sorrow. Yet it was clear that it would also be necessary, in following them through the future, to afford Carlos some freedom from the full responsibility for assuaging his mother's pain and fear. In turning so naturally to her son for comfort, Ana was not so much "parentifying" Carlos as attempting to connect with what remained of their shared family life. Because of the available support of her extended family, Ana was able to turn to other adults for help, easing the burden on Carlos. The violent circumstances of Rafael Gomez's death forced mother and son to share an emotional bond one wishes they could have been spared. The emotional freedom which Carlos may gain later in his development will depend in part on his mother's capacity to integrate what she can of her own trauma and to continue to draw on other adult sources of support.

Although the death of a parent obviously makes a child vulnerable to parentification, the death of a sibling can also force a surviving child into the position of taking care of a deeply bereaved parent. Ellen Abbot, whose mother became so profoundly depressed after the death of her brother Bobby, had always been a responsible caretaker in the family. After Bobby's death, she essentially took on the family functions previously fulfilled by her mother. She prepared the family meals, made sure her younger siblings got to school on time, took care of her father's laundry, and tried to take care of her mother as best she could. Her assumption of several family caretaking functions even before the accident made Ellen feel that much more responsible for the family's well-being after Bobby's death. Like others who suffer the death of a family member through an accident, Ellen was haunted by re-creations of the moment. Agonizingly, she played over and over in her mind the scene of Bobby leaving the house with his friends. Bobby was supposed to have stayed home to help her finish preparations for a family dinner, but he had charmed his way out of this chore and had begged to go off with his friends. Ellen had let him go without a fight, but now in her obsessive replay of the moment she insisted that he stay home with her and help her out. Rationally, she knew her behavior had not been irresponsible, yet she could not avoid a feeling of guilt, which compelled her to make up for the loss by redoubling her efforts to take care of her family. Moreover, her emotionally vulnerable parents were only too glad to make use of Ellen's offers of help and failed to thoroughly question what lay behind her self-sacrifice. Later on in early adulthood, Ellen needed the support of individual therapy to feel free enough of family responsibility to commit herself to a relationship and establish her own married life.

FAMILY BEREAVEMENT
AND DIFFERENTIATION OF SELF

The family therapy concepts of enmeshment (Minuchin, 1974) or differentiation of self (Bowen, 1978) can be useful to our understanding of family bereavement, with the caveat that we must avoid using the concepts as a means of labeling families as pathological in their bereavement experience. Rather, the concept is useful as a continuum on which to measure a family's capacity to tolerate its members' emotional experiences, especially their distinctive ways of grieving. For some families who have lost a member, the maturation process of the children compounds the feeling of family loss and disintegration.

Helen Golden was 45 years old when her husband, David, died from complications caused by the diabetes he had suffered from since childhood. Barry, a junior in high school, was 17, and Claudia and Joel, both living away from home at college, were 20 and 21, respectively. Hilda had been aware of David's potentially debilitating illness when they met in college. She was deeply drawn, however, to his energetic, magnetic personality, and the couple was determined to make a successful life together. The children's young years coincided with their father's grueling years of graduate school and were punctuated by diabetic crises and occasional hospitalizations.

David Golden had a brilliant career as a university professor and researcher, a career that required a great deal of his available energy and Helen's unwavering support. In the last 5 years of his life, renal failure severely compromised his health; his dialysis treatments, which were time-consuming and painful, were of limited success. His family and university community supported his efforts to function with as little interference from his illness as was humanly possible. In the last year of his life, David conducted his classes and supervised his research from his hospital bed. He defied the limitations imposed by his illness until its final stages.

Helen and Barry felt devastated by David's death and exhausted by the painful years of illness that had preceded it. Barry, the baby of the family, had always been a somewhat fearful child who preferred to stay close to his mother's side, exhibiting a pattern of dependency his father felt should be discouraged. Joel and Claudia, although away at college, were also deeply affected by their father's death but in ways made substantially different by their personality styles and relational history with their father.

Claudia was the child most temperamentally like her father; independent and aggressive in her pursuit of achievement, she had strong opinions of her own. She felt that going on with her own challenging career plans as a scientist would be the best way to memorialize her father, who had always approved of and admired her accomplishments. Joel, who was less successful or focused academically, had always struggled with his father over his lack of achievement. Joel felt that his father's death made it all the more important that he prove himself worthy of his father's respect, even though he could not help feeling that he would inevitably fall short of his father's highest standards. All three children grieved in ways that were personally characteristic of them, yet at the same time their reactions reflected a family structure in which David Golden was the dominant figure and his wife and children planets in his orbit.

Helen Golden sought help for her youngest son's depression 8 months after the death of her husband but acknowledged that she too was having great difficulty coping with the death. In initial family sessions Helen and Barry described David as a brilliant scientist and a vigorous and dominant personality in the university community as well as within his family. Both presented him as a strong-willed, wise, objective, and understanding man who insisted on asserting his will in the family but was farsighted enough that, as Barry stated, "He was always right." Both mother and son vividly described David as the sun and themselves as moons that only reflected his brilliance. Without him, all that was of value in the family was gone. The oldest child, Joel, in college at his father's university, was also struggling with profound depression as well as with chronic academic problems. Only Claudia was doing well in school and seemed to have put her father's death successfully behind her. In contrast to Joel and Barry, who had always been seen within the family as overly dependent children and who had always struggled academically, Claudia was, like her father, brilliant in her studies and stubbornly independent, her father's acknowledged favorite.

In exploring her own grief reaction, Helen observed that she had coped well and competently throughout her husband's many years of illness, including the years before he died when he required acute care. Whenever she faltered over the years, overwhelmed by the demands of the family and the professional obligations that were compounded by David's illness, her husband's strength of character had been a resource that kept her going. Helen had felt quite strong after her husband's death, but her adjustment was shattered when her 70-year-old mother died unexpectedly, 3 months after David's death.

For 3 years following her husband's death, Helen described herself as moving like a sleepwalker through the required functions of her life—working as a business administrator, running her household, caring for her son Barry, and fulfilling her social obligations. Going through the motions but emotionally removed from everyone around her, she experienced a constant sense of unreality. It was only at home, where she had a vivid sense of her husband's presence, that she felt most comforted and alive. Helen and David had recently built their dream house, and she kept everything in place exactly as it had been when her husband was alive. Helen herself described the house as a mausoleum in which the dead were more alive than the living.

In the second year after David Golden's death, during the second year of therapy, Helen, Barry, and Joel began to deeply resent Claudia's insistent independence. The trigger of a vicious family fight occurred during a Jewish holiday, when Claudia, unwilling to interrupt the beginning of her academic schedule as well as her plans with her non-Jewish boyfriend, refused to come home. At a family meeting during a later school vacation, Barry and Joel teamed up and attacked Claudia for her heartless behavior toward their mother. Because of the terrible loss they had endured as a family, they felt that it was now of vital importance for everyone to come together and stay together. Helen concurred that their family gatherings were now a great comfort to her, that when they were all together she felt reassured that the family continued to function as a cohesive unit. "Barry and Joel are so loving, so loyal," she said. "Why can't Claudia be a little more like them?"

Claudia, for her part, felt that the family was living a crazy, depressed life in which the dead were more vivid and important than the living. She felt convinced that her father would have supported her decisions and would have disapproved of her brothers' interrupting their lives to comfort their mother. She was unsure of her feelings for her boyfriend, but the more her family disapproved of him, the more she insisted on her right to be involved with him. Joel and Barry countered that their father would never have approved of such blatant disloyalty to the family as Claudia had demonstrated by staying away on the Jewish holidays to be with a non-Jewish boyfriend. Helen worried even more about Claudia's boyfriend's distinct quality as a "lost soul." "What is my very powerful daughter doing with this depressed schlemiel, if not signing up to take care of him in perpetuity?" she asked. "If she is so damn independent, why does she do what he directs her to do, without regard for her family?"

The Goldens' intense focus on family togetherness was meant to be a source of comfort in the face of substantial family loss. Because Claudia's determined independence contradicted these family needs— and in certain ways served as implicit criticism of the rest of the family for interrupting their own ongoing lives—her mother and siblings did what they could to bring her back as part of the family closeness, which included family grieving. Ironically, both sides invoked David Golden's approval of their position. Deepening the irony, Claudia was taking a position that very much reflected their father's habit of putting work over family, a practice the family had never overtly criticized when David was alive but could now, through their criticism of Claudia, struggle with in his absence. The intense energy behind their family grieving, exacerbated by years of struggling with chronic illness and now by the unexpected loss of Helen's mother and disintegration of her family of origin, became focused on the need to stave off further losses by preserving the integrity of their surviving family. Yet Claudia's temperament, her position in the family, and her stage of development all compelled her to contradict the family wish for togetherness. As a family systemic perspective would predict, Claudia was no more free of the family's intense need for shared psychological stability than her brothers. She too was acting on behalf of a deeply felt, collaboratively structured family choreography.

Through family meetings the Goldens negotiated their conflict through open acknowledgment of the enormity of their shared loss and the need to respect different rhythms of living and grieving.

Claudia was afforded somewhat greater freedom of action, if not protection from criticism, while she herself conceded that her insistent separation from the family and flaunting of her unacceptable boyfriend were reactions to recent family behaviors and not necessarily fully representative of her own deepest wishes. In several individual sessions Claudia began to explore how constrained she felt by her boyfriend's neediness. She became alert to the possibility that she might in fact be self-destructively drawn to the project of psychological caretaker, very much in keeping with her mother's role as caretaker to her father's illness.

Discussion

It does seem that the continuum of differentiation of self in family versus family enmeshment is a useful way of looking at the family bereavement experience. However, the dimension of enmeshment or differentiation of self is not simply a pattern of family adaptation that was present prior to the death and that now interferes with the family's reestablishment of equilibrium. Both Minuchin (1974) and Bowen (1976, 1978) suggest that under circumstances of sufficient stress and anxiety, any family may become less differentiated. Clinical experience with bereaved families confirms that for even well-functioning, well-adjusted families, the death of a member is an emotionally overwhelming event that intensifies the emotional reactivity of family members to one another and precipitates an equally intense need to generate new relational structures to reestablish emotional stability. When family members struggle to regain stable self-control and then see their own unbearable grief expressed by other family members, they often communicate, whether deliberately or implicitly, the message that they need help maintaining their own stability through shared family rules about the emotionally safe expression of grief. Families who are ordinarily good at recognizing individual differences between members suddenly become convinced after a family death that there is one proper way to mourn, which someone in the family is violating. Parents who are ordinarily good at bearing their child's pain without having the child's emotions flood them find themselves having to distance themselves from the child because they can't bear the immediacy of the grief. Children in grieving families learn very quickly what their parents will and will not tolerate emotionally, and alter their own expressions of grief accordingly. Parents who enjoyed their children's independence and autonomy find themselves panicking at separations and overprotecting their children. For these families the customary denial of death is eliminated; members describe a painful, difficult-to-repress awareness that every good-bye could be a final one. For families experiencing the overwhelming pain and disruption of death and grief, overly rigid family structures that restrict the flexible exploration of emotional differences often become the only means of providing necessary emotional and functional stability.

Family Cut-Off

A family cut-off is another structural organization that helps a family manage intense emotional reactivity but at great cost to its capacity for ongoing development (Boszormenyi-Nagy & Krasner, 1986; Boszormenyi-Nagy & Spark, 1973; Stierlin, 1977). Family therapists pay close attention to emotional cut-offs in a family as indicating trouble in the capacity for open communication, in family flexibility, and in emotional integrity, all of which characterize healthy or well-functioning familes. Rather than being free from the influence of the family, the cut-off family member is rather deeply involved in some interrupted but intensely present family process. Family cut-offs are often precipitated by family grief reactions and typically reflect a preexisting difficulty in some area of relationship. For example, 45-year-old Barbara Tracy became estranged from both her sister and her mother's extended family at the time of her mother's death from cancer. Her mother had been pivotal in keeping together a group of feuding siblings and cousins. With her death, these squabbles erupted into unmanageable open conflict. While Barbara herself tried to bring these warring branches of the extended family together, she lacked the emotional authority that had made this role possible in her mother's case. At the same time, Barbara found herself repeating the family pattern of feuding when she and her sister tried to divide up their mother's jewelry. Barbara acknowledged that at a time when she felt especially bereft by the loss of her mother, the possession of her mother's jewelry was very meaningful to her. However, the estrangement from her sister following their feud only added to Barbara's multiplying losses.

An especially agonizing kind of extended family cut-off occurs when a parent of young children dies, leaving the surviving spouse to mediate contact with his or her in-laws. When Greg Gauditis was killed in an automobile accident in which his brother was the driver, his widow, Sheila, was left with two young children ages two and five and an overwhelming experience of grief. She and Greg had been inseparable during their marriage, and Sheila was certain that the close-knit Gauditis clan deeply resented her intrusion into their family and the loss of their sense of primacy in Greg's life. Although the accident was not Greg's brother's fault, Sheila was nevertheless left with the lingering feeling that somehow the accident could have been prevented if he had been more careful. The Gauditis family circled their wagons around their surviving son, protecting him from any insinuation by Sheila that he had been at fault in the accident and making her feel that her bereavement response, including her anger, was constrained by her in-laws' family loyalty.

More disturbingly, Sheila found that her in-laws wanted to spend a great deal of time with her children, their grandchildren, far more than she felt was right for them at such a vulnerable time. Her in-laws kept insisting that the two children visit them overnight, a separation Sheila would not allow, because of her concern about the children and also because of her own difficulty separating from them. The situation degenerated into a court battle over the grandparents' right to visitation, a battle fueled by grief and by the earlier struggle over where Greg's greatest loyalty belonged.

For other young parents who lose a spouse, such as Susan Bates, whose husband, John, died of Lou Gehrig's disease after a 5-year illness, leaving her with a young daughter, the relationship with in-laws may deteriorate because the latter may be totally unable to tolerate ongoing contact with their child's spouse and children. The discomfort the Bates family felt when Susan married John had had no opportunity to abate, as John had become ill almost immediately after the wedding. The maintenance of full extended family ties without an emotional cut-off, even if a daughter- or son-in-law later remarries, requires that families of origin face their grief at the loss of their child.

Extended family situations are even more volatile and complex under circumstances of remarriage, where the new family needs to incorporate in some way the deceased parent's extended family. Deborah, who had married Steve Yeats after his wife committed suicide and who lovingly parented his daughter, Linda, fully appreciated the importance in Linda's life of her connection to her maternal grandparents. Yet on family visits to the grandparents' home, Deborah had to endure sitting in their living room under an enormous wedding portrait of Steve and his first wife. Deborah, like many stepmothers, needed to contend with the presence of her predecessor, a process made much more difficult by the painful bereavement process Linda's grandparents were still engaged in. The presence of the ghost from the previous marriage can significantly interfere with ongoing development in the new family. Yet children need the help of all adult members of both their nuclear and extended family in order to maintain a living, evolving image of their dead parent as a resource in their ongoing development. The challenge of maintaining this developmental access to an evolving image of the dead parent requires a great deal from all the adult survivors and can often be interfered with by unresolved family-of-origin difficulties, which are often placed under even greater strain with the death of a family member.

SYMPTOMS IN INDIVIDUAL FAMILY MEMBERS AS COMMUNICATIONS OF SHARED ADAPTATION

Family therapists, especially strategic and systemic therapists working from Bateson's theories, emphasize the organizational and transformational nature of communication in ongoing family development. They see communication as the means of coconstructing a shared reality through which family members adapt to changing circumstances. From these perspectives, symptoms are viewed as communicating a family's best adaptational strategy for stable self-organization at a particular moment in the family life cycle (Haley, 1973; Madanes & Haley, 1977). From a systemic developmental perspective, a grieving family member who becomes symptomatic is communicating a wider family problem. The symptom is an attempt, albeit an unsuccessful or awkward one, to both address and disguise the family problem, such as unresolved grief. For example, Alice Abbot, who kept a shrine to her dead son, Bobby, in the couple's bedroom, might have been indirectly representing the impossibility of preserving her marriage without Bobby as an ongoing physical presence.

Since any symptom, even if dysfunctional, nevertheless represents the family's best attempt to resolve its problem at a particular moment of shared family development, a strategic family therapist would respond to this family impasse by prescribing the symptom, that is, by encouraging an even greater focus on the symptom, with increased devotion of time and energy, as a means of mobilizing a shift in the family's use of the symptom. In discussing the symptom of unresolved grief with the family, a strategic family therapy approach might reframe the symptom as a positive contribution to the family's life. For example, Alice's grief would be seen as serving a necessary function on behalf of the whole family, and a strategic family therapist would affirm the importance of sustaining Bobby's presence in the household as much as possible, perhaps even prescribing additions to the shrine or more frequent visits to the cemetery or a greater portion of family time deliberately scheduled for remembering Bobby. With this intervention the therapist would hope that the family would become freer to explore the alternative possibility of allowing Bobby's ghost to fade into the family background rather than inviting it to occupy center stage.

In contrast to practitioners of strategic family therapy, systemic–epistemological family therapists would not attempt to manipulate a symptom directly, out of the conviction that a family therapist cannot assume to know what is best for a particular family. They would, for example, respond to Alice Abbot's symptom of extreme grief, the shrine in her bedroom, with an exploration of every family member's perspective on the family's commemoration of Bobby (Hoffman, 1981, 1990; Keeney, 1983; Keeney & Thomas, 1986; Selvini-Palazzoli et al., 1978). Rather than assume that a particular means of resolving the conflict, such as lessening the family focus on Bobby or moving the shrine to a less central position, would reflect improvement, systemic therapists are more likely to believe that the family's unaccustomed exploration of alternative perspectives would disrupt family homeostasis and force the integration of a new adaptive resolution. Thus, by acknowledging the family's need to keep things as they are they support the family's need to maintain stability.

In working with the Abbot family, I explored the ways Bobby continued to remain an enduring, supportive presence for every member of the family, as well as the ways the spotlight on his commemorative shrine was rendering other important family relationships and functions all but invisible. Steven, 2 years older than Bobby but still an adolescent himself when his brother died, told both his parents how alone he had been feeling since Bobby's death, having lost not only his brother but also his parents, because of their consuming grief and preoccupation with Bobby. I affirmed the importance and appropriateness of Alice's need to keep Bobby a central presence in her life at that point in her bereavement process; at the same time, I encouraged her to consider the impact of her intense relationship with Bobby's ghost on the rest of the family. Any symptom, like any creative symbolic form, is multifaceted, revealing our human conflicts and ambivalences. If we try to directly do away with the symptom, we are simply intensifying the overwhelming needs the symptom was addressing in the first place. In all likelihood, we are probably also duplicating a relational context in which important aspects of the complex, collaborative self had to be sacrificed in adaptation to a more powerful partner's reality. If we, as therapists in a position of power, recognize and acknowledge the importance of emotional needs, such as the need to preserve contact with the dead or to freeze the passage of developmental time, we free people to explore those other aspects of their emotional life they are neglecting by their devotion to the symptom. As Alice began to shift her unremitting focus on Bobby back to the emotional life of the family, she and Ed were forced to face their enduring marital problems more directly. Four years after Bobby's death the couple decided to end their marriage.

Memorializing the Forbidden Grief

While current symptomatic bereavement reactions such as those in the Abbot family can be addressed strategically, techniques that affirm the importance and meaning of the symptom can also be used effectively to evoke "operational mourning" (Paul & Grosser, 1965; Paul & Paul, 1989) under circumstances of unacknowledged historical grief. In many of these families a symptomatic family member chooses symptoms designed to commemorate the uncommemorated dead and to underscore a family's unfinished grief work. Jack Mavrides, the youngest child in a large Greek family, was psychiatrically hospitalized at age 20 for a violent psychotic episode. His father, an immigrant who had once worked as a fruit peddler, had worked his way through business school and now ran an extremely successful, visibly prestigious law practice. Jack had become resentful, volatile, and threateningly belligerent within his own family, in dramatic contrast to his earlier role as the affectionate, beloved baby of the family. Jack had been behaving in a manic-like way, staying out all night prowling the streets of Boston and staging violent confrontations with strangers. He had become incapable of functioning at the local college where he was enrolled. He was lucky, we remarked as a staff during the intake, that he had not already managed to get himself killed, as he seemed determined to do.

An initial family interview revealed that Jack's older brother, Andy, had been a heavy drug user and had been killed at age 20 during what could only retrospectively be considered a drug deal gone wrong. Jack, only 12 at the time of Andy's death, had respected his father's injunction that Andy's deteriorating life and violent death, a shameful stain on the family's honor in their lifelong struggle out of poverty, never be discussed again. Yet for Jack, Andy's death had represented the loss of a much-admired older brother, and he had mourned his brother silently and intensely in the ensuing years. As Jack approached the age at which Andy had died, he began to wear Andy's clothes, visit the cemetery, and seek out situations in which he might end his life through the re-creation of Andy's violent end. In family therapy during Jack's hospitalization, we reframed his symptoms as symbolic representations of the family's inability to discuss Andy's life and death, which Jack desperately needed to do in order to resume his own development. While the rest of the family had attempted, unsuccessfully, to forget Andy and his presence in the family, Jack had become more and more concrete in his evocation of Andy's presence. Jack became his dead brother in every way he could. At the time of his hospitalization his condition had become so volatile and his reaction to his family so violent that for the first full family session, in which I planned to talk about Andy's death, I had a hospital guard posted outside the door. I wanted to ensure that there would be someone available to restrain Jack if he became unable to control his rage with his family. Reframing Jack's symptom as a positive contribution to the family's unfinished grief and focusing the family's energy on remembering the impact of their disassociated traumatic grief reaction served to immediately and dramatically change Jack's mental status. He became cognitively clearer, less violent, and less driven to live (and, if necessary, to die) by the need to commemorate his dead brother. The family's capacity to acknowledge the impact of Andy's death and their initiation of a process of shared grief and commemoration relieved Jack of a burden that had threatened to permanently distort his own development.

COCONSTRUCTING A NEW FAMILY NARRATIVE

The systemic conceptualization of family therapy as an opportunity for intervening in the family's meaning-making process by coconstructing an alternative family narrative (Hoffman, 1990; Laird, 1989) is an extremely useful approach to family bereavement, as is well illustrated in the Ackerman Institute's AIDS work (Walker, 1991). Walker and her colleagues recognize the pressure that both families and society place on individuals who, through homosexuality or substance abuse, are believed to have "brought AIDS upon themselves." In their therapeutic work they aim to construct with the patient a narrative of pride and connection rather than of shame and isolation, a narrative that acknowledges the disproportionate burden of blame people with AIDS carry on behalf of the larger society.

The efficacy of creating a new family narrative that deconstructs those enduring shared assumptions about family relationships that were at one time stabilizing but are now destructive can probably be illustrated by almost any successful family therapy. Dorothy Singer, a 35-year-old teacher, and her 65-year-old mother, Janet, explicitly requested help working out a reconciliation in their relationship, which had been distant since their pitched battles over independence during Dorothy's early adolescence. Mother and daughter engaged in a brief but intensive therapy that allowed them to resolve family relationship issues that had been caught in a 40-year-old intergenerational time warp. The distance established between them during the storm and stress of the early adolescent phase of the family life cycle had been exacerbated at the time of Dorothy's father's death from heart disease 10 years later (and 10 years before the start of our current work). Richard, a hard-driving, brilliant, but moody man who was obsessed with his work, had never recovered from a profound depression precipitated by the failure of his company and the collapse of his career during Dorothy's elementary school years. He alternated between vicious criticism of his wife and children for their failures and equally vicious self-criticism. Dorothy left home to enter college, distancing herself from both parents because of her fear that her relationship with them was fraught with psychological danger to her self-regard.

When Dorothy was 25, 10 years prior to our work together, her father suffered a severe heart attack from which he never fully recovered, dying of a subsequent heart attack 3 months later. In those 3 months Dorothy renewed her relationship with her father. She believed they had successfully reached back to a time in their relationship when he had been more psychologically available, and she felt an intimate connection with him. She felt profoundly guilty about this connection, however, and believed she had taken her mother's rightful place at her father's deathbed. Following the death, Dorothy's relationship with her mother continued as before, with very little contact and an enduring sense of mutual resentment, until a crisis in her mother's health moved them both to reconsider how they might renew their own relationship before they ran out of time.

When Dorothy and Janet entered my office, it was clear they had avoided each other all those years because they felt their anger at each other was too hot to handle. The moment they began to talk about their relationship and the history leading to their estrangement, the anger that had been ignited between them during Dorothy's adolescent rebellion flared up again, fresh and intense as ever. Janet was unshaken in her belief that Dorothy had been a difficult, out-of-control teenager who had to be monitored at all times. Dorothy, for her part, was enraged that Janet still refused to consider her own crazy projections and ridiculous demands for control as a factor in her adolescent rebellion; at the same time, she was intensely frustrated with herself because she remained so reactive to what she considered her mother's distorted projections.

A number of important family developmental moments and their meanings were examined and collaboratively reconstructed during this brief (three session) mother–daughter therapy. As Janet and Dorothy expanded the context of their own relationship to include problems in the marriage and unresolved grief in Janet's family of origin, they arrived at a very different understanding of their anger at one another. Janet was able to acknowledge that her husband had been a terribly troubled man whose fluctuations between destructive rage and withdrawn depression had touched them all deeply. She had tried to make things better at home by attempting to prevent his violent explosions, working hard to correct herself and her daughter in anticipation of his criticisms. Janet had married Richard shortly after the death of her brother in a car accident, a tragedy she still could not talk about 40 years later without bursting into tears. Her brother's death had left her feeling that her loved ones could be arbitrarily snatched from her at any time.

As Janet and Dorothy fought, wept, and remembered, Janet began to reconstruct her own life story, picking up fragments that had been disassociatively warded off because they engendered so much pain. But these fragments, loaded with so much unacknowledged feeling, were the very elements in Janet that Dorothy was most reactive to as an early adolescent. For example, Janet would, as Dorothy reminded her mother, become panic-stricken if she did not know her daughter's whereabouts every minute of the day; she preferred to keep Dorothy home from school rather than face the daily separations and would call her in as sick with almost any minor, if not invented, ailment. As Dorothy related these incidents, her mother responded as if she were trying to see across a street enshrouded with a veil of fog. Janet could barely make out the incidents; she had to listen closely to the details Dorothy related and work hard at remembering them. Janet was also stunned to see the way a coherent pattern linked together the death of her brother; her panic at separations, which she had considered life endangering at the time but which she now clearly saw as overreactions on her part; and Dorothy's intense adolescent rebellion, which she could now see as an appropriate response to her own dissociated grief. Janet then remembered a story of her own, which Dorothy only vaguely knew but which had exacerbated Janet's worry about the health and safety of her children: A friend of hers had lost a child to cancer, and for years afterward Janet worried that every cold or flu symptom portended a similar tragedy. Through this process of exploration of the past and discovery of lost connections between overwhelming experiences, Janet could begin to understand the effect on Dorothy of her own enormous difficulty with separations from the children and of her terror of any conflict that might result in abandonment by her husband. Janet's acknowledgment of her own contribution to their battles enabled mother and daughter to review some of their fights with less rancor and more mutual acceptance.

This rewriting of the family developmental narrative to include excluded aspects of Janet's family history—especially her unexamined psychological response to her brother's death, which had continuously haunted her and had found expression in her profound anxiety over separations—enabled mother and daughter to explore again the scene at Richard's deathbed, which Dorothy had remembered as a source of deep satisfaction but even deeper guilt. Dorothy revealed what she remembered of her father's death and expressed her sense of guilt over having a better relationship with him than her mother did. Janet, now less embattled with Dorothy and more sympathetic to the difficult position her daughter had been placed in during her growing-up years, said simply and genuinely that she had in fact been very touched by the visible affection and sense of reconciliation between father and daughter. She pointed out that she had had a great deal more time with Richard over the years and a great deal more time to say good-bye to him after his first heart attack than Dorothy had. With this affirmation from Janet and her realization that her mother did not begrudge her the few good memories she had salvaged from a lifetime of difficulty with her father, Dorothy began to examine for herself her deep loyalty to her mother and her fear of causing her any additional suffering through her actions. Janet and Dorothy rediscovered a buried but important past theme in the story of their own relationship: their mutually satisfying attachment from Dorothy's childhood, before her adolescence made separation issues between them so intensely troubling. The problems between them during that stormy adolescence, exacerbated by marital and family difficulties, had obscured their memories of loving attachment and mutual loyalty and replaced their multifaceted history with an overarching narrative of anger and distance. The re-creation of a shared developmental narrative, which more fully included the burdens in both Janet's and Dorothy's developmental histories, helped mother and daughter overcome the barriers and achieve a mutually satisfying relationship.

CONCLUSION: PRESERVING THE CAPACITY FOR ONGOING FAMILY DEVELOPMENT AFTER A DEATH

The death of a family member precipitates radical developmental transformations and the creation of new structures that will support family stability and ongoing family development. Two dimensions of family restructuring in response to family bereavement stand out in the family stories in this chapter: first, the importance for families of establishing a new basis for homeostasis, even if the equilibrium is based on a rigid intensification of previous patterns of emotional regulation and, second, the existence of a greater permeability of family boundaries, in which mutual emotional reactivity is heightened, requiring more extreme means of shared emotional control. Fundamentally, bereaved families are families under extreme stress. Even for previously well-adjusted families, the challenges of new adaptation to the crisis of a family death require structural solutions that might well appear to outsiders as, at best, rigid or, at worst, morbidly disturbed. Yet inevitably, these adaptations represent a family's best attempt at generating the new family structures that will support their ongoing shared development. From a systemic developmental perspective on family bereavement, a therapist needs to acknowledge and support a family's struggle to establish growth-promoting stability while searching with them for sources of stability that will not interfere with the family's ongoing development.

Families in the initial stages of overwhelming grief may respond with rigid structures or rules for relating as a means of reestablishing functional and emotional stability. These overly rigid structures may leave them ill prepared to face the demands of subsequent stages of the family life cycle or to use new family developmental experiences as pathways toward integration of the previously overwhelming grief. Families, like individuals, establish the best reorganization they can with the tools of a particular developmental moment after the shattering blow of grief. Yet if they create overly rigid strategies for stability, they lose the opportunity to learn from experience that the originally overwhelming pain and distress might now be more manageable. While such rigid adaptations are extremely costly for all family members, they interfere the most with the ongoing development of children, who may be significantly burdened with emotional responsibility for unacknowledged grief in ways that become intertwined with their ongoing development. At the same time, both children and families show an extraordinary capacity for resilient new adaptation with new sources of support. With new sources of safety and stability, families can review and reorganize responses to the family death and loss in ways that gain them greater freedom for the work of ongoing family development.

CHAPTER 10

The Death of a Child

ITS IMPACT ON ADULT AND

FAMILY DEVELOPMENT

THE DEATH OF A CHILD AS A CRISIS
OF ADULT DEVELOPMENT

Both the child bereavement and family systems literatures have emphasized how much parental grief reactions set the stage for the permissible range of reactions from family members to the death of a
member (Baker et al., 1992; Bowlby, 1980; Furman, 1974; Silverman
& Silverman, 1978; Silverman & Worden, 1992; Stephenson, 1985;
Walsh & McGoldrick, 1991). Most of the limited attention to the
impact on children and families of parental grief reactions has focused
on the death of the spouse and the challenge of parenting grieving
children when adults themselves are bereaved. In this book earlier
chapters on adult bereavement focused on the application of a systemic developmental model in understanding how the death of a
spouse impacts on adult development, namely, by precipitating the
exploration and reconstruction of those aspects of the adult self that
were invested in the marital partner and by stimulating a developmental process that accommodates a new sense of self and a new internalized relationship with the spouse. The death of a child can also be
usefully conceptualized as a developmental crisis. With the death of
a child, the adult's grief experience is centrally connected to the experience of self as parent.

The death of a child was an expected occurrence in the lives of
families before the turn of the century (Leavitt, 1986). Nevertheless,
even under circumstances of high infant mortality, whether in this
culture in general in the last century or under current conditions of
poverty and poor prenatal care in this and other countries, it is clear

that parents grieve for their children (Eisenbruch, 1984a, 1984b; Scheper-Hughes, 1990, 1992). With improvements in maternal and child medical care, infant and child mortality have decreased so substantially that they are now viewed as events that are against the natural order of life. Parents now expect their children to outlive them, an expectation that adds to the shattering blow and profound self-blame that grieving parents experience.

In order to use a systemic developmental perspective to understand adult grief after the death of a child, it is important to understand the role of parent–child relationships in the process of adult development. Parenting is itself an infrequently studied area of individual and family development. Parental functioning has mainly been studied in the child development literature, which assesses parenting as a contributing factor in child developmental outcomes (Belsky & Isabella, 1985; Bronfenbrenner, 1979). As the adult bereavement literature on the impact of the death of a child suggests, grieving parents, unlike a grieving spouse, who can proceed with relinquishment of the lost relationship and reinvest in new relationships, have invested important aspects of self in their children that in many instances cannot be relinquished. Rando (1986) argues that the imposition of spousal bereavement models on parental bereavement accounts for the mistaken diagnosis of grieving parents as suffering from interminable or pathological grief and that, in fact, the normal bereavement following the death of a child most often involves a lifelong process of grief that requires integration into the ongoing course of family development.

Rando (1986) suggests that it is necessary to understand parental bereavement in terms of the important aspects of the self and hopes for the future that adults invest in their children. Parents who outlive their children feel devastated in their basic competence as parents, for they have failed to fulfill the vital parental function of protecting their children. Grieving parents are likely to experience substantial survivor guilt. Although bereavement in general involves a rumination over the circumstances of the death and a search for a loophole that might have changed the outcome, grieving parents are especially vulnerable to obsessing about the circumstances of the death in an attempt to gain control over the outcome and restore their sense of competence as parents or to search for understanding and meaning (Rando, 1986; Sanders, 1989). In instances of anticipated grief, when death follows an incurable childhood illness, parental grief is diminished if the parents feel satisfied that they did all they could to contribute to their child's care and well-being (Koocher, 1986; Mulhern, Lauer, & Hoffmann, 1983). On the other hand, parents who were very involved in the care of a terminally ill child may face an even greater sense of emptiness when the child's death ends a phase in which they had a heightened sense of purpose as parents. The age of the child does not seem to alter the severity of parental grief, although it does change the family developmental issues that are stimulated by the death and loss (Rando, 1986; Sanders, 1989).

For grieving parents, fresh experiences of grief are stimulated by new milestones in family development. Grieving parents track the age the child would be had he or she survived and find their grief stimulated by their realization of what they have missed out on in their family lives. Parents find they have to "grow up with the loss" as they pass these new developmental milestones. The renewal of family life after the death of a child depends on the adult mourners' capacity to accept the loss and find a regenerative use for the pain (Pine & Brauer, 1986; Rando, 1986; Sanders, 1989). For many grieving parents, spiritual or religious beliefs provide an important source of comfort and meaning (Cook & Wimberley, 1983).

Because a couple has gone through an agonizing experience together, the marital relationship itself is an important resource after the death of a child. Yet the death of a child can also leave couples profoundly estranged, as they retreat into private and often discordant grief experiences. The literature on the loss of a child has been contradictory in reporting divorce rates after the death of a child (the divorce rate in the general population of parents with young children is itself high), but research and clinical bereavement literature do suggest that marriage is significantly stressed by the burden of grief. Because the centrality, activity, and meaning of parenting differs for men and women, significant gender differences in parental grief have been reported in the literature (Cook, 1984; Rando, 1983, 1986). The highly polarized gender roles and accompanying gender differences in syle of emotional coping seem to contribute to a sense of discordance and mutual misunderstanding on the part of grieving couples. Grieving mothers are especially likely to report that their husbands do not understand their grief and cannot adequately provide support (Cook, 1984). Grieving fathers are unaccustomed to the emotional intensity involved inasmuch as it is a capacity for emotional control that is our cultural expectation of men. The marital relationship, which is ordinarily a source of emotional and social support for adults, becomes heavily burdened by the shared task of grieving the death of a child.

The integrity of the family system is shattered by the death of a child. Although couples with surviving children have continuing responsibilities in their roles as parents, they frequently become preoccupied with the attachment loss to the dead child and the implications of the death for their injured sense of self as person and parent. While surviving children are an important source of emotional comfort to their grieving parents and provide them with a sense of purpose in going on in spite of their agonizing pain and grief, relationships with surviving children do not alter the anguish of the parents' grief. Emotionally depleted grieving parents are likely to feel overwhelmed by the realistic demands of ongoing parenting, especially since their surviving children have themselves lost a sibling and are suffering their own grief experience. A parent's relationship with and view of surviving children may become burdened with his or her attempts to regulate vulnerable self-esteem in the area of parenting (Hogan & Balk, 1990). These adult attempts at self-regulation through the medium of the parent–child relationship are likely to affect the course of both child and family bereavement (Bowen, 1976; Bowlby, 1980; Herz, 1980, 1989; Walsh & McGoldrick, 1991).

The reality that relationships with surviving children do not diminish adult grief contradicts the cultural assumption and expectation that grieving parents will count their blessings and focus on their attachments to their living children. In the case of neonatal death of a first child, parents are often encouraged to assume that the child was defective and to look forward to the birth of a new child instead. Many grieving parents who are unable to accept such prescriptions feel like social outcasts. Moreover, because most parents of young children find it agonizing to consider the possibility that they might themselves lose a child to death, they may react toward grieving parents in ways that increase their sense of banishment from their social network. For this reason, Compassionate Friends, which offers peer support groups for grieving parents, has become an important source of support for adults who have lost a child (Rando, 1986; Videka-Sherman & Lieberman, 1985).

What can a systemic developmental model, which locates adult parental development in a shared family life cycle, contribute to our understanding of the collapse and rebuilding of life structure after the death of a child? The death of a child takes place at a particular moment in developmental time, for both the individual adult and the family as a unit, in the developmental process of creating and stabilizing a shared identity, a collaboratively created self. In Chapter 4 I focused on Gail Kaplan's experience as a widow and described the reconstruction of her sense of self after the loss of her husband and the required reorganization of her life, including the integration of overwhelming emotions and the construction of new family relationships and family functions. One important part of Gail's integration of her grief experience was a relational life review, which allowed Gail to explore how she had formed her adult life structure in response to her relationship with Stuart and how she now wished to structure her new life circumstances to accommodate new areas of expansion in the development of her complex adult self.

Far more than child development, with its physically determined neuromaturational milestones, adult development is coconstructed through a process of collaboration between the realistic demands of social roles and the needs of a subjective, more private process. Cultures differ enormously in how they choose to balance the process of individuation, which can be conceptualized as the dialectical balance between adaptation to group norms, both familial and cultural, and individual self-expression. In our culture we emphasize far more the individual invention of the self, idealizing the pioneer or frontiersman who has cut loose the bonds to both family and community. Yet as human beings we cannot do without the connections to family and community that create the supportive context through which we construct a uniquely private as well as interdependent self. Adult life structure is relational structure, and development for both men and women is collaboratively constructed over the course of the family life cycle.

Optimal or ideal human development would permit the exploration and integration of the many aspects of a complex, contradictory self that are negotiated in changing relationships over the course of the family life cycle. Yet most of us lack the social supports or the personal courage to radically invent ourselves outside of socially sanctioned and practical possibilities. Beginning in adolescence and young adulthood, the stability required by individual and family growth is gained by some constriction of avenues of development for the self. Most couples in this culture rely on gender-stereotyped roles for a great deal of guidance in determining the course of adult development. Most couples substantially increase their gender specialization with the birth of children and the demands of child care. Over the course of the family life cycle the constriction or simplification of the potentially complex self is compensated for by the opportunity to find expression for aspects of the self in relationships to spouse and children. It is often only when children become more independent and leave home to lead lives of their own creation that parents are offered the developmental opportunity to reexamine their own individual and marital lives and to reintegrate aspects of the self that were earlier denied or that could not be developed.

The death of a family member brings the delicately balanced process of shared family development to a crashing halt. From a systemic developmental perspective, parenting is an essential component of the collaborative self, and the death of a child shatters the organization and stability of adult identity. The death of a child stimulates in the parents a radical life review, as the developmental pathway through which they arrived at their enduring life structures now suffers an irreversible collapse. For adults, aspects of the self that were invested in the child are suddenly, abruptly, lost to the self and need to be reintegrated into the self or into new relationships. The radical discontinuity of a death forces individuals into an initial state of shock and denial with the result that not only the overwhelming emotions of distress and terror but the unstabilizing disruption in the sense of self are assimilated slowly.

In order to illustrate the impact of the death of a child on adult development I will describe the grief reaction of the adults in two families, the Johnsons and the Shaws, whom I briefly described in Chapter 9. I will elaborate the impact of these adult responses and of the adults' attempts to reestablish a secure equilibrium and sense of self on the mutual adaptation and interweaving of child and adult developmental processes over the subsequent course of the family life cycle.

Each child has a unique place in the inner life and in the self-organizing structure of the parent's own development. A lost child is mourned by a parent in a way that reflects aspects of the self invested in that particular child as well as the way that adult fulfills the parenting role in particular and conducts relationships more generally. The death of a child launches a painful reexamination and reintegration of these aspects of the self at a time when the emotional burden of loss is enormous. The death of a child initiates a radical adult and family developmental crisis and requires equally radical techniques for reestablishing a sense of shared stability, as the following two family stories illustrate.

PARENTAL GRIEF AND THE COLLAPSE
OF ADULT LIFE STRUCTURE
Background

Steve, age 36, and Denise, age 34, requested treatment within hours after their son Tim, age 16, was brought dead on arrival to their local hospital after an automobile accident. The other children in the Johnson family (already mentioned in Chapters 5, 6, and 9) were Eric, age 15; Greg, age 10; and Suzie, age 5. The Johnsons sought therapy unusually quickly after the death of their son because they were worried about the effect of the death not only on their children but also on their marriage. Parenting was the central focus of their successful shared family lives, and they realized that their marriage was less a source of intimacy than a resource for managing their busy, extremely satisfying family lives as the parents of four thriving children.

The 17-year-old Johnson marriage, which had functioned successfully as the base for their normal family development, could not survive the catastrophic emotional stress and life structure collapse triggered by Tim's death. Steve and Denise separated at the 1-year anniversary of Tim's death and subsequently divorced. The parents' adult and family developmental histories suggest the developmental vulnerabilities that were exposed by their attempts to cope with their shattering grief. The following discussion is based on therapeutic contacts consisting of six family sessions at the time of Tim's death, five couples' sessions 4 months later, eight individual sessions with the father 5 months after the couples' sessions, and one couples' session at the 1-year anniversary of the death. The family and couple's sessions were conducted with a cotherapist, Esther Gross, a licensed social worker.

Steve and Denise were relatively young parents of adolescent children. Both described themselves as insecure, socially isolated young people who had been relieved to find each other and to start a family of their own. They were introduced by mutual friends when Steve was in college completing a business degree and Denise was working as a secretary. Since Steve and Denise had married and begun their family when they were so young, there was only a short interval of time between their being children in their families of origin and being parents themselves. They went from living at home with their parents to living with each other.

Steve described himself as having a close relationship with his mother and a distant, eventually quite hostile relationship with his father. Although Steve had aspired to a career in psychology or the humanities, his father had pressured him to make a more practical choice and he settled for a career in business. At the time of Tim's death, Steve had been employed for the 15 years since his college graduation by a local company as a project manager.

Denise described herself as coming from a large, close-knit, happy family. Her father had been a somewhat unapproachable figure, but she was quite close to her mother and her brothers and sisters. Her own and her family's expectations for her as a young woman had been that she would marry and have a family. Denise was aware that her parents encouraged her brothers in their schoolwork and career aspirations more than they did the girls in the family, but she felt no rancor about that.

The Johnsons had been married for only a year when Tim was born; thus, they had little experience being marital partners without also being parents. Eric was born a year after Tim, Greg 4 years after Eric, and Suzie was born the year Greg started kindergarten. The Johnsons described themselves as a very child-oriented family, and both parents were actively, meaningfully involved with their children. While the death of a child is a shattering experience for any parent, the Johnsons may have been especially vulnerable because of the centrality of parenting in their lives and the neglect of other aspects of their adult identity.

Tim was described by both his parents as a charming, handsome, sociable boy who was successful at both traditional academics and creative writing and as the child who could make everyone laugh. Although both parents denied that they would ever play favorites, they each acknowledged that they felt Tim was something special, with a brilliant future ahead of him. He had just begun high school the previous year, and because he had initiated the typical adolescent struggles over independence, he was the focus of some conflict with both parents at the time of his death.

Eric, age 15, had long been designated the family's problem child. As therapists it seemed to us that Eric had decided he could not compete with Tim as the family's good son and that he might as well give the bad son identity his all. Although an intelligent and fundamentally affectionate boy, Eric tended to be more interested in his friends than in either family or academic activities. With the family he tended to be sullen and distant, feigning obliviousness to the adverse observations that were inevitably made, implicitly or explicitly, about his failure to measure up to the high standards set by his older brother. Even when Tim began to oppose his parents for the first time, he managed to do it so diplomatically that his parents allowed him to get away with more defiance than they tolerated from Eric.

Greg, age 10, was seen by his parents as very intelligent but extremely private and not nearly as emotionally expressive and accessible as Tim. Suzie, age 5, the family's only girl, was protected from the "golden boy" comparison to Tim that plagued the more rebellious, underachieving Eric and the academically successful but socially withdrawn Greg.

Steve and Denise had become specialized and radically different in their emotional styles of marital communication, with Denise being typically expressive and Steve being typically private. In the early weeks after Tim's death, Steve withdrew from the family in his grief, intensifying his customary pattern of distancing from the family and keeping his emotions private, and Denise felt unable to ask him directly how he felt since this would have violated their implicit marital agreement that she protect his privacy. Sharing his emotional reaction would have brought Steve closer to his own feelings, as well as to the feelings of other family members, a painful process his numb and isolated state was meant to avoid.

The Johnsons understood the problems inherent in their avoidant style of communication, and each partner struggled to engage the other more. Yet the overwhelming blow of their grief heightened their need to rely on established patterns in managing their overwhelming emotions. The problem was most dramatically apparent for Steve, who longed to withdraw into a numb state where he felt and remembered nothing. Without meaning to, the couple often displaced their marital and personal conflicts by focusing on Greg's lack of emotional expressiveness, an emotional style explicitly viewed in the family as similar to Steve's.

After Tim's death, the established family pattern of relationships, in which each of the children bore a relatively stereotyped set of family expectations, was radically altered. Eric, who under the shadow of his older brother's favored position had become the disappointing or problem son, responded to Tim's death with a successful redirection of his own adolescent pathway. This left Greg, who had been relatively protected by Eric's position as the disappointing older brother, as the child who showed the most evident problems in his response to Tim's death. In contrast to Eric, who was working so hard to turn his life around and achieve the successes that might bring comfort to his parents, Greg appeared indifferent to the death and untouched by the family's great sadness. If anything, he was provoking fights with his mother over insignificant things so that she would become furious with him and reprimand him. Greg was especially vulnerable in the family because his emotional and interpersonal style was the most difficult for his parents as they struggled to deal with their own grief.

A Father's Unbearable Grief

Tim was exactly the kind of child Steve had always wanted to be, the kind Steve's father had wanted *him* to be. Steve's father was a talented writer who had been forced by his family's economic needs to give up a writing career and become an advertising executive. Steve stated ruefully that he had never shown any talent as a writer, much to his father's deep disappointment. The talent had skipped a generation and emerged in Tim, whom everyone had expected to accomplish special things as a writer. Steve and his father had never been close and had suffered a breach in their relationship several years earlier, when Steve's father left Steve's mother for another woman. Steve had been furious at his father's unethical conduct, had not spoken to him for 4 years, and had also limited his contact with the grandchildren. After Tim's funeral, mutual friends insisted that father and son end their animosity and talk with each other. Steve found the opportunity for reconciliation with his father a relief; at the same time, he grieved for the lost opportunity Tim had represented for a deepening relationship over the years between grandfather, father, and son.

Tim represented for Steve the opportunity for reparation in his own self-esteem as well as in his relationship with his father. Whereas Steve had been isolated, private, and awkward, interested in science rather than sports, Tim was gregarious, graceful, and talented as a writer. Tim had a gift for engaging people, something Steve's own father could do. Steve was much more the kind of child Greg was now; he sometimes looked at Greg and painfully remembered his own unappealing, unhappy childhood self.

Steve became aware during the course of therapy that he was grieving his now lost hope that fathering a son like Tim, who had made it so easy to be close, would give him an opportunity to have the relationship he had missed with his own father. Steve remembered that his grandfather had disapproved of his father's aspirations as a writer and had discouraged him from pursuing a writing career. Ironically, Steve's relationship with his own father had repeated the same unfortunate pattern of a father and son who couldn't appreciate and admire each other. Steve realized the importance of his unconscious wish to break the pattern and heal three generations of alienation between fathers and sons through his relationship with Tim. Without Tim, he felt the dreams of himself as a successful father would never be realized.

Whereas before Tim's death Steve had felt satisfied with the balance of choices in his life, he now found himself angry at everyone's high expectations and overburdened by responsibilities at work and at home. He felt that his life was in a rut, that he was too caught up in doing correct and conventional things. He found that he could no longer tolerate his previously tolerable career as a business manager in a large company. In the 6 months following his son's death, Steve slipped into a deeper and deeper depression.

As hard as Denise worked at keeping Steve involved with the family, he became increasingly more withdrawn and more depressed. He functioned well at the office, and in fact in the year after Tim died he successfully changed his work responsibilities, gaining a promotion into a higher-level management position. At home, though, he found himself unable to spend any time at all with Denise and the children, preferring to sleep late on weekends and to go out by himself. Steve could not bear doing things with the family and realized that it was because he was then forced to remember that Tim was no longer there.

Nine months after Tim died, Steve requested individual therapy for his severe depression. He began to talk in more detail than was possible for him during his acute grief state about the circumstances of his son's death. As often happens in the bereavement experience after an unexpected death, Steve focused on his final words with Tim in an anguished, self-reproachful way. He remembered that in their last conversation, as Tim prepared to leave a cousin's birthday party to go out with his friends, he had provoked a fight with his son about his failure to complete his chores, and Tim had promised to go right home and finish them before heading out for the evening. Steve remembered that when he and Denise returned home after the birthday party, he walked into the house and observed not only that Tim had failed to complete his chores as he had promised but that he had left his clothes strewn all over the living room and had left a mess in the kitchen as well. Fuming with frustration, Steve was prepared to deliver an angry lecture to his son when he received the call from the police that Tim and his friends had been in a car accident and that Tim, who had not been wearing a seat belt, had been thrown from the passenger seat through the front window and had been killed instantly.

Steve's internal struggle with his adolescent son over chores and responsibilities was still very intense and constituted a much more easily evoked, reassuring reality than the new reality of loss and grief. Yet he felt terribly burdened by the memory of his angry last words toward his son, and his angry feelings were now unacceptable to him because they spoiled his final memories of their relationship. Steve's exploration of his unavoidable feelings of anger and regret enabled him to begin to move forward in time and to experience his profound grief directly, that is, with less incapacitating numbness and depression.

Steve bitterly resented losing his favorite son; his bitterness was all the more intense because he and Tim had begun to view each other as companions. Steve had enjoyed wilderness camping when he was single, but Denise did not share his interest (she considered it a risky sport). He had given up this activity after they were married but had lately had hopes of resuming it with his oldest son; in fact, he and Tim had been planning a trip together. Somehow, Steve could never picture himself enjoying a camping trip with the rebellious Eric, who so clearly preferred his own buddies to the company of his father, or with Greg, who was too withdrawn and uninterested in outdoor sports, and he did not expect to share that closeness with his daughter. After the difficult and self-sacrificing years of early parenting, Steve had been counting on sharing activities with his son at a time in his own life cycle when he was still young and vigorous enough to enjoy them. With Tim's death, he felt he had been deprived of one of the important rewards of being the young father of an adolescent son.

Steve noticed that when he spent any time at all with the family, he would become flooded with images of Tim. Gradually, he began to participate in more activities with Greg and Eric and found himself painfully aware of their own sadness at losing Tim. Steve realized that both Eric and Greg tried hard, each in his own way, to please him and that each son experienced his father's disapproval or avoidance of him as terribly rejecting. Empathically aware of his sons' feelings and remembering how he as a child had felt rejected by his own father, Steve resolved to work harder at giving more to his surviving sons. In order to do so, though, he had to overcome his anguish in remembering his lifelong avoidance of pain in his relationship with his father and in acknowledging his low self-esteem in response to his father's rejection of him. In addition, his closeness to any of his children, but especially a son, forced Steve to not only face his own grief at losing Tim but the grief of each child at the loss of a brother. Parenting, previously so rewarding an experience, one that had always provided Steve with a means of compensating his childhood losses with a more positive future as a father to his own children, had now become an emotional minefield. Moreover, it seems that Steve, more than most parents, had felt his success and satisfaction as a father completely in terms of his relationship with only one of his children.

Although Steve initially felt he could work toward renewing his emotional investment in his surviving children, he found that his relationship with Denise remained extremely distant. The only person in his life he felt he could get close to was a young woman colleague. He worried about the effect of this deepening relationship on his family, but he could not keep from pursuing his involvement with the only person who made him feel more alive. He had never known a woman like her—so self-confident, aggressive, and successful in her career. Through their conversations, he began to think about his own potential for further education and career advancement.

Ten months after Tim's death, Steve was identified as the most severely impaired member of the family. Even after his serious depression began to lift, his marriage continued to be in serious trouble. Steve's decision to initiate a new relationship and turn to an outsider for comfort served multiple purposes in his coping with his overwhelming grief reaction. First, because he found it too painful to be close to family members, who in too many ways reminded him of his painful loss, Steve found it a relief to become intensely involved with someone who did not remind him in any way of Tim and his death. Second, because he found himself questioning all his life choices after Tim's death, including his career and marital decisions, Steve turned to a woman who was completely different from Denise and who encouraged him to return to an earlier time in his life, before he had closed off career choices owing to his own lack of confidence. Third, his relationship with another woman represented a repetition of a family-of-origin pattern in which the husband becomes involved with another woman. Although Steve had consciously disapproved of his father's infidelity, under the stress of bereavement he found himself reverting to an unconscious identification with his father through a similar behavior.

At the first anniversary of Tim's death Steve told Denise that he wanted out of the marriage, and he moved into his own apartment. Denise desperately reproached him for his abandonment of the family, asking him how he could compound the loss each member had suffered in this way. "Even a criminal deserves a second chance," she said to him. "Why can't you give me a second chance to make things better between us?" Denise invoked Tim's support for her side of the argument, saying to Steve, "If Timmy could see what was happening to us, he would be terribly upset. Remember how much he worried when we fought and how he would plead with us never to get a divorce?" The more Denise called on Tim to invoke Steve's guilt, the more he withdrew from her in stone-cold fury.

Summary

Even though therapy was sought very early in the family's attempts to cope with the loss of a child, the marriage was not able to survive the death. The Johnsons had entered a preventative therapy in part to avert just such a serious impact on their marriage, yet previous marital and family difficulties were exacerbated by their bereavement reaction in a complex way that resulted in the dissolution of their marriage. Steve had vowed to be a different kind of father to his children than his own father had been to him, and he had been a successful, empathically involved father prior to Tim's death. His adult life structure heavily emphasized his role as a father, and the construction of his identity as a father, his ongoing sense of competence and esteem in that role, was powerfully focused on his relationship with Tim and on the intergenerational reparation made possible by this relationship. Under the disequilibrating stress of bereavement, Steve painfully struggled to rebuild a collapsing life structure and to redefine his identity as a father, so central to the organization of his emotional life. Steve attempted to reestablish a sense of inner balance by turning to a relationship outside the family, one that would provide a radically new avenue for emotional and identity stabilization. He seemed to hope this new way of life could help him avoid, as much as possible, the profound grief and bitter disappointment that were now set off by his relationships with his wife and children. More unconsciously, Steve seemed to respond to Tim's death by forging an identification with his father, who had also turned to another woman as a way of dealing with marital problems.

A Mother's Grief

For Denise, Tim had been the son who would strive for and achieve special accomplishments in the world outside the family, a direction she herself had never attempted. She resented bitterly the loss of Tim's future and her opportunity to watch him make something special of himself. Denise's older brother had a child exactly Tim's age, and the cousins were good buddies, already planning to room together in college. Denise now looked at her nephew and felt the grief of her own son's lost opportunities in life. Yet in spite of the significance of her identification with Tim's potential for achievement, Denise did not find his death as personally shattering as did her husband. She was able to remain invested in the development and accomplishments of her surviving children and to find solace in her relationships with them. Denise's identity continued to center on her role as the mother of still dependent children. After Tim's death, she found some comfort in the idea that now she would never lose the child Tim had been, for he would never grow up; her other children would grow up, leave home, and become adults with their own families, all in the natural course of things, while Tim would always stay with her in her memories as a child.

Denise was also more identified with and involved with Eric's remarkable personal changes. She had been worried about Eric's struggles to escape from the shadow of his brother's glory even before Tim's death, and she found his successes a source of genuine joy.

While she realized with regret how much Eric had suffered as the second son in comparison to Tim and worried that she might burden him too much with the expectation that he would take Tim's place, she also welcomed the opportunity to forge a new kind of relationship with the now more accessible Eric. Denise was initially as shattered as Steve by the suddenness and finality of the loss of their son. It was in the established balance of their marital relationship, though, that she very quickly reorganized in an attempt to keep her grieving family afloat. She avoided talking to Steve about Tim, because he looked so stricken when she did so. She talked about him with the children, though, and put all her considerable energies into their family life. She had always thought Eric was not living up to his full potential, and when Eric responded to Tim's death by straightening out his own life, Denise was able to take an interest in his blossoming. As Steve became more withdrawn, Denise found herself turning more and more often to Eric for opportunities to reminisce about Tim. She found she could now count on Eric as they shared attempts to keep the family's spirits up. Suzie, an affectionate and expressive little girl, was also a source of enduring pleasure for Denise, who felt she had to keep a grip on her own depression in order to provide Suzie with the semblance of a loving family life. Greg continued to be the problem Denise focused on, since she found him hard to read and hard to reach. Nevertheless, she felt better able to reach Greg than to reach Steve and sought opportunities to be close to Greg that were activity oriented and therefore more acceptable to him as a way to feel close. Thus, she was able to maintain a close relationship with Greg also and could appreciate his special intellectual gifts. Denise's identification with Tim did not seem to involve the same early childhood difficulties that affected Steve, and perhaps this accounted for her more full investment in all the children.

Finally, Denise may have been forced to overcontrol her own intense grief reaction because she was concerned about Steve's extreme depression and isolation and its impact on the family. Concerned that Steve was withdrawing in his pain and that he seemed unable to bear any reminders of Tim, she tried to help him express his grief more directly, as she felt that was the root of his depression. At times during the course of their couples' therapy, Denise would compare her more successful bereavement to Steve's. She would tell him that she was doing better than he because she was able to express her feelings whereas he was holding his in. However, Denise's approaches and suggestions only made Steve withdraw even more. Steve, over the course of their mutual adaptation, may have been expressing the deepest depression felt by the whole family; the family became organized toward cheering him up but to no avail.

Conclusion

While the focus of this discussion of the Johnson family has been the adult developmental crisis initiated by the death of a child and its impact on parenting and the marital relationship, it is clear that the development of the children and also of the family as a unit was radically redirected by Tim's death and by the family's attempts to reestablish a manageable stability. I have focused especially on the adult developmental crisis provoked by Steve's grief reaction because his experience of grief illustrates the way a life structure and self-organization can collapse at the death of a child and the loss of this developmentally crucial attachment. The divorce in the family exacerbated the family's losses, for Steve maintained almost no contact with the children after the divorce. Shortly after the divorce became final, Steve married the young woman coworker he had turned to for comfort after Tim's death. He successfully competed for a promotion in his business firm, requiring that he and his second wife relocate to California. After the move, Steve continued to send regular child support payments but made no effort to maintain regular contact with his children.

Yet Steve's absence did free Denise and the children to express their grief over Tim's death directly and to eventually go on with their lives while putting the loss in perspective. Their open expression of grief would have been necessarily more constrained if Steve had remained in the family and they had continued to shape their family relationships in response to his overwhelming depression, emotional withdrawal, and intolerance for reminders of Tim.

For the Johnsons, the loss of Tim was compounded by the loss of father and husband as well. Denise was forced to return to school and to work. While she was initially terrified of these life changes, she found herself expanding the sources of her pride and satisfaction as she successfully managed the dual blows of death and divorce. She worried about the impact of the divorce on her children and their ongoing development. Several years later, with the children doing very well with the tasks of late adolescence and young adulthood, Denise continued to wonder what price they would have to pay for the loss of both brother and father over the course of their own development, a price only the evolving range of their own adult developmental futures could fully reveal.

EARLY ADOLESCENCE AS A DEVELOPMENTAL CHALLENGE TO A GRIEVING FAMILY'S POSTBEREAVEMENT ADAPTATION

Background

Sally and Bill Shaw (introduced in Chapter 9) requested treatment 7 months after the death of their 15-month-old daughter Mary, who was killed in a bicycling accident during the family's summer vacation. Bill, age 36, and Sally, age 34, felt that it took them 6 months after the trauma of their daughter's death to be ready to talk to someone (a more typical situation than that of the Johnsons, who asked to be seen immediately after Tim's death). The Shaws were worried about the effect of Mary's death on their surviving children, Laurie, age 7, and Josh, age 4. In addition, Bill, who had been terminated from his job as a business manager for a financially troubled company in the previous month, described himself as severely depressed since their first Christmas after Mary's death. My initial work with the Shaws, consisted of grief work beginning 7 months after Mary's death, and was comprised of five family sessions, one session with the children, and eleven couples' sessions, all over a period of eight months.

Seven years after Mary's death, the family recontacted me for a consultation on their difficulties with Laurie, who had just entered early adolescence. In this phase of work with the family, I met with both the parents and children for an initial evaluation, and then worked with Laurie in individual therapy. I met with Laurie weekly for about 6 months, and met with her parents separately every 2 to 3 weeks during this time.

Immediately after Mary's death, the Shaws as a family endured so many stresses and tragedies that they had begun to feel persecuted by fate. A month after their daughter died, Sally's mother was diagnosed as having breast cancer and underwent a mastectomy. Then Sally's younger sister suffered an acute illness and moved into their house so that she could be treated at a local teaching hospital. Bill commented that if life had any fairness or balance, they were due to win the lottery, because their luck had been so abysmally terrible. Sally fought the feeling that they were being punished for doing something bad, a feeling very much shared by 4-year-old Josh. Seven-year-old Laurie, preoccupied with cheering her parents up, vigilantly searching for signs that her parents might be feeling sad; when she detected such signs, she would attempt to distract her parents by changing the subject.

In contrast to the Johnsons, who were isolated from each other by their grief, Sally and Bill found themselves clinging to one another after the death of their child. Bill said that he found himself rethinking his life's values since Mary's death. He had been on a high-finance business track since graduating from the New England college where he and Sally had met, having worked his way up through the corporate ladder while getting an MBA at night. Although the family shared activities during weekends and vacations and Bill was an active and concerned father, he acknowledged that he had been primarily preoccupied with establishing himself in his career during the family's early years.

Bill had been driven not only by his own need for achievement but also by his experience in his family of origin. He was the older of two brothers in a family with a powerful intergenerational legacy of male irresponsibility in the family. Bill's mother had been separated from her father, because her mother's family disapproved of his irresponsibility and drinking and had separated the young couple. Bill's younger brother became heavily involved in drugs as a young man and remained dependent on his parents; he had married and had fathered two children, but his wife left him, taking the children with her and refusing to allow them any contact with their father or grandparents. Bill felt that the happiness and success of his own family had been an important source of solace for his often depressed mother. With the death of his daughter and the loss of his job, he felt that he too had disappointed his parents.

In the first months after his daughter's death, Bill found himself wanting to be home as much as possible, resenting any claims on his time that took him away from Sally and the children. He found his job terribly discouraging and felt he had lost all interest in or ability to do his work. He was actually relieved when he was called in by his boss and told that the company was in financial trouble and would have to close his department. Bill had been feeling responsible for the confusion and chaos at work and was relieved to discover that the company was going under and that the problems in his department were symptomatic of that. As he began looking for a new job, Bill hoped to find work that would give him a greater sense of purpose and meaning. During the job search, which was a difficult and protracted one for an executive at his level of experience, he found himself fantasizing about staying home with his family rather than working outside the home.

Sally felt especially shattered by Mary's death. First of all, she felt responsible for the accident, both realistically and psychologically: The family had been on a bicycle trail together; Sally had Mary in a backpack and was leading the group—Laurie, on her new three-speed bike, a babysitter behind her, and Bill and Josh bringing up the rear. As Sally turned around to check on Laurie's progress, she missed seeing a pole that had been placed to mark a road junction. She and the baby fell over, and Mary hit her head on the pole and lost consciousness. Although the baby appeared unscathed, she began having convulsions in the ambulance and died a few hours later of severe internal injuries.

While Bill reassured Sally that he would have done the same thing and that she had no reason to blame herself for irresponsibility, she nevertheless felt that she had failed horribly in her protective functions as a mother. Although any mother would have such a feeling under these circumstances, Sally was particularly vulnerable to feelings of failed responsibility, guilt, and self-blame. Her mother was a self-involved, highly anxious, hypochondriacal woman who had made Sally and her younger sister feel responsible for her physical well-being. Sally had never found her family particularly remarkable and had been haunted all through her childhood by insecurity and feelings of little self-worth. It was only after she married Bill, when she was 22 and he was 24, that he began to point out to her how self-centered and manipulative her parents, especially her mother, could be.

Sally had earned a master's degree in education and had taught early education at the beginning of the marriage; she then decided to devote herself to her children and to community activities that involved them as a family. She described herself as terribly overextended and admitted that she felt guilty when she was asked to do something and had to say no. Sally was aware that she was a hovering, overprotective mother; she knew she was the talk of the neighborhood because she would not let her children play outside their yard. Sally's sense of safety in the world was sustained by proximity to the people she cherished, and she profoundly believed that if the children were within sight, she could protect them.

Given Sally's psychological vulnerabilities, Mary's accidental death was an especially cruel blow. During their bicycle trip, she had felt that it was Laurie, who was far behind her and on her own bicycle, who was the vulnerable one of the children. She fully believed that Mary, who was close to her body, was protected by her. Not only did Sally feel terribly responsible for Mary's death, but she now felt that there was no safe place for her children and no way to protect them from danger.

The pain of losing Mary was especially acute for the family because of her status as the beloved baby. Both Bill and Sally felt that they had learned from their difficult experiences with the older two children and were now well qualified to parent this baby. Sally described Mary as a relaxed, happy, trusting baby whom she had been able to take care of in a relaxed, successful way. Laurie, an overactive child with a short attention span and some learning difficulties, could not easily respond to Sally's own needs for meticulous organization; the tensions between them were evident in their relationship. Sally found Josh a complicated little boy, although she appreciated his ability to become absorbed in independent play for long stretches of time and his love of order and organization. With Mary, her baby, she felt her parenting was everything she wanted her relationship with a child to be.

Bill, too, felt a special bond with Mary: People said she looked more like him than either of the other children, and he had devoted more time to her as a baby than he had with the others because he was no longer involved with the consuming combination of career development and school during her first year. His father had been distant and emotionally withdrawn during Bill's growing up, and his relationships to his children offered him a great deal of satisfaction. Mary's death left him with a profound feeling of failure.

Both Bill and Sally had devoted enormous energy to establishing a sense of competence as parents, and Mary's death shattered their sense of effectance in the world. During a therapy session after Easter Sunday, when they had visited Mary's grave, both described fantasies that attempted to repair their shattered images of themselves as parents. Bill described feeling enormously comforted by visits to the grave. When he was there, he would concentrate on the carving of a baby girl that they had commissioned for a headstone, fantasizing that there was something he could do, something he could fix, that would infuse the stone image with life. Sally, on the other hand, derived no comfort at all from visits to the cemetery; instead, she found them physically wrenching and disturbing. Her fantasy when she visited the cemetery centered not on the headstone but on the grave: She imagined that Mary was cold and lifeless but that if she could dig out her body and hold her close, she could warm her back to life.

Two weeks after the Easter Sunday visit to the cemetery, Sally became pregnant. The Shaws had felt terribly conflicted about having another child, fearing the emotional burden of replacement the child would carry, but they had stopped using birth control shortly after the lonely and depressing Christmas holidays. While the couple continued to feel the loss of their daughter with acute pain, they felt glad that they would once again have the opportunity to give life to a baby and thankful that their time for nurturing an infant was not yet over. It was clear at the time that the pregnancy gave Sally and Bill an opportunity to renew their sense of competence and purpose as parents. During the pregnancy, though, Sally was already anticipating the painful memories of Mary that the new baby's development would inevitably evoke.

The Shaws worked their way through the painful process of restabilization and reconfigured their family development by having a fourth child, who would allow them to complete as a family the ongoing process of caring for a young child. When Danny, a feisty, active, demanding baby, was born, both Sally and Bill were relieved that he was so distinctly himself that they could never confuse him with Mary and inadvertently pressure him to psychologically replace her. During Danny's infancy, the family had to further absorb the loss of Sally's mother, who died of cancer. After that experience, Sally and Bill felt they had reached a clearing during which their energies could once again be directed toward the rhythms of work and care of their developing children instead of crisis and tragedy.

A Daughter's Sacrifice

Following Danny's birth and Sally's mother's death, the Shaws went through a relatively stable family developmental phase during which they recognized and resonated protectively to each other's emotional fragility and need for stability, a phase that corresponded to Laurie's remaining elementary school years. In Chapter 9, I described Laurie's role in a family triangle which supported the family's need for stable structure in recovering from the instability and distress following Mary's death. Sally's relationship with Laurie, which had been fraught with the tension between Sally's perfectionism and need for control and Laurie's more impulsive, expansive style, now went into a period of quiescence as Laurie did everything she possibly could to fit her parents' image of a good, devoted daughter. Artistically creative yet impulsive and disorganized, Laurie threw herself into the many activities in which she excelled, following a rigorous, regimented schedule that included academics, sports, music, theater, and dance. The family conflict over independence and separation, which had begun to emerge during Laurie's early elementary school years, was resolved through a shared family decision to cherish their closeness and be emotionally responsive to each other's vulnerabilities.

The Shaws made an excellent and courageous recovery from the tragic death of little Mary. It is only in retrospect that we can review their mutual family developmental adaptation and identify the possible sources for Laurie's developmental difficulties, which resurfaced during her explosively troubled entry into adolescence. The Shaws contacted me again, when Laurie was in the eighth grade, because she had become engaged in a series of behaviors she seemed unable to control. In the summer before eighth grade, she had begun to menstruate; she had initially experienced a great deal of bleeding, which could only be controlled with hormonal therapy. The family, after years of financial struggle, found their dream house in a neighboring community; the relocation required that the children change schools. While both suburban school systems had comparably good reputations, the Shaws discovered that the atmosphere of the two schools differed somewhat; the new school required Laurie to make her way among a group of children who were more conformist and less academically oriented. Laurie became obsessed with her appearance as a route to peer acceptance and popularity and was inconsolable if she could not find exactly the right clothes to wear. She pushed her parents to take her on shopping trips to secure precisely the right item; she felt desperate if they refused. She often plundered both parents' closets in search of something to wear that might help her feel more confident about her appearance. Inevitably, her relief at finding the right item was brief at best.

Laurie had always been a child of extreme emotional intensity, but close family supervision and a rigidly regulated schedule had kept this intensity within manageable bounds. Suddenly, her routines and rituals began to totally fall apart. Laurie began to secretly cut music classes so she could hang out after school with friends. She struggled with an eating disorder, compulsively eating her way through the kitchen (and leaving a total mess), then secretly vomiting in the bathroom so she could control her weight. Introduced by her father to a commercial on-line service on their computer and oblivious to the fact that access to this network was extremely expensive, Laurie racked up a thousand dollars in computer line and telephone bills before her parents were forced to restrict her use of the line. She started to get telephone calls from men she had "met" through the computer lines who were trying to arrange to meet her in person. Her academic performance, which had been stable, plummeted from A to C and D work.

After years of responding positively to her parents' demands and expectations, Laurie became extremely resentful of their attempts to control her actions. The reactivity about issues of control was shared, as the Shaws struggled to help Laurie contain her clearly out-of-control behaviors through intensification of their demands and expectations. The rage, when it erupted between Laurie and either of her parents, felt explosively hot. The escalations in their arguments seemed more abrupt and intense than could be explained by the ordinary family developmental stresses of a member's entry into adolescence and a family move.

Laurie's struggles over her appearance evoked Sally's sympathy, fear, and anger; she indulged Laurie's anxiety by taking her on expensive shopping trips, then became anxious and enraged when Laurie would dress in ways that made her look too sexy or old for her years. Sally was simply furious when Laurie would trash her closet to borrow a sweater that would eventually resurface, along with her new, expensive clothes, in the heap at the bottom of her closet. The focus of Bill's concern over Laurie was his fear that she would dissipate her brilliant talent and promise through undisciplined behavior and self-indulgent manipulations of the sort that had characterized his talented younger brother, who had squandered his gifts.

In trying to understand Laurie's adolescent developmental crisis and the family's response, the parents and I reviewed together the family's adjustment to Mary's death and tried to understand the shared family adaptation from a new angle. Had the arduous process of recovering from Mary's death inadvertently submerged issues that were now resurfacing with the new demands of Laurie's early adolescence? Sally could remember how much anxiety she had felt when the children were out of her sight after Mary's death and how vulnerable she had felt to the possibility that an accidental death could strike her family again. Because of her own mother's disproportionate anxiety and overcontrol, Sally had struggled even before Mary's death with how much distance she could allow the children. After Mary's death, it became important to her to control, as much as possible, the children's comings and goings. Bill felt more distance from the mother–daughter struggles over appearance, but he was very concerned about Laurie's decline in achievement and the potential danger she faced at the hands of predatory young men. Both Sally and Bill could look back over the course of Laurie's development, remembering the temperamental vulnerabilities that were clearly evident in her preschool years, and recognize that after Mary's death Laurie had tried very hard to successfully comply with their high expectations of her.

At one level, we could all see Laurie's crisis as an exaggerated but still recognizable early adolescent response to her parents' hovering attention and high expectations. Laurie was shattering a hard-won emotional equilibrium, and the Shaws responded with an emotional intensity that they had not experienced since Mary's death. It helped them regain a better sense of proportion toward Laurie's excesses when they appreciated the difficulty of her family position. Sally and Bill often unfavorably compared Laurie, their talented but erratic oldest child, to their studious, considerate, exacting son Josh, whose temperamental style fit much better with their own personality styles and expectations. While Sally had achieved a sense of distance from Danny, an impetuous, independent little boy, she had yet to achieve this with Laurie. As their oldest child, Laurie kept introducing Bill and Sally to the growing edge of their new experiences as parents.

I had been meeting with Laurie in individual therapy sessions, trying to help her sort out her own private struggles with her complex conflictual desires and intense emotions from her battle with her parents. In exploring her resentment of her parents and in trying to sort out her reactivity to them from her more private struggle to make her own way in life, Laurie could see right on both sides. Revealing an intriguing mix of sophistication and insensibility, Laurie could often articulate aspects of her experience and behavior in the family that she could identify as both problematic and compelling. "I can see," I told her, "after all these years of compliance and silence, why you feel so angry, embattled, and entitled to your rage."

Laurie and I explored together the consequences of Mary's death for the family, and especially for her in her position as oldest child. Laurie, remember, had been riding a new three-speed bicycle on the day that Mary was fatally injured. Sally had Mary in a backpack and was riding her bike up front while Bill and their babysitter followed with Laurie and Josh. Sally had turned around for a moment, wanting to see how Laurie was progressing on her bike; she did not see the cement pole marking the intersection until she collided with it. Laurie, for the first time, acknowledged that she had been intensely angry at her mother for allowing such a moment of carelessness to happen at all, a moment that had cost Mary her life. At the same time that she felt this intense resentment, Laurie, knowing that her mother was consumed by her own guilt, strove to keep her anger to herself. Submerging her angry accusations out of consideration for her mother's vulnerability, Laurie turned her attention away from her anger and devoted herself instead to adapting as much as possible to her parents' expectations. Her seven-year-old's accusation against her mother had never been exposed to the light of later developmental understanding and experience, and because it had not undergone the erosion afforded by the wear of discussion and reexamination in the light of a more mature understanding of accidents and causality, Laurie's anger resurfaced intact. Forbidden thoughts have a terrible way of growing into greater importance because of their seclusion rather than shrinking from lack of attention.

Laurie's anger at her mother and her suppression of her angry thoughts in all likelihood added fuel to the developmental crisis over her autonomous rights, a crisis that might have been intense under ordinary developmental circumstances in this family, given the parents' tendency to equate independence with danger. For example, an observer might have interpreted the source of the sequence of events leading to Mary's tragic death as Sally's overprotective attention to Laurie, who was riding her new bike, a three-speed model that required new skills to operate. The Shaws, however, had ignored that dimension of the accident and had instead interpreted the source of danger as Laurie's emerging independence, represented by the new bicycle. And the Shaws remained a family that associated independence with danger.

After discussing Laurie's secret anger directed against her mother in individual therapy, Laurie and I talked about the best way we could open up the exploration of this subject between her and her parents. Laurie was reluctant to introduce the subject herself because she was afraid she would hurt her mother by essentially accusing her of causing the accident. She gave me permission to talk about her feelings with her parents during one of our regularly scheduled meetings; this would provide a safer way to start the conversation. I met separately with her parents to review this submerged but intense family grief issue. I also preferred to bring up Laurie's anger in a couple's session because I wanted to protect the parents' privacy and to concentrate on supporting them emotionally.

Bill and Sally were taken aback, yet not fully surprised, by Laurie's angry blaming of her mother for Mary's death. After all, they had struggled with the same thoughts at the time of the accident, as had everyone who heard their story. (I remember when I presented the Shaws at a case conference: Each of my colleagues who was also a parent in turn declared why he or she would never be so foolish as to allow such an accident to happen. I had to confront them with their self-protective attribution of control over unpredictable fate, as if they had forgotten that an accident is the result of an unlucky configuration of unpredictable events.) Bill felt confident that he had deeply searched his soul for feelings of blame; he knew how vulnerable we all are to accidental tragedy. Sally knew that her ability to suppress her own tendency toward self-blame for causing the accident was always precarious. No matter how much perspective she had acquired —with time, with therapy, with Bill's supportive understanding, which was genuinely free of blame—she could even now hardly bear the weight of her own self-blame and self-recrimination. Crying from the deepest part of herself, where she carried her still fresh grief, Sally told Bill and me, "No matter how well I put my grief aside, I can still reach into it anytime, as if it happened yesterday." Sadly, Laurie had chosen silence as a way of protecting her mother from accusations that Sally, herself, could never escape. Yet at this stage in her own grief, with more distance from her early remorseful feelings, and with more trust in her own ability to cope, Sally felt ready to talk to her daughter about the circumstances of the death.

We resolved to open up family discussions of grief as much as possible, while preserving the feelings of safety of family members, to allow Laurie an opportunity to verbalize her disappointment and anger at her sister's death. Sally felt anew her resentment of the terrible tragedy that still interfered with their pleasure in their family, that still stirred so much pain. She also understood Laurie's sense of isolation in having feelings she could not possibly share with her emotionally fragile, overwhelmed parents. Bill and Sally sat down together with Laurie at home and talked about her, as well as their, shared struggle to put the tragic fatal accident into perspective. Once Laurie could talk freely about her feelings of resentment that Sally's moment of carelessness, resulting in Mary's death, had caused, she was freer to apply her more mature cognitive perspective to understand the circumstances in which the accident had occurred. She was relieved to hear that her parents had also struggled with these concerns and did not consider her thoughts disloyal.

The work of reexamining the family grief reaction was only one small part of the work now required by the new family developmental crisis. The work of tracing the impact of Mary's death on the family's adaptation and subsequent development was undertaken to help them identify their own strategies for stability that had helped them survive a tragic crisis point—as well as the price paid for that stability. The aim of therapy was to reconfigure these strategies in new, more flexible ways in response to the new demands of Laurie's adolescent development.

In her school-age years Laurie had acquired developmental burdens not only from her struggles to cope with her own considerable emotional loss with the death of her sister but also from her attempts to support her parents' coping. Her parents, protected by Laurie's successful, if temporary, control of her spontaneity and independent will, were taken by surprise when the old family issues of independence and self-assertion erupted again. These issues, now intensified by the developmental transition of puberty in their oldest child, were intertwined with the family's shared attempts to cope with a traumatic grief reaction and were made even more difficult to confront by 7 years of suppression. Bill and Sally responded to Laurie's intensified adolescent separation needs with their own intense confusion about the difference between normal separation processes and their own fantasies equating death with self-assertion, independence, and separation.

The Shaws turned their attention to Laurie's unique needs and began the hard work of responding with greater self-awareness and flexibility to her age-appropriate needs for more autonomy. A transfer to a private school, where she received more individual attention and could safely express her individuality among supportive peers, helped Laurie substantially in coping with her own attempts to make her way along a new developmental course.

CONCLUSION: THE ADULT AND FAMILY DEVELOPMENTAL IMPACT OF THE DEATH OF A CHILD

A family is frozen by a death at a moment in real time, with the imagery of the particulars of the death constantly reviewed, magnified, and elaborated as family members struggle to accept and integrate the reality of their loss. The bereaved family is also frozen in developmental time, as family members are halted in their developmental progress and are forced to focus their resources on establishing a sense of equilibrium in the face of enormous stress and regressive disorganization. The work of grieving requires that a family accept the death in a way that promotes their continuing commitment to their shared lives. Parenting challenges the individual's capacity for maturity under the best of circumstances; with the assault on the self experienced when a child dies, parents often become preoccupied with establishing equilibrium within the self and lack the resources to maintain their caring relationships with spouse or children.

For Steve and Denise Johnson, the loss of an adolescent son inextricably intertwined his death with their ongoing struggle to establish themselves as a family with increasingly independent children—yet within a marriage that had itself never matured. The work of grieving requires that a family accept the death in a way that promotes their continuing commitment to their shared lives. The Johnsons had made choices in early adulthood that led them to form a successful child-oriented family. Yet the marital relationship did not have the resources to enable the couple to withstand the severe impact of the loss of their child. Steve and Denise may have suspected their own vulnerability, since they sought therapy so soon after Tim died, as if it was too hard for them to be alone together in their grief. For Steve Johnson, his son's death generated an immediate life cycle crisis; he reorganized his life so as to radically restrict his enduring contact with his family as a means of coping with the emotional impact of his grief, a reorganization that involved a major modification of a life structure centered on parenting.

For the Shaws, the immediate grief reaction after Mary's death did not generate a marital crisis. The Shaws, like the Johnsons, were married at about the same age, the year the husbands graduated from college. However, the Shaws had been more actively involved than the Johnsons in the development of their individual lives and careers and had postponed childbearing to allow more time for both career development and their marital relationship. Because of the different decisions made early in marriage, the Shaws and the Johnsons, although equal in age, were involved in different stages of the family life cycle. The fact that the Shaws were at an earlier stage of the family life cycle gave them the freedom to consider coping with their loss by deepening their commitment to parenting and having another child. The Johnsons, too, considered having another child but decided not to do so because of the age of their older children. Moreover, because they had lost not an infant but an adolescent child, a son well on his way to becoming a successful young man, it may be that they sensed that the birth of another child would not have given them a sense of restoration or comfort, as it had for the Shaws.

These two couples married as young adults, but they took different courses in the development of their adult selves outside the marriage and in the development of their marital relationship before the birth of children. These choices in early marriage became extremely significant when the death of their child initiated an intense, painful review of them. In the face of death, it is natural for adults to question the meaning and purpose of their lives. With the death of a child, the loss of aspects of the self invested in the particular child and in the marital and parenting roles requires reorganization of the self so as to achieve a new stable definition of the collaborative self.

While the Johnsons faced their most disequilibrating life crisis within a year of Tim's death, the Shaws faced their own family life cycle crisis when Laurie entered early adolescence, 7 years after Mary's death. The Shaws' strategies for stability following Mary's death included the requirement that Laurie submerge her already emerging needs for independence, a requirement that made it more difficult for them to respond to Laurie's entrance into early adolescence with the necessary flexibility and freedom for creative collaborative change. The circumstances of Mary's accidental death, on the day Laurie acquired her first three-speed bike, a tool of independence and separation, had inadvertently served to entangle mother and daughter more deeply in a struggle that confused separation with tragedy and proximity with safety.

Both the Shaws and the Johnsons will continue to face the family developmental consequences of the death of their child as they enter later stages of the family life cycle. These families were forced to shoulder an overwhelming emotional burden that absorbed the energy they would otherwise have channeled into their active, loving family relationships. Ironically, it was in part because parenting was so much the heart and soul of both these families, because their relationships to their children were so central to the meaning of their lives, that the death of a child dealt them such a crushing blow. Yet each subsequent stage of the family life cycle presents these and other grieving families with creative new opportunities to rework their earlier adaptation, and to emerge with new sympathy for their own vulnerabilities and appreciation of their own considerable strengths.

PART IV

CULTURAL AND SOCIAL FACTORS IN FAMILY BEREAVEMENT

CHAPTER 11

The Sociocultural
Context of Grief

Carol Gray, a 21-year-old Irish Catholic nursing student, entered a bereavement and social support group (Shapiro, 1975) after her mother's death from cancer. The illness, while anticipated, had an extremely rapid course. Carol experienced herself as far more grief-stricken than she was "allowed to be" by her classmates, family, and friends. A few months after her mother's death, Carol visited her father and younger siblings at their home and found herself arguing with her father over dinner preparations. Carol wanted to preserve the dinner ritual as her mother had done it, because it allowed her to feel her mother was still with them. Her father wanted to change everything about the way they ate dinner, from meal preparation to eating arrangements, because he found the reminder of his wife's absence too painful.

In reviewing the argument with the group, Carol acknowledged that she was far angrier at her father than the situation warranted. Exploring her feelings, she realized she resented her father because he, as her mother's husband, occupied the acknowledged position of "chief mourner." "It's not fair," she said, "that everyone treats him like it's the worst thing that ever happened to him and treats me like I'm too old to be so affected by my mother's death. After all, he can always get another wife, but I'll never again have another mother." For Carol, the experience of bereavement highlighted a problematic cultural assumption about appropriate grief reactions: A man who loses his wife has more priority as a mourner than a grown daughter who no longer lives at home.

Not only was Carol struggling with her overwhelming feelings, but she was also trying to figure out how her feelings fit with what was normatively expected of her by her Irish Catholic family and by her university peers. Her family was unaccustomed to displays of intense feeling of any kind. Carol's comment concerning the possibility of her father's replacing her mother with a new wife reflected her expectation that her father would "forget" the painful memories of her mother. Her college-age friends did not want to discuss her feelings either, in part because they were trying to manage their own developmental progress out of the parental home and could not bear the regressive pull of Carol's frank acknowledgment that her life would not be the same without her mother. Carol found that, except in the support group, she was unable to express to others her deep feelings of sorrow and resentment, because these feelings contradicted social expectations. Had she been a member of a different ethnic subculture, one that did not emphasize a college-age young adult's separation from family or the strict control of emotions, Carol might have had a very different framework for understanding her own grief as well as for receiving social support.

Carol's grief experience illustrates how much individual bereavement is given its organization, support, and meaning by the social expectations of a particular culture. While patterns of family relationship are powerful determinants of the collaborative self, these patterns are themselves organized in a social context that reflects the given culture. Carol's family and peers conveyed a clear expectation that young adults reach a certain age and have no more need for their parents. Further, her social environment defined the marital unit as the central family relationship, thus giving it emotional priority over the relationship between adult child and parent. In our culture families have come to rely enormously on the nuclear family rather than the extended family because of greater geographic mobility, work demands, and the high value we place on individual autonomy. In other cultures, as well as in ethnic American subcultures, intergenerational or extended family relationships remain important resources for emotional and instrumental support throughout the life cycle (Rossi & Rossi, 1990).

As we can see from this case example, the sociocultural and individual practices of bereavement are not necessarily in harmony. Mourners' responses vary enormously in their goodness of fit with prevailing cultural norms regarding the length of the grieving period and the pattern of reentry into whatever roles are sanctioned for the postbereavement phase. Acceptable patterns of behavior differ by gender and age. Cultural circumstances determine the flexibility with which social roles can be challenged by the individual or family for whom prescribed behaviors do not provide a good or harmonious match. The conclusion that an individual's grief reaction is inappropriate or pathological is based not only on the nature of that individual's grief reaction but also on the range of and tolerance of differences in grief reactions allowed by his or her culture.

THE SOCIOCULTURAL PERSPECTIVE
IN CLINICAL WORK

Our clinical work with grieving families, then, can best be understood in the light of these social patterns and expectations that help to organize family bereavement reactions as emotional crises and as psychosocial transitions of identity. From a sociocultural perspective, grief is a crisis of life structure in which habitual interactional patterns and role relationships need to be reestablished. Social norms prescribe certain ideal solutions for the management of grief feelings, for the re-creation of life structures, and for the reestablishment of a meaningful sense of identity in connection with surviving family members and members of the wider community.

Therapists in the United States who work with grieving families from different minority culture backgrounds encounter significant cultural differences in the management of grief and search for resources that might teach them the ritual, practices, and beliefs of families from different cultures. Although such resource materials for therapists are valuable in understanding the experience of grieving families from different cultural backgrounds, they can be misused. The cataloging of culturally different grief practices can parallel the dilemma in multicultural education, namely, the tendency to stereotype or trivialize an extremely complex culture by having teachers present a few isolated items of language and culture (Darder, 1991; Nieto, 1992). A family's dependence on cultural beliefs and practices varies enormously with its culture, immigration status, and socioeconomic class, as well as with many other dimensions of family circumstances and history (Falicov, 1988). A systemic developmental perspective that includes larger social systems as they impact on family coping can help therapists achieve a more multidimensional and dynamic view of a particular family's unique circumstances. Moreover, families differ in their individual interpretation and unique integration of minority culture practices with majority culture beliefs, in general and with respect to their grief work. We therapists ourselves are located within our own ethnic subculture, our individual and family grief history, and the mental health profession, all of which define the dimensions of the interpretive lens through which we understand and respond to grieving families.

Therapists working with grieving individuals and families need to remain sensitive to cultural bereavement traditions and to assess a family's location relative to its own culture-of-origin practices. At the same time, we need to help families evaluate when these traditions facilitate and when they impede the optimal growth-enhancing adjustment to the death and its consequences. This is an especially difficult task for therapists in a diverse cultural milieu like that of the United States, in which many grieving families present not only with different cultural backgrounds but also with varying degrees of acculturation to mainstream American culture (Eisenbruch, 1984b). If therapists respect family members' own cultural self-assessment, we are more likely to support a family's best use of its cultural resources as part of its grief experience. If we assume the position of a therapeutic expert who can draw the line between culturally appropriate grief practice and pathological grief, we may miss important cultural variations. Whatever their cultural background, families often need our help to discover their own best use of cultural traditions as supportive resources.

Different cultural traditions approach the following social and personal issues of bereavement differently: defining the relationship between the dead and the living, describing the nature of life after death, and enabling the social reconstruction of the ruptured relationships within family and community. Each culture defines the processes of bereavement and reconstruction in ways that are consistent with its beliefs regarding life, death, and an afterlife, emphasizing certain aspects of the broad range of human experience while diminishing the importance of others. In addition to designating accepted bereavement practices, cultures differ in the social roles they assign to bereaved family survivors. When a member of the community dies, the community is first and foremost concerned with preserving its own continuity and integrity; it mobilizes symbolic rituals that dictate the appropriate roles and expression of feelings for the bereaved in the immediate family, the extended family, and the larger community.

The goodness of fit between these prescribed social roles and the experience of grief and recovery for any particular grieving family varies, depending on the family's own history, structural organization, and emotional style. I have worked with widows who find the American way of grief, in which widows are often asked within the first year of a husband's death when they plan to start dating, extremely intrusive and offensive. The 2-to-5-year timetable that most widows seem to require is very much at odds with our cultural beliefs, to the profound discomfort of these women. Some widows in our culture would find more congruent and personally supportive the older Greek and

Italian traditions that require a widow to wear black for the remainder of her life and do not permit her remarriage.

Grief is a fundamental expression of our social constructions and values. At the same time, it is an experience that places us outside our existing social constructions and categories while we reclaim and reestablish our place in the social world. The experience during a transitional period of being outside of accustomed social structures and marginal to them is an important element of the grief experience. The transitional location of bereaved people in the social role structure, including their greater symbolic and spiritual proximity to the world of the dead, corresponds closely to their sensation that they live in a world where the dead have a greater immediacy and psychological reality than do the living. The experience of being dissociated from the flow of lived experience, of feeling frozen in time, is a psychological reflection of this altered social and spiritual state. Cultures differ substantially in the process they prescribe for bridging this psychological and social transition. In the dominant North American culture, which emphasizes the centrality of the isolated individual; minimizes the importance of spiritual, as compared to scientific, explanations; and stresses the value of "letting go" and "moving on," social sanctions are likely to pressure the bereaved into reentering the flow of ordinary life long before they feel psychologically ready.

In this culture the bereaved often find themselves in the unsought and unwelcome role of social critic, having been confronted with the discrepancy between their real feelings and the projections or attributions to which they are constantly subjected by well-meaning but self-serving friends, relatives, and members of the community. Most of us, quite understandably, wish to turn away from full empathy with the bereaved, as this would mean imagining the unimaginable pain of suffering such a loss in our own lives. Social isolation may be especially intense for parents who have lost a child, who frequently report that friends who are parents avoid them because they cannot bear the reminder of the parents' enormous loss and grief (Rando, 1985, 1986). The irritable social withdrawal of many bereaved people has most often been explained as a function of their difficulty facing a world in which their loved one no longer exists. In accounting for the social isolation of bereaved people, though, we must include their acute sensitivity to those social expressions of sympathy that reduce the mourner's experience to something other people can more easily manage. "Don't worry," people say, "you can always have another child." Or "Don't give in to your grief; you already have two beautiful children to live for." Or "You don't have to be alone; you can remarry."

The bereaved become especially sensitive to the defensive operations we use to get through our daily lives without the painful recognition that our lives could be shattered at any time, through no fault of our own, by death.

In addition, when they are thrust out of normative family life and must begin a painful process of exploration and reconstruction, the bereaved become more aware of the social construction of family life and of our cultural assumptions about how families operate. This process is perhaps most evident for widows and widowers, who are forced to become aware of the polarized gender arrangements of our culture under circumstances where they are now missing the necessary, complementary partner (Silverman, 1986, 1987; Stroebe & Stroebe, 1987). And with the death of a child, men and women are forced to confront the emotional and functional arrangements under which we make children and emotions the business of women and financial providing the business of men (Cook, 1984).

The Study of Cultural Traditions of Bereavement

What I am calling a sociocultural perspective in this chapter is really distilled from what can be considered two separate literatures: cultural anthropology, with its emphasis on different cultural arrangements (e.g., Marcus & Fischer, 1986; Rosaldo, 1989), and sociology, which emphasizes normative social constructions within a particular culture (e.g., Rossi & Rossi, 1990). In addition, the fields of psychology and mental health have begun to address cross-cultural issues (Harwood, 1981; Stigler, Shweder, & Herdt, 1990) and to make a contribution to our understanding of bereavement experiences cross-culturally. The sociocultural perspective on bereavement can heighten our clinical awareness of diverse cultural arrangements as they frame the family developmental process and shape the social reconstruction of the collaborative self following the death of a family member.

While we therapists will naturally be most immersed in considering the experience of bereavement from the perspective of our own culture, the field of cultural anthropology has an extensive literature that challenges our own culturally embedded point of view of the grief experience. The sociological and cross-cultural perspective on bereavement can give those of us who work with families a much-needed widening of our culture-bound assumptions about bereavement. In fact, some authors have argued that the medical and mental health industries are themselves subcultures with their own norms and assumptions about the proper way to grieve, subcultures families are forced to struggle with in their encounters with these institutions

(Stephenson, 1985). We may be less likely to identify a particular family's way of grieving as pathological if we become better acquainted with the extraordinarily wide range of beliefs and rituals through which different cultures recognize the losses brought about by a death while continuing to affirm life.

Traditionally, cultural anthropologists have been drawn to the study of funeral and death rituals across different cultures as an avenue toward understanding the central values and social structures of those cultures. Most pragmatically, the burial sites and skeletal remains are often the only signs of ancient cultures that survived for millennia. More substantively, though, the bereavement rituals and emotional expressions of grief that are permitted by a culture highlight sociocultural organization and values more generally, and often form the core of anthropological theory about a given culture (Huntington & Metcalfe, 1979).

In addition, the perspective of the anthropologist has been applied to American grief practices in both the dominant culture and in ethnic or religious subcultures (Eisenbruch, 1984b). This cross-cultural perspective serves as a means of exploring the embedded cultural assumptions in American ways of grief as well as of highlighting the distinct beliefs and practices of different subcultures. The presence of culturally diverse groups in the United States, each with a distinct immigration history and degree of acculturation to the dominant culture, creates in this country a wide assortment of bereavement practices and assumptions about the nature of grief (McGoldrick et al., 1991).

Anthropologists have asked the question, Are there any universal human principles associated with the experience of death that are given expression across different cultures? Does the experience of bereavement contain any commonalities in different cultures, or is the expression of grief culture specific and culturally determined? We intuitively attribute a great deal of universality to the grief experience, which is in fact experienced and expressed very differently in different cultural contexts. The benefit of cross-cultural comparison is that it not only highlights the culture-bound nature of the grief experience but also serves to clarify aspects of our grief experience that are so culturally embedded we take them for granted.

In addition, a smaller literature on bereavement in the United States has examined bereavement beliefs and practices within different racial, ethnic, and religious subcultures. Writers exploring ethnic minority bereavement practices and traditions have been especially interested in the process of cultural transition for American immigrants, such as Mexican-Americans or Indochinese, and in the goodness or poorness of fit between American legal and commercial regulation of the funeral industry and the distinctive cultural practices of various ethnic groups (Eisenbruch, 1984a, 1984b).

The emotions of grief, especially in its acute phases, often feel to the bereaved as if they are occurring in spite of themselves and their wishes; it is as if their bodies are taken over by a rush of sorrow that ebbs and flows in waves. If grief is universal, then it must have developed through biological mechanisms of evolutionary selection and must be in some way adaptive. Bowlby's (1980) work on an attachment theory approach to grief indicates that attachment is essentially a biological process made necessary by our primate dependence on a web of social relationships and that separation of an individual from the group is an extremely serious event. Attachment theory suggests that grief is the mobilization of this biologically determined sequence of sadness and angry protest in the face of separation, the adaptive purpose of which is to restore the presence of the caretaker. These separation responses persist even when they cannot serve the function of returning the lost person.

The Universality of Death versus the Diversity of Bereavement Ritual and Belief

If there is a biological foundation to the separation processes mobilized by the irreversible loss of death, what is the role of culture and its diversity of rituals and beliefs in the organization of the grief experience? Eisenbruch (1984a) argues that the diversity of cultural grief reactions is not incompatible with a biological foundation to the grief reaction. He asserts that every culture has its own distinct way of easing the suffering of grief by offering the bereaved an explanation for the meaning of the death and a prescription for how to proceed with life.

For example, the Western belief in the finiteness of the individual life cycle, especially with the decline of religious beliefs and their replacement with secular or scientific values, makes us more likely to view death as a final separation and heightens our feelings of protest and denial. In Buddhist culture, with its belief in the eternal cycle of being and its insistence that the ego or self is an illusion, the death of a family member is viewed as less final and the suffering or loss associated with a death is more likely to be accepted as part of a spiritual cycle (Stroebe & Stroebe, 1987). Members of American subcultures that retain their spiritual beliefs are more likely to derive comfort from their belief that there is spiritual or divine purpose to the death and spiritual continuity with the deceased (Cook & Wimberley, 1983).

While bereavement seems to have a biological foundation, the diversity of meanings and social constructions associated with it are extraordinarily diverse. In their review Huntington and Metcalfe (1979) describe a wide range of funeral rituals:

> What could be more universal than death? Yet what an incredible variety of responses it evokes. Corpses are burned or buried, with or without animal or human sacrifice; they are preserved by smoking, embalming, or pickling; they are eaten—raw, cooked, or rotten; they are ritually exposed as carrion or simply abandoned; or they are dismembered and treated in a variety of these ways. Funerals are the occasion for avoiding people or holding parties, for fighting or having sexual orgies, for weeping or laughing, in a thousand different combinations. The diversity of cultural reactions is a measure of the universal impact of death. But it is not a random reaction; always it is meaningful and expressive. (p. 1)

The funeral ritual, which is the immediate response to the departure of life and the ritual disposing of the corpse, is almost universally treated as an opportunity to affirm life and the continuity of community ties. The ritual can include everything from expressions of celebration and vitality, such as the vigorous, stylized dancing among the Nyakusa of Tanzania, to the highly ritualized self-mutilation, with the degree of severity prescribed by the bereaved's relationship to the deceased, practiced by the Warramunga of Australia (Huntington & Metcalfe, 1979).

Emphasizing the Anger Component of Grief. Renato Rosaldo, an anthropologist who for many years studied the headhunting Ilongot tribes of the northern Philippines, describes the profoundly cultural construction of the grief experience through an extraordinary analysis of his own grief after the accidental death in 1981 of his wife, anthropologist Michelle Rosaldo. In an article entitled "Grief and a Headhunter's Rage," Rosaldo (1989) describes his attempts to understand, over many years of fieldwork, the matter-of-fact equation among the Ilongot between grief, its accompanying rage, and the relief brought by the activity of headhunting. Ilongot men depart on headhunting raids into the territories of enemy tribes in which they ambush the first person who comes along, kill their victim, behead him and toss away the head. "In tossing away the head, they claim by analogy to cast away their life burdens, including the rage in their grief" (p. 16).

While he was able during fieldwork from 1967 to 1969 and in 1974 to transcribe the words of informants who described the importance of headhunting as a means of coping with the heart-wrenching mix of sorrow and rage evoked by the death of a loved one, Rosaldo felt himself unable to understand this process. (Over the course of Rosaldo's fieldwork with the Ilongot, he witnessed a period of cultural transformation during which the practice of headhunting was strictly outlawed by the Philippine government. The Ilongot turned to evangelical Christianity as a means of finding an outlet for their feelings of grief when their traditional means of coping with the rage and sorrow of grief had been blocked.) At the time of this fieldwork, Rosaldo found the Ilongot explanation of the relationship betwen grief, rage, and headhunting lacking in depth or cultural texture and tried to find "deeper" explanations, such as anthropological exchange theory, in which taking the life of a victim could be seen as balancing the loss of a loved one. He realized at the time that the Ilongots themselves felt he was totally missing the essential point, but he still had no entry, through his own cultural or personal experience, into the Ilongot way of grief. It was only in analyzing his own reaction to the death of his wife, who fell to her death during a field expedition in 1981, that Rosaldo fully understood for himself the depth of rage evoked by death.

Rosaldo expresses concern that the traditional anthropological emphasis on ritual in the study of bereavement can serve to obscure a true understanding of the grief experience. He argues that while the stylized rituals in funerals might bring the broader community into closer contact with their sense of loss, they can only serve to distance the bereaved themselves from their depth of feeling. At best, funerals catalyze a process of emotional response that will unfold over subsequent months and years.

Rosaldo concludes that one's own particular cultural and disciplinary perspective, which he describes as the "positioned subject," determines the features of any experience, one's own and others', one is able to identify and analyze. He further notes that while the therapeutic culture in the United States encourages the bereaved to explore the anger provoked by death—anger at the loved one who has died for recklessly abandoning them, anger at agents of the culture implicated in or insensitive to the death—the broader culture essentially ignores the rage in grief, thus restricting the grief experience. While grief cannot be reduced to rage, he asserts, neither can the compelling component of rage be overlooked. Rosaldo feels that his field experience with a radically different culture whose practices had so fully given voice to the dimension of rage in grief enabled him to understand a key dimension of the violent physical force behind his own grief experience. Once he had experienced the rage of his own grief, a central aspect of Ilongot life, the interweaving of grief, anger, and the emotional relief associated with the head-hunting ritual became clear to him for the first time.

Bereavement as a Social Transition: The Concept of Liminality

In addition to defining the expression of sanctioned emotions, the cultural construction of bereavement serves the purpose of creating a social transition in which the bereaved acknowledge their separation from ongoing social structures, exist outside of these structures for a period of time, and then reenter the community in a new social form. Van Gennep first introduced this concept of transition, or *liminality*, to the anthropological literature, a concept that has been elaborated by others (Huntington & Metcalfe, 1979).

The concept of liminality is used, first and foremost, to indicate a spiritual transition period between being alive and being dead, in which the spirit of the person resides in an altered, sacred space. Every culture needs to come to terms in its own way with the reality of death and its people's fear and horror of it. The uncertainty concerning the nature of life after death preoccupies most cultures in some fashion. In many cultures the rituals of the funeral are attempts to help the spirit of the deceased make its way to the next form of spiritual life, and the community is given the responsibility for making this transition a good voyage or passage. Because of their proximity to the spirit of the deceased, the bereaved are also considered to be in this transitional space, which they enter through rites of separation and emerge from through rites of reintegration into society. Eisenbruch (1984a) quotes Van Gennep as follows:

> During mourning, the living mourners and the deceased constitute a special group, situated between the world of the living and the world of the dead, and how soon living individuals leave that group depends on the closeness of their relationship with the dead person. Mourning requirements are based on degrees of kinship and are systematized by each people according to their special way of calculating that kinship. . . . During mourning, social life is suspended for all those affected by it, and the length of the period increases with the closeness of the social ties to the deceased, and with a higher social standing of the dead person. If the dead man was a chief, the suspension affects the entire society. (p. 290)

Émile Durkheim, the French sociologist, and his students, Van Gennep and Herz, all writing at the beginning of the century, viewed the ritual mandate of grief and mourning on the part of kin as serving the function of enhancing the solidarity of the group, which has been threatened by the death of one of its members. According to Herz, the death of the individual is not just a biological event; the deceased is "a social being grafted upon the physical individual" whose "destruction is tantamount to a sacrilege against the social order" (in Eisenbruch, 1984a, p. 291).

In sum, then, the concept of liminality can be used to address the dual nature of the bereavement rituals and reactions prescribed by a particular culture: (1) They create avenues for the public articulation of deeply felt emotions such as sorrow and anger and provide community comfort for those emotions and (2) they help restore the social order disrupted by the death. Death disrupts the community in a number of ways: (1) through the loss of one of its functioning members, a loss that must be accommodated; (2) by altering the social roles of bereaved kin, roles that must be redefined; and (3) by forcing the community to confront the existential reality of death, a reality to which it must respond by creating meaningful spiritual or symbolic rituals to address the eternal cycles of birth and death and thus to renew and affirm life.

The Cultural Construction of Bereavement in the Death of a Child

The fact that grief is at the same time a biological reality and a socially constructed process is well illustrated by the circumstances following the death of a child in different cultures. In our culture the death of a child is an unexpected event that adults experience as so deeply shattering that they do not necessarily expect to recover. More and more of the current bereavement literature in fact documents the conclusion that the grief experience following the death of a child is one from which adults have an extremely difficult time recovering (Rando, 1986). Increasingly, the grief experiences associated with second- or third-trimester miscarriages or stillbirths are also being identified as far more profound for parents than the medical field was at one time willing to acknowledge (Leon, 1990, 1992). One argument mentioned in historical and cross-cultural studies is that these devastating bereavement experiences after the death of a child exist precisely because in our world of advanced medical technology and commitment to public health most children are expected to survive to adulthood (Leavitt, 1986). The advances in childhood survival generated by a high-technology medical industry have been accompanied by a health services mentality in which death is to be fought against in each and every case with all the technological means at hand (often prolonging life without consideration for its quality). This has led to the explicit belief that all out-of-life-cycle deaths, especially those of young children, are preventable by alert-enough parents and doctors.

The cross-cultural literature has asked the question, What is the nature of parental bereavement in different cultures, especially in those where social deprivations create circumstances in which infant mortality continues to be high? Eisenbruch (1984a) considers it a condescending Western belief that in societies where infant mortality is high "life is cheap. This myth is a tendentious distortion of a complex human reality" (p. 293). It would be more accurate to say that for the painful loss of a child under harsh life circumstances, where such an experience will be endured by a couple at least once and possibly many more times, a society and its individuals collaborate to create belief systems and rituals that will offer parents some emotional shelter from their pain.

For example, the Yoruba of Nigeria and the LoDagaa of Ghana treat the corpse of an infant very differently from that of any other child or adult, believing that it has special demonic qualities and may come back to haunt the parents. The Yoruba call babies who die in infancy *abiku*, or "born to die," and believe that these children are really demons who can be born again and again to the same mother, always dying to rejoin the other demon spirits at a predetermined time (Eisenbruch, 1984a). In parts of West Africa, babies cannot be buried for fear that this will offend the Earth shrines, which protect fertility and survival.

In an anthropological study of maternal bereavement under conditions of high infant mortality, Scheper-Hughes (1990, 1992) argues that both maternal feelings and maternal bereavement are complex socially constructed processes that take into account the social realities under which women and their families live. She studied families in a shantytown of Northeast Brazil, Alto de Cruzeiro, where infant mortality ranges from 30% to 40% of all live births. Historians of childhood have speculated that circumstances of high infant mortality might make children interchangeable or replaceable inasmuch as the mothers might have limited attachment to their children or might be willing to practice infanticide on fragile or undesirable offspring with limited chances for survival. Scheper-Hughes challenges these hypotheses as applications of our own historically and culturally biased conceptions and argues that maternity itself is a poorly understood experience that we both idealize and denigrate through culturally biased distortions and contradictions.

Scheper-Hughes found that in this Brazilian shantytown, under the extraordinarily poor conditions of endemic malnutrition, contaminated drinking water, and exploitative work conditions, mothers are intensely attached to some of their children but are, at the same time, likely to severely neglect those infants who do not seem likely to survive, the latter are identified as "wanting to die," and it is considered an interference with their fate to intercede on their behalf or to give them precious resources. Mothers are permitted to show a great deal of attachment to their older children, in contrast to their attitude toward infants, and can be altogether devastated by grief after the death of an older child, especially one who appeared to be destined for life.

Scheper-Hughes further found that while mothers were aware of the social circumstances that caused so many babies to die in their shantytown, and specifically blamed their living conditions for the devastatingly high rate of infant mortality, they attributed the death of their own infant to "child sickness," a naturally occurring illness that just happens to a child. She speculated that these mothers were exercising necessary denial in order to cope with their helplessness to change the socioeconomic conditions under which they were forced to live. Mothers felt it was an injustice to care for offspring with "child sickness," since care might prolong lives that would never be "right," that is, fully livable, especially under circumstances of such economic adversity.

In order to limit maternal attachment to the fragile ones, this culture views all infants as incapable of having feelings, a capacity for understanding, or intrinsic value as persons, all of which children are assumed to have once they survive to the toddler years. The discouraging of mothers from crying at the funerals of their infants, a particularly poignant cultural practice that reflects this emotional detachment, is based on the belief that the infant's spirit has to make its way to heaven and a mother's tears will make the path slippery and impede the way.

Scheper-Hughes attributes these maternal experiences not to the selfishness of mothers but to the brutal, economically determined social conditions of exploitation, in which human beings are considered expendable. Forced to adapt to such conditions, these Brazilian mothers maintain a dual consciousness in which they are both aware of their abysmal life circumstances and forced to dissociate this awareness in facing the constancy of death in their own family lives. As a result of this tragic cycle of social injustice and the corresponding psychological defense it necessitates, the infants themselves are dehumanized and blamed for their own deaths.

APPLYING A SOCIOCULTURAL PERSPECTIVE
TO GRIEF PRACTICES IN THE UNITED STATES

Socioeconomic factors, which are an important dimension of cultural experience, are often not considered in discussions of the bereavement practices in a culture. Our American urban poor and minority communities have their own experience of unacceptably high infant mortality rates and murder rates among young men, which we explain and address in terms that blame the communities themselves, for example, by focusing on drug use or gangs. We are not ready, as a culture, to declare these death rates among minority children unacceptable, because such an awareness would make it necessary for us to address the conditions of poverty and racism that these families endure and that are the social context for these deaths. Yet we are fully capable of making a concerted commitment to prevent other conditions leading to childhood death, as is shown by the implementation of laws requiring the use of infant car seats. The deaths of unrestrained infants in automobiles, which were once viewed as accidents of fate, are now labeled by law and by cultural practice as deaths caused by parental neglect (Garbarino, Dubrow, Kostelny, & Pardo, 1992).

The Impact of High Technology

Because the economics of our high-technology society demands it, our culture is becoming more and more committed, without evaluating human priorities and consequences, to expensive medical procedures that prolong life. While we can be grateful for the extraordinary feats of medical treatment that restore life and health to the ill or injured, we also need to look critically at medical practices that promote the use of expensive high-technology procedures without acknowledging the human relational context in which patients live. The hospital experience is becoming more salient for many bereaved families, who live an intense, significant period of their own lives as participants in the treatment process but who have no official relationship of any kind to the hospital and medical team once the patient finally dies. Studies of family adjustment following the death of a child from cancer find significantly better adjustment and fewer symptoms of psychopathology in parents and siblings who participated in home care as compared to those whose family member received hospital care (Koocher, 1986; Martinson, Nesbitt, & Kersey, 1984; Mulhern et al., 1983). Although families who choose home care may have preexisting strengths, these findings suggest the possibility that the opportunity to provide direct care to the child at home may enhance parental, sibling, and family adaptation to the death of the child by increasing family intimacy and communication.

The practice of high-technology medicine in the United States, with its emphasis on the involvement of many specialists who are relatively isolated from each other and from the family of the dying patient, is hard on all families but is especially culturally discrepant for minority group families. Families from Latino cultures, for example, accustomed to familism, often bring many members of the extended family for hospital visits, express the wish to stay overnight with the patient, bring gifts of food for the patient and the hospital staff, with whom they desire a sense of intimate connection, and offer the hospitality of their home to the care providers. The American emphasis on professional efficiency and clear boundaries between treatment and family life violates the cultural expectations of Latino families and deprives them of a culturally congruent supportive relationship with the physician and the treatment team. These differences between the culture of hospitals and the culture of many minority families can lead to profound misunderstanding of a family's grief experience on the part of providers. Ana Margarita Cebollero, a Puerto Rican psychologist and Director of the Latino team of psychiatry at Boston Children's Hospital, described an incident in which the Puerto Rican family of a girl who had died in the hospital sent a photograph of their daughter in her coffin at the wake as a final memento to every member of the treatment team. Most of the staff, who were Anglo-Americans, were shocked at what they considered an action by the grieving family that was at best inappropriately morbid, at worst pathological. Cebollero, translating across the gulf of cultural differences, reassured the staff that the family was simply gratefully including them in the family process of sharing the deceased's last moments before burial.

Therapists who work with grieving families need to be aware that hospital and medical communities function as subcultures that for their own economic, legal, and psychological reasons emphasize the limited goal of exhausting every possible means of prolonging life. Families may need help critically assessing these medical goals for themselves. They may also need help managing the consequences of extreme medical interventions, even when these are a family's choosing. New approaches to the care of dying and terminally ill patients, including the hospice movement and the honoring of living wills, show an emerging awareness of possible alternatives families might choose in collaboratively constructing a shared experience of death and bereavement.

For ethnic minority families, especially those whose primary language is not English, the process of negotiating with a physician, who is typically viewed as an unquestionable authority, may be especially difficult. In cultures that do not encourage assertiveness in relation to medical authority, providers may need to help empower patients and their families so that they are able to say no to optional medical procedures that run counter to their religious or cultural beliefs. Medical units need to make available competent translation and other culturally sensitive services so that families will have appropriate access to the information they need to make complex medical decisions. Treatment decisions for critical care have both medical and moral consequences and can have an enormous impact on a family's subsequent grief experience and attempts to come to terms with the death. Confusion because of cultural or linguistic differences and misunderstandings can be extremely costly to the recovery process for grieving families. It is simply unacceptable for us in the treatment field to inadvertently add to the emotional burdens of grieving families.

Bereavement and the Tension of Acculturation

The fit between an ethnic minority individual and society is influenced by many complex factors, including exposure to other subcultures through acculturation. When dealing with the diverse ethnic and cultural backgrounds of the significant immigrant population in the United States, clinicians encounter a wide range of variations in the interweaving of majority culture institutions, such as the funeral industry or the medical profession, and an individual family's ethnic and religious background.

In addressing the serious lack of ethnic or cultural awareness in the mental health system's response to patient symptomatology in general, and grief responses in particular, a number of recent writers have attempted to catalog ethnic practices in order to raise clinician awareness of normative ethnic diversity (McGoldrick et al., 1991). It has become customary in traditional mental health practice to create diagnostic norms for the designation of health and illness and even to measure the wide range of human reactions to distress in terms of norms. These norms do not reflect the impact of gender, cultural, racial, or ethnic differences; developmental circumstances; or social and situational context on the symbolic or symptomatic representation of distress. This overall problem in the field of mental health is perhaps best exemplified by the absence of consideration of such variables in the American Psychiatric Association's *Diagnostic and Statistical*

Manual of Mental Disorders (3rd edition, revised), or *DSM-III-R* (Pope & Johnson, 1987). The new edition of the *Diagnostic and Statistical Manual of Mental Disorders* (*DSM-IV*), while noting these problems of social and cultural context, has not yet changed its basic approach (American Psychiatric Association, 1994).

Writers in the field of cross-cultural psychiatry have attempted to address this problem by documenting the cultural beliefs that guide the distinct responses of members of different cultural groups to circumstances of extreme distress. One typical illustration of this approach is the documentation that members of such subcultures as the Hispanic or Portuguese are more likely to somatize their distress, that is, present their psychological anguish in the form of physical symptoms. Another culture-bound syndrome discussed in the mental health literature is the Puerto Rican *ataque*, characterized by a seizure-like fit with no organic basis. Of course, it is our own culturally biased perspective that views somatization as more "primitive" and pathological than mental symptoms. Yet it might be just as accurate to say that the aforementioned cultures, unlike more technologically oriented ones, recognize more clearly the interrelatedness between emotional states and physical health. Just as tears are viewed as a physically direct, appropriate expression of sadness, so too may the more physically wrenching experiences of grief, such as pain in the chest and heart or difficulty breathing, be viewed as appropriate.

There are other grief responses that would be labeled as pathological by mainstream American clinicians and as normal by members of minority groups. Hallucinations of the deceased, which are often experienced by the acutely bereaved (Bowlby, 1980), are thought in American mainstream culture to diminish after the early, acute bereavement reaction, but members of other cultural groups report hallucinations of the deceased more frequently and more persistently. For example, the Hopi describe hallucinations in the bereaved as commonplace for a long period after the death (Eisenbruch, 1984b).

The simple cataloging of cultural differences, while a useful initial means of combating the tendency to judge all cultural groups by majority norms, can itself lead to ethnic tribalism in which groups that are complex, evolving psychosocial organizations are reduced to a few stereotypically generalized features (Seedat & Nell, 1990). There is a danger that clinicians may feel they have learned about a culture once they have mastered knowledge of these stereotyped characteristics— or, equally unfortunate, they may conclude that only another member of the same culture can contribute to improving the mental health of a minority patient or family. An overly great emphasis on cultural characteristics can also obscure the complicated interweaving of cultural features with the highly individualized subjective interpretation of those features by any particular individual or family.

Addressing the impact of political structures on family therapy in South Africa, Seedat and Nell (1990) point out that cross-cultural psychology can be used to justify racist or colonial thinking. Segregation practices are justified in terms of race-based differences, a technique that inevitably places the politically subjugated group in a lower category in terms of mental health needs or capacity for growth. These and other writers suggest that the therapist who wishes to help patients who fall outside of (and therefore, implicitly, below) the dominant culture's standards needs to address not just cultural differences but socioeconomic and gender differences as well. Moreover, the exploitation and relational problems that result from sociocultural tensions affect the psychological health of members of both dominant and oppressed groups (Lerner, 1986). Power asymmetries are preserved through the dominant culture's control of the definitions of successful functioning and optimal mental health and its tendency to view these as inborn characteristics of the individual rather than as consequences of a society's unjust distribution of power and resources (Prilleltensky, 1989).

Finally, ethnic minorities in the United States are not static groups with unchanging cultural traditions and values. Rather, we are groups of people in cultural transition and evolution, groups with complex immigration histories, from Mayflower Puritans to Vietnamese boat people, and different patterns of relating to the U.S. "melting pot" ideology. The area of bereavement therapy may, in fact, be one of the areas of mental health work in which assessment of a family's relationship to ethnic cultural traditions is especially important, even when that family appears acculturated to the secular American culture. Theorists and mental health practitioners frequently observe that under circumstances of life cycle transition, stress, or loss, individuals and families are more likely to draw upon what has been called their "ideological ethnicity," that is, those customs and beliefs that are not fundamental to the person's daily life but that provide a deep reservoir of understanding with which to make sense of important life events (Eisenbruch, 1984a, 1984b; Harwood, 1981). With the death of a family member, when the sense of continuity with the past is most severely disrupted, even families who are highly assimilated to mainstream culture often seek out funeral rituals that will enhance their sense of continuity with an ancestral past.

Eisenbruch (1984b) notes that many American families who are in some state of transition to the mainstream culture find themselves wishing to create a funeral ritual and other bereavement observances that affirm their ancestral cultural history even though they lack knowledge of these customs and their strands in the complex interweaving of cultural traditions that inform our ritual approach to bereavement. Even in the traditional cultures of other countries, for example, in the East African and the Australian aboriginal cultures, the process of Westernization and the destruction of traditional sources of education that provided for continuity of ancestral knowledge represent losses in the individual's capacity for dealing with death and grief that may leave the bereaved with increased vulnerability for ill health.

LIMITATIONS OF THE MENTAL HEALTH FIELD'S OWN ASSUMPTIONS

The loss of embeddedness of individuals in a culturally supported web of connections with church, community, and family traditions has left a social vacuum that many observers believe has been filled by mental health providers, an outcome that has many advantages as well as some largely undiscussed disadvantages. While the field of mental health has a great deal to contribute to our understanding of grieving families, their experience, and their pathways toward recovery, it is clear that we therapists are still substantially in the dark about the complex individual, familial, and social processes that are stimulated by the death of a close family member.

Mental health practitioners have operated with unexamined biases and values, contributed by our field's own assumptions, that dictate our advice to and attitude toward grieving families. I have already discussed the assumptions made by psychoanalytic theory about the "decathexis" of the lost object and the assumptions initially made by crisis theory about the 6-to-8-week limit on acute grief. The mental health field continues to assume that the open, direct verbal expression of the emotions of sorrow, anger, and anxiety is in all instances the appropriate way to resolve grief in a healthy or well-adjusted way. The field of family therapy, too, has made its assumptions about the benefits of open rather than closed communication in the grieving family system. Unfortunately, what we fail to understand as being part of the field's development, we are more likely to see as pathological. Currently, we are more realistic as a mental health field about the long-term nature of recovery from grief and the importance of maintaining connections to the deceased. We do, however, emphasize grief feelings as a step in letting go and moving on.

Yet recent studies suggest a much more complex relationship than we have assumed in the clinical literature between confrontational (open) versus avoidant (closed) strategies for managing grief. The work of Polak and his collaborators (Polak et al., 1975), who provided immediate intensive interventions with families who had experienced a sudden, unanticipated death, found upon evaluation and follow-up that the families who participated in the intervention were in fact more symptomatic and troubled than the families who had received no services at all. On the basis of their research these writers suggest that families may in some ways benefit from closing down or avoiding the subject of grief—or at least opening it up at their own pace. Stroebe and Stroebe (1991), in a study of avoidant versus confrontational styles of mourning in widows and widowers, found that self-reported avoidance of memories of the deceased was correlated with depression in men but not in women. They suggest that for men, whose cultural roles make it possible for them to be more effectively distracted from grief, avoidance may be more of a handicap than for women, who are more likely to be confronted with their loss as a natural outcome of their instrumental and emotional social roles.

In a paper provocatively entitled "The Myths of Coping with Loss," Wortman and Silver (1989) also question the assumptions made within the mental health field about the nature of healthy, appropriate grieving. They note that there is a wide range of behaviors in the expression of distress or depression both immediately after and several years after the death of a family member. While many family members do experience deep sadness and directly express this dimension of their grief, there is a substantial proportion of the population that does not react to the death of a family member with profound sadness or depression. Wortman and Silver conclude that we know very little about the grief experiences that are adequate for the resumption of healthy functioning, and they question the assumption made most frequently by mental health practitioners, namely, that it is imperative for healthy mourning that family members mourn and "get it out" immediately after the loss so as to "complete" their mourning within a specified period of time. Similarly, Leon (1992) argues that parental grief reactions after a stillbirth vary widely across individuals and cannot be prescribed either by mental health professionals or by the culture at large.

Silverman and Worden (1992), in a preliminary report from a longitudinal study of school-age children's grief reactions following the death of a parent, note that parents of grieving children often express concern that their children are not openly and directly expressing grief at the loss of the deceased parent. These authors find that at the point in the bereavement process they are currently analyzing—4 months after the death of a parent—children express their grief by frequent references to the missing parent rather than by expressions of sadness and loss. Silverman and Worden argue that the process of remembering and reestablishing direct ties to the now missing parent may in fact be the more important and useful grief process for the child's ongoing developmental work of reinternalizing the missing parent. Yet clinicians and the culture at large recommend direct expressions of grief and often see elaborate reminiscences of the dead family member as an indication of a child's failure in "letting go."

The involvement of the mental health field in bereavement work also runs the risk of professionalizing and stigmatizing a normal developmental process that would ordinarily be taken care of by families using ordinary resources of social support. Many families, in fact, turn to each other in self-help or mutual support programs, such as the Widow-to-Widow program (Silverman, 1986) or Compassionate Friends (Rando, 1986; Videka-Sherman & Lieberman, 1985). Although these groups at times use professional consultation, they tend to emphasize the shared experience of recovery and the help the recently bereaved receive from those who have already "been there." While the self-help group format is not for everyone—and some participants experience the groups as creating their own culture of assumptions about the stages of good grieving—these groups provide an alternative to the professional support of bereavement.

One example of the professionalization of bereavement is the creation of rituals for the commemoration of the lost loved one. In the field of family therapy in general, therapists have been addressing the loss of traditional rituals that were once embedded in everyday life, and bereavement therapists have noted that the absence of ritual for completing the psychological work required in mourning has adverse consequences. Grief therapists have been recommending the collaborative creation of bereavement rituals as part of the therapy process; rituals that feel psychologically meaningful are decided upon and actualized (Imber-Black, 1991; Rando, 1985). For many of those patients who have lost continuity with their family history and who lack a knowledge of ritual observance, the therapeutic creation of ritual is a beneficial process. Therapists who recommend the creation of such therapeutic rituals to commemorate a person who has died or to mark a significant turning point in the grief process advise that this process should be cocreated by therapist and patient rather than prescribed by the therapist. Otherwise, the therapist may begin to occupy the precarious role of high priest or priestess in an as yet unarticulated new religion.

A family developmental perspective recognizes that during times of overwhelming change due to family life cycle transitions families attempt to balance the discontinuity of their current lives with a continuity with past traditions and identifications. Because a therapist with this perspective interprets a family's turning to family-of-origin beliefs and rituals and their revival of "ideological ethnicity" (Harwood, 1981) as an attempt to create intergenerational continuity so as to balance the disorienting process of rapid change, he or she might find it most constructive to help such a family identify resources consistent with their cultural background that could help generate meaningful rituals to enhance the family's cultural and ancestral ties.

The complex participation of the mental health community as a culture with its own assumptions and its own vested interests is itself a complex subject and cannot be treated fully in this chapter (Cushman, 1990). Therapists are, after all, in the business of treatment, and we might find that economic incentives lead us to underestimate how much families can do on their own through their own available resources (Albee, 1992; Prilleltensky, 1989).

Attention to cultural constructions of the bereavement experience, including an awareness of the mental health field as a subculture with its own assumptions about "good," or "healthy," and "bad," or "sick," grief, is crucial in designing intervention strategies for supporting optimal family adjustment to the grief experience. An analysis of grief as a culturally embedded relational developmental process can be used to help families themselves examine the match between their own cultural and family assumptions and traditions concerning grief and their own needs for supporting the ongoing development of their family relationships. The most growth-enhancing bereavement practices support a balance between the comfort of family traditions that affirm a sense of intergenerational continuity and the value of exploring and encouraging individual expressions of unique reactions and needs. From a family developmental perspective, the creative integration of cultural or family tradition and personal innovation promotes the most flexible adaptation by family members to the overwhelming sense of loss and encourages their shared reconstruction of a satisfying new family life. In promoting this arduous and creative family developmental process, we as therapists cannot afford to impose our own views of cultural traditions. Instead, we need to help families become aware of these tensions at the interface of historical, cultural, familial, and individual experience so as to resolve them in a way that best suits their own needs and current life circumstances.

CHAPTER 12

The Interweaving
of Cultural Background
and Family
Developmental History

THE STORY OF A DAUGHTER'S GRIEF

BACKGROUND

The complex interweaving of cultural and family developmental factors in a family's bereavement experience is illustrated by the Ruiz family, originally from rural Puerto Rico and now living in Boston. Gloria Ruiz, a 50-year-old mother of 11 children, was described as a vital, energetic and charming woman who was adored by all her children. She was a dominant figure in all their lives, and insisted successfully on having things done her way. At the time of Mrs. Ruiz's death from a brain tumor, the household consisted of Carmen, a 32-year-old unmarried daughter; her brother Mario, age 24 and drug dependent; and her two half siblings, Roberto, age 16, and Luisa, age 11.

Carmen, the third oldest of the 11 children, had helped her mother take care of her younger siblings from the time she was 8, when her alcoholic father was hit by a car and killed. Mrs. Ruiz was pregnant with Mario at the time her husband was killed, and Mario remained her "baby" in the family, along with the later-born Roberto and Luisa. Carmen, compliant and close to her mother, was chosen as her mother's helper over her older sister Vilma. Carmen remained at home as her siblings grew up and left the household to raise their own families, always helping with the care of the household and family, although never directly in charge.

The older siblings agreed that Mrs. Ruiz "spoiled" the three young-

240

est children, the poor results of which were already evident in Mario's unemployment and drug addiction. However, all family members agreed that there was no stopping Mrs. Ruiz from having her way. As much as Carmen remained devoted to the care of her family, she was treated as a somewhat marginal or ridiculous figure by her older siblings, perhaps because of her very willingness to remain devoted to her mother without setting off on a life of her own. There was a distinct Cinderella quality to Carmen's central, and thankless, role in the family.

The family was referred for treatment because the two younger children, Roberto and Luisa, were refusing to accept the authority of their older sister Carmen, now their legal guardian, and were behaving in a rebellious and angry way when she attempted to discipline them. Most of the married siblings lived in the neighborhood, and Luisa would often run away to the home of one of her other sisters, complaining that Carmen was mean and crazy, an accusation the older siblings had no difficulty believing to be true.

While the grief experience was intense and powerful in this family, the initial clinical concern was the reorganization of the family's caretaking system. Vicky Borres, a Puerto Rican family therapist, worked with Carmen to help her make the transition from a somewhat denigrated delegate of her mother's unquestioned authority to the role of appropriate parental authority in her own right. Initially, treatment consisted primarily of family sessions in which Carmen was helped to establish a better sense of her own authority as the parent in charge and to set stricter limits with her siblings. At the same time, the difficulty Roberto and Luisa were experiencing in accepting their sister in the role of mother when they had just lost their mother was acknowledged. After 6 months of these family sessions, a year after Mrs. Ruiz's death, family relationships were greatly improved. Carmen was providing more consistent authority without being domineering, and Roberto and Luisa were responding with more appreciation for and less resentment of their sister's new role. However, the clinical team felt that Carmen, who had always been so attached to her mother, would need individual therapy to help her go on with her own life as someone other than a caretaker to her siblings.

ATTACHMENT BEYOND THE GRAVE: RENEGOTIATING THE BALANCE BETWEEN SELF-ASSERTION AND FAMILY LOYALTY

When she began individual therapy with me, a year and 3 months after her mother's death, Carmen disclosed that she saw her mother every day. She interpreted the nightly dreams in which her mother came and spoke to her as real visitations from her mother and believed that her spirit was still literally present in the household. In addition, she kept her mother's room exactly as it was at the time of her illness and death. Although it was now officially Luisa's bedroom, Luisa was too terrified to sleep there, and both she and Roberto slept in Carmen's bed. The clothes her mother had worn before she died were still in the room, unwashed, and Carmen would often enter her mother's room to smell them because they so vividly evoked her physical presence.

The siblings differed in their relationship to their mother's spiritual presence and in their attitude toward Carmen's intense, enduring relationship with their mother's spirit. Roberto and Luisa agreed that their mother continued to be a physical presence in the household, since sounds would emanate from her bedroom, especially during the night, and they would also sometimes see her. Luisa maintained that a music box with a moving clown on top could sometimes be heard playing at night, when no one was in the room, and she understood this to be her mother's spirit wishing to hear her favorite music. Unlike Carmen, who welcomed her mother's enduring spiritual presence, Roberto and Luisa were terrified by this ongoing haunting sense of their mother's restless spirit. Roberto and Luisa's fear of their mother's spiritual presence may reflect, at least in part, their greater exposure and acculturation to majority cultural beliefs in the United States, on the basis of which these otherworldly visits would be viewed as spooky and menacing rather than as a culturally congruent dimension of the spiritual relationship with a deceased family member.

The older siblings who lived outside the household at first supported Carmen's belief in the enduring physical presence of their mother's spirit. After their mother's death, several of them had experienced these spiritual visitations or dreams of their mother. The family found these visions of their mother to be understandable and appropriate manifestations of her spirit. However, during the second year after their mother's death, the siblings began to insist that Carmen was preventing their mother's spirit from gaining the freedom from this world and release into heaven that it deserved. They complained that Carmen was preventing their mother's departure by so urgently maintaining her earthly contact with her, by so desperately needing her. They believed that Carmen's close relationship with their mother's spirit was no longer appropriate and that their mother's spirit was responding to Carmen's needs rather than its own. They insisted that only if Carmen was willing to let go of this unnatural attachment would their mother's spirit finally be released.

Because of her many years of personal sacrifice and devotion to the family, it seemed to me only fair that the siblings grant Carmen the right to release their mother's spirit at her own pace, through an exploration determined by her own emotional and developmental needs rather than the needs and expectations of others. Consistent with a family developmental model, I assumed that Carmen's enduring relationship with her mother reflected vitally important dimensions of that relationship that Carmen needed to maintain her own psychological stability.

Our therapeutic work, then, began simply with an acknowledgment of her mother's specialness and importance in her life. Initially, Carmen needed to remember and grieve her mother, whom she described as a beautiful, loving, generous, magnetically charismatic figure who had died a long and undeservedly painful death. During her mother's last months Carmen had been especially pained by the loss of her mother's vitality, exemplified by her full figure, which was tragically reduced during her illness to a skeletal shell. Because Carmen had not understood the course of her mother's illness, we reviewed and translated the medical record from the hospital for her. Carmen had simply not believed that her mother, who was so vibrant a person, could succumb to this mysterious disease, and she had clung to the hope that she would recover, a hope bolstered by the fact that her mother continued to be, until the very end, fully aware and in complete psychological control of herself and the family. For this reason, Carmen experienced her mother's death from cancer as sudden and unexpected.

As with anyone who experiences the grueling ordeal of a loved one's slow death from cancer, Carmen existed in the last months and weeks of her mother's life in a world that had become narrower and narrower. Carmen's mother was home during a good deal of her illness, and Carmen took responsibility for her physical care. Carmen, like most family members who experience the death of a loved one from cancer, was preoccupied with the medical process that extends life as long as possible, and perhaps this aided her own process of denial. In addition to the psychological dimension of denial, Carmen's cultural and linguistic differences from the medical staff involved in her mother's care made it difficult for her to understand the progression of her mother's illness and the rationale for the medical interventions, such as surgery and chemotherapy, which often seemed to be so much worse than the illness itself. Carmen's experience of confusion concerning the basic medical facts of her mother's illness and treatment highlights the importance of maintaining on medical units family services that are linguistically appropriate and culturally sensitive.

While the anticipation of a death is considered helpful to a good outcome for survivors, the beneficial effects seem to accrue only if the illness is of a relatively brief duration, no more than 6 months. If the illness is longer, family members who share caretaking are likely to be left exhausted by the physical care of the terminally ill. Further, they must endure the psychological burden of watching their loved one physically deteriorate, becoming a shadow of his or her former self. After such an experience, most family members describe themselves as being preoccupied with images of the final scenes of the illness, at home or in the hospital, in much the same way that an image of sudden trauma is difficult to surmount. For a period of months—and in some instances for years—family members describe themselves as having difficulty retrieving memories of the loved one that precede the traumatizing experience of their physical illness and decline.

Carmen had her own developmentally compelling reasons for holding on to her mother and refusing to prepare for her death. Most mourners, though, find that even when they anticipate a death with a great deal of forewarning, they experience it as sudden and shocking and that even when their loved one has already long been inaccessible owing to heavy sedation, delirium, or coma, they nevertheless experience a sense of the person as present right up to the moment of the death. Once a person has finally died, a new level of grief work is undertaken that I myself have never heard families describe as part of their anticipatory grief.

During Carmen's exploration of the circumstances of her mother's death, her idealization of her mother was not confronted. In doing the work of retrieving more complete memories of her mother from before her illness, Carmen began to slowly explore and remember their multifaceted relationship. She began to consider that her mother's control of the family was not always for the good. During the growing-up years of Mario, Roberto, and Luisa, she had often complained that her mother set no limits with the children. Mrs. Ruiz, in turn, accused Carmen of being cruelly competitive and harsh with her younger siblings. Carmen felt that her mother had never acknowledged how much she had sacrificed to help care for her siblings. Carmen, who after 5 years in the United States still spoke little English, enrolled in an English program at a local Latino advocacy center. In addition, she began dating—something she had never done before—a man who had been known to the family but whom she had never before considered as a boyfriend.

The exploration of her own independent identity created an enormous psychological upheaval for Carmen, who began to experience extraordinary psychological distress. First, she began to have dreams in which her mother's spirit was angrily reprimanding her for neglecting her younger siblings. In these dreams Carmen would feel stricken with pain, guilt, and remorse that she was displeasing her mother and failing to properly fulfill her responsibilities as her siblings' guardian. Rather than confront Carmen in any way that would challenge her carefully protected, and very much needed, image of her mother as a supportive, idealized presence, I began to work with her on how she might present her own side of things to her mother in a way that affirmed the enduring nature of their relationship and her continuing obligation to fulfill her filial responsibilities. After all, Mrs. Ruiz had managed to care for her family as a devoted mother while still maintaining an active social life of her own, which included relationships with others outside the family circle and, after her husband's death, with boyfriends as well. It seemed to me that Carmen could, in her presentation to the spirit of her mother, help Mrs. Ruiz understand that her need for a life of her own should be considered along with the needs of her siblings. Carmen was very relieved to find that as a result of these discussions of her contribution to the family and her need for a life of her own, her mother's criticisms during her "visits" ceased. Carmen's images of her mother criticizing her for neglecting her family responsibilities gave way to images of her mother mournfully wishing she could rejoin the family, who looked so happy and *gorditos* ("plump"). In these images Mrs. Ruiz was complimenting Carmen for being a good, caring "mother" whose children were thriving.

Carmen continued to feel that living a life of her own was a serious challenge to her ongoing family responsibilities on behalf of her mother. She placed this family tradition of a daughter's responsibility in an intergenerational context, because her grandmother had been similarly taken care of by a daughter, Mrs. Ruiz's younger sister, Rosa. Aunt Rosa had married and had children of her own, but she had always lived with her mother in rural Puerto Rico. Rosa had a "breakdown" after her mother's death, and at the time of my treatment of Carmen she was still seeing her mother's spirit in her home, as was one of her daughters. In telling this story, Carmen was torn between admiration of her aunt for her loyalty to her mother and pity for her because her life was still haunted by disturbing visitations from her mother's restless spirit.

In her daily life Carmen struggled between her sense of obligation to care for others and a growing sense of entitlement to attend to her own needs and live her own life. She began to experience moments of intense rage, the first she had given expression to in her life, when she felt particularly exploited by her family or by her boyfriend. She gradually began to modulate these intense responses as she became more aware of this behavioral pattern in which she would take care of other people at her own expense and then give way to an overwhelming sense of rage. Carmen began to set limits earlier in the cycle of self-sacrifice and subsequent rage and to give her own needs more consistent consideration, a development that brought new luxury to her life.

DISCUSSION

While Mrs. Ruiz's death was very painful for the entire family, it was experienced by each sibling in a way that was determined by his or her age and position in the family system. Although the younger siblings, especially Luisa, could be seen as potentially the most developmentally affected by the death of their mother, the family's history and developmental circumstances generated an extremely vulnerable position for Carmen. In fact, the distortion of Carmen's development in response to the family's bereavement experience began not with the death of her mother but with the death of her father. After her father's death 8-year-old Carmen was withdrawn from school and called upon to help as a family caretaker, thus altering whatever developmental course she might have followed. Carmen was selected, in contrast to her older sister Vilma, because she showed herself to be closer to her mother and more cooperative with her mother's needs. Mrs. Ruiz remained very much the head of the household, with Carmen functioning as a satellite in her orbit rather than as a person in her own right.

Carmen's grief work of developmental integration in response to her mother's death was all the more monumental because she not only had to take on the authority of the family's primary caretaker but also had to discover how to consider her own needs after a lifetime in which they had a very low priority in the family hierarchy. While the first stage of Carmen's therapy addressed the change in family caretaking structure, the second stage needed to address the developmental processes that had been interrupted when Carmen became an assistant family caretaker after her father's death.

As has already been discussed in previous chapters, the death of a family member generates a period of denial during which the mourner attempts to slowly assimilate the reality of the death and incorporate the many changes, both in daily routine and in the inner organization of emotions and identity, that the loss of the loved one precipitates. For Carmen, the developmental work of grieving her mother and rebuilding a sense of self in her mother's absence was initially overwhelming, for Carmen had from a very early age relied on her mother for her sense of self. In addition, she felt herself to be within a family tradition of devoted daughters who could not live their own lives without their mothers.

Carmen's position in the family system as the unappreciated Cinderella and the interruption of her own development required by this position made her all the more developmentally fragile at the time of her mother's death. Because the task of rebuilding her identity required a shift in both the family organization and her own individual developmental course, Carmen needed a moratorium during which she continued to keep her mother by her side. Since the Puerto Rican culture is more comfortable than the secular American culture with the idea that the deceased continues to exist in the family as a spiritual presence, Carmen was able to make use of this cultural belief to extend the time she needed to absorb the reality of her loss. However, out of her own developmental vulnerabilities she remained involved with her mother's spiritual presence beyond the time deemed appropriate by the rest of her family, who believed her overly intense involvement was interfering with their mother's spiritual peace.

The most pivotal maturational process for Carmen, for which she needed therapeutic support, was the development of the capacity to recognize and consider her own emotions and to act in ways that were determined not simply by the needs of others but by her own needs as well. In Carmen's experience this degree of autonomy contradicted her mother's wishes, wishes made all the more powerful because they were first voiced at the time of her mother's bereavement after the death of Carmen's father. Carmen could not give up the feeling that living her own life meant abandoning the responsibilities that her mother had delegated to her and that had become her reason for living. Because of these developmental conflicts, Carmen needed to create an especially lengthy transitional or "liminal" period during which her mother was still present. We used that transitional period to therapeutic advantage by encouraging Carmen to present to her mother's spirit her arguments for setting more limits with her younger siblings, for her own benefit as well as theirs.

While Carmen made considerable progress after her mother died in venturing out into her own life, she continued to be quite emotionally vulnerable for two reasons. First, she was trying out psychological experiences and life activities that were quite new to her and that she was unaccustomed to modulating on her own. Second, she had to struggle with the sense of guilt that her evolving autonomy was a violation of her loyalty to her mother and that it was severing the very connection that had been so important to her throughout her life. It was important to respect Carmen's definition of the therapy process as one of helping her work out her ongoing relationship with her mother through her dreams, rather than confront her with her need for "letting go" (which, as therapists bound by our own personal and cultural perspective, we might have been tempted to do).

On the other hand, as Carmen's therapist, I was not willing to accept a restricted definition of her developmental course, in which remaining loyal to her mother's memory meant continuing to sacrifice any opportunity to live her own life on her own terms. I felt that it was quite possible for Carmen to balance her family loyalty and obligations with a consideration of her own needs and that her initial difficulty in doing so represented a maladaptive family adjustment rather than the expression of a culturally determined family pattern.

I fully realize the intrinsic difficulty in judging the value of different cultural traditions and the terrible problems that can arise when we therapists impose our own culturally or personally determined values on vulnerable patients who depend on us for responsible objectivity. As therapists we must never presume to know which dimensions of the experience of a family whose culture differs from our own constitute a useful or appropriate cultural tradition and which dimensions constrain optimal family health. At the same time, I believe it is important and necessary as a responsible member of any group—family, professional community, or culture—to critically assess beliefs and assumptions about family functioning so that we do not support potentially destructive practices simply because they are normatively held by a particular group. While some cultures might hold to traditions in which they negate the active selfhood of women or the emotional expressiveness and dependence of men, it seems to me that a climate of social justice that promotes optimal health must grant the full rights of personhood to all its members. At the same time, we have to remain sensitive to the ways individuals and families need to remain connected to their cultural context and to support moves toward independent self-definition that do not disrupt or sever the individual's ties to a very much needed web of family and community relationships. The best safeguards against the arbitrary imposition of one's own values are created by upholding the highest standards for respectful listening and close collaboration with our patients and their families. Carmen's increased independence was in fact supported by her family and viewed as a long-overdue process of maturation and personal growth.

If we listen respectfully to our patients with a willingness to learn about our own embedded cultural assumptions and our points of difference as well as points of convergence, we stand the best chance of helping families work out their own best—that is, most emotionally satisfying and most growth-promoting—response to the tragic reality of family death and loss. We therapists may inadvertently promote our own closely held, self-protective personal and cultural beliefs at the expense of the families we work with. Our only protection from this unconscious and all too human abuse of our power as practitioners is to remain as self-aware and as self-critical as possible. This attitude of open, respectful listening is extremely difficult to maintain, given the emotionally overwhelming and disorienting experience of truly listening to the pain of grieving families, especially when attending to cultural differences threatens to expose aspects of our own belief systems which are part of our ongoing, unexamined life adaptations. Attendance at a Latino Catholic or African-American Southern Baptist funeral, with their far greater acceptance of detailed reminiscences and open, often dramatic expression of grief, could leave a member of our mainstream culture with the disturbing impression that our funeral practices are relatively barren and painfully devoid of a deep, emotion-laden remembering of the deceased. Yet with an attitude of open, respectful listening and a willingness to tolerate the painful disorientation of new learning, we can make our work with grieving families a resource for the expansion of our own growth.

CONCLUSION: EXPANDING OUR CULTURE-BOUND NOTIONS OF FAMILY BEREAVEMENT

What have we learned about a sociocultural perspective on bereavement from our discussion of the literature and the extensive case description of Carmen Ruiz and her family that can inform our ongoing clinical work with families? First, I believe that awareness of sociocultural influences is vital to our understanding of family bereavement. Our deepest emotional experiences, our attachments to beloved family members, are lived out within the mundane work of day-to-day family living. The death of a family member disrupts the work of the family, which must reorganize the ways members fulfill family work roles as well as family emotional functions. Our family relationships provide the stability and continuity necessary for ongoing family development. When a close family member dies and we face the destabilizing discontinuity of the intense sorrow, rage, and confusion of bereavement, we turn to rituals as a means of establishing some sense of stability, social support, and continuity with cultural and family traditions.

The death of a family member exposes our culture's social arrangements, since the bereaved are forced to recognize the social losses precipitated by the death of a pivotal member. This is perhaps most acutely experienced with the death of a spouse. The price widows pay for our culture's polarized gender roles is pointed out by the examples of Gail Kaplan (Chapter 4) and Helen Golden (Chapter 9) who have had to struggle to reclaim lost aspects of their family role and personal identity that they had invested in their husbands. Even the death of a child, though, exposes and challenges our social arrangements, although a child cannot be said to fulfill family work role functions the way an adult member does: In culturally promoting isolated nuclear families; polarized gender roles; and intense relationships between parents and children, especially between mothers and children, our society creates social circumstances in which the death of a child becomes a life event from which many people fear they will never recover. Men are forced to experience overwhelming feelings for which their gender role arrangements did not prepare them, and women are forced to face the centrality of parenting in their lives at a time when the loss of the opportunity to parent feels unbearable.

Our cultural assumptions—that death severs all bonds to the deceased; that people recover from the loss of a close family member relatively quickly; that people become free to form new attachments; and that the feelings of grief, while initially intense and acute, can be handled privately—do not fit the experience of most of the bereaved. Other cultures accept more continuity than ours does between the spiritual and material worlds and provide more freedom for emotional expression, yet each culture can be seen to have its costs and benefits in promoting the adaptation and ongoing development of any particular family.

Carmen Ruiz and her grief experience illustrate the complex interweaving of individual and family history, family structure, and cultural factors in determining the bereavement experiences of its members. Carmen's grief experience is best understood as her own creative, psychologically supportive, and personally integrative interpretation of cultural practice in the context of her own life history and family relationships. We minimize both her pain and her creative attempts at mastery if we view her grief as an example either of psychopathology or of typical cultural practice. We can best help families from any cultural background by appreciating the importance of their cultural practices and beliefs as living, evolving traditions that provide continuity with community and with family history at a time when they desperately need to balance the discontinuity of change. As therapists we should always be prepared to hear the ways our patients contradict our personally, professionally, and culturally determined ideas about the nature of psychopathology, the relationship between the living and the dead, the emotional experience of grief, and the length of time it takes to recover one's social functioning. If we are willing to be humbled and surprised by what our patients know about living with death and grief, we are in a much better position to support their own best efforts toward growth and change.

CHAPTER 13

The Circumstances of the Death and the Structure of Grief

A VIOLENT DEATH: THE MURDER OF RAFAEL GOMEZ

I met 7-year-old Carlos Gomez and his 32-year-old mother, Ana, 10 days after the murder of their father and husband, Rafael Gomez, who was shot in the living room of their home (The grief experience of the Gomez family was described in Chapter 9 when discussing the bereaved child's increased burden of responsibility for a grieving parent). Two men, strangers to the family, had entered their home, tied up Carlos and his mother in the adjoining bedroom, fired a series of shots, and then left the house. Ana was able to free herself and Carlos, and the two of them entered the living room to find that Rafael had been killed, shot in the head and body. Although the murder had the appearance of a drug-related crime, Ana insisted that her husband, who ran his own small-appliance repair business, was a deeply religious family man who could not have had any dealings with criminals. She had to assume that there had been some confusion, a matter of mistaken identity, so little did her husband's violent death reflect the quality of his life.

Ana had taken Carlos and fled from their now violated home in the city, a home where they had lived together as a family but that was now indelibly seared in their mind's eye as the scene of Rafael's murder. While Ana, fearing the murderers would be looking for her and Carlos, concentrated her energies on their need to find safety, 7-year-old Carlos struggled with a different fear: If he and his mother left their home, where they had always lived, how would his father know where to find them? Ana sought shelter in her sister's home in a nearby community, where she immediately enrolled Carlos in school, and both mother and son began the long, arduous process of putting back together their traumatized psyches and shattered lives. Ana's sister, Maria, herself profoundly grieving her brother-in-law's death, was all the more alarmed by the frightening changes she saw in both her sister and her nephew; it was she who insisted, 10 days after the death, that the whole family seek a therapeutic consultation.

At the time I met them, Carlos and Ana were sleeping together on the fold-out couch in her sister's crowded apartment, their reaction to the loss of husband and father characterized by what we would diagnostically term posttraumatic stress disorder. Accompanied by Carlos and her sister, Ana came to the first evaluation session in a numb state of profound depression easily penetrated by panicked fearfulness. Carlos, in contrast, was all raw, exposed nerves. If I had not known the nature of his recent traumatic experience, I would have described him as the most hyperactive of children with Attention Deficit Disorder; his movements were frenetic, his attention easily distracted, his speech and actions a rapid-fire flow of intrusive, violent images and compensatory bravado. In the joint interview he was keenly focused on his mother's mood; he remained standing, as if in the interests of protecting her safety, and put his considerable charm into soothing and entertaining her. In an individual play-therapy interview conducted by Esther Gross, Carlos immediately let her know that he was eager to tell his story and explore the vivid details of his father's violent death. Carlos, as most young children would have been, was both horrified and fascinated by what he had seen. He (like most of us) had no idea how much blood a single living body could spill. Carlos's family was deeply religious, and he had been reassured that his father had gone to heaven. But where is heaven? he wondered. Was going there like going to another city, as he and his mother had? Did this mean his father had gone someplace else to live permanently? Could they find him and persuade him to come back? Could his father, like Elvis Presley, be sighted again in spite of reports of his death? During play therapy Carlos engaged in a compelling fantasy game in which he called heaven on the toy telephone and talked to his father. At another time, enacting his fantasy, he cavorted around the therapy room and down the hallways impersonating Elvis Presley by playing an imaginary guitar and singing into an imaginary microphone; he was trying, at one and the same time, to lift his mother out of her depressed stupor and to identify with a powerful celebrity who was reportedly dead yet seemed so alive on television and in the public's imagination.

Ana, in contrast to Carlos, who discharged his overwhelming

anxiety through vigorous, driven compulsive action, longed for sleep and peace, for escape from the intolerable horror of the violent imagery that intruded on her waking thoughts and shattered her sleep, for respite from her memories of the terror and helplessness she had felt as she and Carlos waited in the next room listening to the shooting and fearing they might be killed as well, of the struggle to loosen her ties and those of Carlos, and of the nightmare vision when they entered the living room of floor and walls covered with so much blood and bits of tissue that it was impossible to clean. Her state of numb shock was nevertheless easily penetrated by all kinds of images that triggered a sequence of disturbing associations that led to the very images she was trying so hard to obliterate.

STRESSORS SPECIFIC TO THE CIRCUMSTANCES OF THE DEATH

The distinctive traumatic grief reactions of the wife and son of Rafael Gomez to his violent death dramatically illustrate the importance of understanding the impact of the circumstances of the death in creating an individual's and family's grief responses. A number of researchers have concluded that the circumstances of death generate profoundly different responses in structuring both individual and family grief responses (Bowlby, 1980; Eth & Pynoos, 1985; Furman, 1974; Kliman, 1986; Leenars, 1991; Parkes & Weiss, 1983). Rather than talk about grief as a monolithic process, we find instead that we have to consider the particular circumstances of a death and of the mourners. We must ask not only who died and who they were to the family in terms of their actual day-to-day as well as psychological significance but also how they died and how much the death itself disrupted ongoing family functioning. We must ask what resources the family had available at that particular moment of the family life cycle to counterbalance the stresses that accompany a particular way of death.

A family developmental model of family bereavement emphasizes the reality of the circumstances of the death in constructing the grief experience at every level—from the social, to the family interactional, to the privately psychological. In assessing a family's grief experience, it is important to understand who died, who they were and how they contributed to the construction of the collaborative self within the family; how the current family developmental moment collides with the circumstances of the death so as to shape the family's bereavement reaction; and how the realistic balance of stress and support, continuity and discontinuity, enhances or impedes the family developmental process of growth-enhancing integration.

The death circumstances themselves frame aspects of the family grief reaction and evoke predictable reactions. For families who survive the murder of a loved one, terror and fear may take priority over other responses, as they did in the Gomez family. For families whose member died as a result of the irresponsible behavior of others, for example, a hit-and-run driver, the grief reaction involves overwhelming rage and a deep need to bring the murderer to justice. Clinical work and research in fact suggest that a successful outcome for families of murder victims depends in part on their satisfaction with the judicial outcome of the murder case (Amick-McMullan, Kilpatrick, Veronen, & Smith, 1989; Getzel & Masters, 1984; Poussaint, 1984; Rynearson, 1984).

Although the details of the circumstances of the death are enormously important in understanding grief, they are surprisingly difficult to focus on, in part because they make the experience of the death and of loss so agonizingly vivid for both the teller and the listener. The nature of the death—whether anticipated or unexpected, due to illness or accident, acute or chronic, peaceful or violent—affects the family's grief reactions in two powerful ways: through the actual accompanying stresses of a particular way of death and through the intense emotions and meanings provoked by the death's circumstances. These two dimensions of loss—one at the level of behavioral reality, the other at the level of subjective meaning—present distinct though interrelated tasks for a family's coping, organization, and integration.

With the death of Rafael Gomez, Ana and Carlos Gomez lost much more than a husband and father. Ana's means of financial support was disrupted, and her sense of safety in her own home was violated. Because she had not been able to identify the murderers and did not understand the motivation for the murder, she began to view herself as especially vulnerable in a world filled with danger.

The death of a family member, even an out-of-life-cycle death, will not necessarily be traumatic for the survivors, as was the case for the wife and son of Rafael Gomez. There is a common conception in this society that any death in the family is traumatic. However, death accompanied by violence or abrupt, unexpected disaster introduce an additional dimension of overwhelming stress and the need for more serious coping mechanisms. Traumatic grief reactions occur when a death's violent or physically overwhelming circumstances themselves force survivors to give priority to coping with their overwhelming feelings and perceptions. As Ann Burgess (1975) described it in her pioneering work on family reactions to homicide, anxiety about safety, or what she calls victim-oriented thought, takes priority over grieving the loss of the family member. In these instances of traumatic grief, which is what Ana and Carlos Gomez suffered, a posttraumatic stress disorder response takes emotional priority as the only means of managing the overwhelming horror of witnessing a violent death; the terror that such a death could be inflicted again, by anyone at any time; and the profound helplessness at having been completely overpowered and incapable of taking any action to prevent the murder (Eth & Pynoos, 1985). The emotional exploration of the loss and the psychological work of transforming the internal relationship to the deceased may need to be postponed until much later. Psychoanalytically oriented writers in the grief literature have often referred to all instances of bereavement as "psychic trauma," trivializing the violence involved under circumstances of true traumatic stress. Overuse of the designation *traumatic* obscures the radical difference between the grief reaction of Carlos Gomez and that of, for example, 7-year-old Alan Kaplan, whose father collapsed from a heart attack. Alan's work in understanding the circumstances of his father's death did not include the need to confront the reality of mutilation, deliberately malevolent physical violence, and overwhelming horror and helplessness and did not involve a sense of enduring physical danger. While faced with an agonizingly painful loss and terrible grief, Alan could confront his father's death and ask questions whose answers he could make sense of and process.

Even though traumatic grief reactions in the wake of violent death are unique and distinctive, it is important to note that many circumstances of death that would not ordinarily be thought of as traumatic, such as the last days of a terminally ill family member, can be extremely stressful for survivors. Terminal illness can result in enduring symptoms of traumatic stress in family members, who may alternate between a numb sense of unreality and vivid, intrusive ruminations or dreams reliving the terminal phase of the illness or the period just prior to the death. The circumstances of death generate particular constellations of stresses, some of which can best be described as affecting families on a continuum of stress and support. Others can only be described as creating a discontinuous leap into the domain of traumatic stress reactions, and these grief reactions will be characterized by the alternation between intrusive and numbing symptoms of a posttraumatic stress disorder. The nature and specific circumstances of the death, whether anticipated or unexpected, due to illness or accident, peaceful or violent, creates a powerful organizational event to which family members react in both their emotional responses and in their striving for understanding of the death's meaning.

Discussion of Stressors in the Child Bereavement Literature

The role of the circumstances of a death in constructing the grief reaction has been discussed in great detail in the literature on childhood grief. Erma Furman's (1974) seminal book, *A Child's Parent Dies*, was among the first to explore the importance of the actual circumstances of the death in determining the psychological organization of childhood bereavement. She pointed out that the death of a parent with still young children at home is inevitably an untimely death, whether it is violent or due to disease: "Each form of death entailed its own frightening, frustrating, overwhelming experiences for the family" (p. 101). According to Furman, the details of the death itself may coincide and become interwoven with the child's fantasies of a particular age; for example, a mutilating accident may stimulate castration anxiety in a preschooler. In Chapter 6 I described the experiences of 5-year-old David Green and his 2-year-old brother, Joshua, whose mother died in an airplane crash. Each boy incorporated the details of the accident into his fantasy life with the tools of his own developmental stage. Joshua, at a preverbal phase of development, played at jumping down from a great height. David elaborated private fantasies for warding off physical aggression, which he had connected with his father's explanation that his mother had lost consciousness prior to the fatal crash owing to a blow to her head. In addition, both boys accepted their father's explanation of their mother's death in a way he hoped would make it more tolerable for all of them: They considered the true horror to be a blow to the head rather than the conscious awareness of one's own imminent death.

Children who lose a parent are dependent on the surviving parent for an account of the death and its circumstances that they can process at their developmental stage and level but that does not flood them with unmanageable or incomprehensible imagery or information. The details of the death itself, for example, in cases of illness, may be too complex for a child with limited capacity for reality testing and a primitive understanding of causality. Because young children require so much help from adults in understanding and interpreting important life events, the adult's capacity to communicate about the death becomes extremely important to the child's understanding and coping:

It is not surprising that the child's surviving parent and other adults close to him find it difficult to help the child with his anxieties. They may not yet have mastered their own anxieties or may hope to shield the child from a similar dread. This sometimes leads a parent to deny to his child the real events and the concreteness of death. In some cases the parent attempts to alter the facts by presenting the child with an untruthful but more palatable version of what happened. (Furman, 1974, pp. 102–103)

Perhaps a parent is most likely to distort the circumstances of a death when it is a violent suicide. Cain and Fast (1966) suggest that an adult's distortions of the circumstances of death, especially when they contradict the reality of the child's own independent observations, may seriously compromise the child's capacity for ongoing reality testing.

Discussion of Stressors in the Adult Bereavement Literature

In the adult bereavement literature, the role of the circumstances of death in the construction of the grief experience has been discussed in comparing sudden death to anticipated death of a spouse (Parkes & Weiss, 1983; Stroebe & Stroebe, 1987) and in evaluating the impact of different circumstances in the death of a child on adult symptomatology (Rando, 1983; Raphael, 1983; Sanders, 1989). The circumstances of death shatter different assumptions about the safety or stability of the world; they generate different disruptions of ongoing life structure for managing the activities of daily life and evoke different intense emotions in the attempt to make sense of the death and loss and re-create a coherent understanding of one's life and the place of the death within an ongoing life structure.

Just as a child's understanding of the circumstances of a death relies on adult support for sorting out confusing dimensions of the death and its implications and meanings, so too does the adult's understanding and integration of overwhelming or traumatic life events rely on—for better or for worse—a higher authority, namely, the culture (Herman, 1992; Lebowitz & Roth, 1992). Society has its own investment in the definition of certain kinds of death, and this definition in turn most powerfully influences the family's own process of meaning making. The soldier killed in a socially defined "good war," such as World War II or the recent Gulf War, leaves his grieving family the solace of his heroism, very much in contrast to the experience of families whose men fought in the Vietnam War. During the Gulf War, Vietnam War survivors and the families of soldiers killed in the war were in fact subjected to President Bush's statement that with the Gulf War victory we had finally licked the "Vietnam syndrome," once again reinforcing the disqualification of these families and their enormous sacrifices.

Suicide survivors and, more recently, families with a member dying of AIDS are those whose bereavement experiences are regarded negatively, because of the assumption that the deaths were caused by the individual's disturbed or immoral behavior. The Life After Murder Program at Roxbury Comprehensive Medical Center, which serves an urban African-American community, was initially told by its funding source that it could only provide services to families whose murdered member was an "innocent victim." Such a distinction would have promoted a cultural definition of the meritorious dead and the guilty dead and would have completely undermined the program's credibility in a community ravaged by drugs and violence in which no such categorizations can possibly be made (Spark, 1992). Clinicians and researchers who work with family survivors of suicide and AIDS emphasize the importance of addressing the social response to the family's situation. Clinicians can help these families write an alternative narrative in which they arrive at a more positive sense of the death and its meaning (Dunne, McIntosh, & Dunne-Maxim, 1988; Walker, 1991).

Stressors and Family Bereavement

In order to understand the reality of the grief experience undergone by a particular family we need to understand not only who died and how but how much disruption to the family's stability the death caused. The circumstances of the death create the circumstances for the grief reaction, both in the specific challenges and stresses required by the process of coping with a particular way of death and in the emotions and meanings that are evoked by a particular way of death. Not only the impact and meaning of the moment of death and its details but also the circumstances of the death contribute to the particular ways life is disrupted for a family and to the multiple stresses that accompany the death and its aftermath. In his work on bereavement after chronic illness, Rolland (1987, 1991) referred to the specific patterns of deterioration associated with a type of fatal illness as the psychosocial characteristics of the illness, which themselves evoke particular emotions and demand that families cope with distinct tasks. An understanding of family bereavement requires a thorough inquiry into how the specifics and consequences of the death have radically altered the course of ordinary functioning in a family's daily life. These changes in the conditions and requirements of life are often the most immediately stressful components of family bereavement. Most families place their attention and energy first on the requirements of coping with the demands of restructuring a new, stable life in the aftermath of death. It is in the emotionally textured detail of living a transformed life that the full emotional meaning of a loss emerges for a family. This attempt at reestablishing stable functioning is accompanied by attempts to reestablish stable relationship patterns for regulating shared family emotions. Finally, new shared family meanings that make sense of the loss will need to be generated, again drawing on the specific circumstances of the death and its consequences.

When a Death in the Family Means the End of a Way of Life

Silverman and Worden (1992) poignantly and accurately describe the death of a parent as the death of a way of life. Gail Kaplan's story in Chapter 4 illustrates the enormous consequences of parental death for the circumstances of daily living, with so many details of everyday life being associated with the deceased and reminding the survivors of all they have lost. When Stuart Kaplan died, leaving Gail with a 6-year-old and a 1½-year-old son, multiple details of everyday life for the family were altered. Gail was aware of this every morning when she packed the lunches and drove the children to school; before, Stuart would have taken their older son Alan to school while she took care of the baby. The routines of everyday living, previously shared in somewhat gender-typed ways, now required that Gail incorporate many of Stuart's functions as husband and father. After increasing her work hours, Gail had a new appreciation for the difficulties faced by single parents; she now had the feeling that she had many more responsibilities than one person could possibly handle. Some tasks, such as planning a family vacation, were harder than others psychologically, because they meant a deeper confrontation with losing Stuart; for example, Gail realized, with a profound sense of loss, that the family could no longer go camping because she could not manage the physically rigorous task of loading up the car with camping gear.

   The tasks of reorganizing daily living are entirely different when the mother of a young family dies (statistically, children are more likely to lose a father than a mother). The family loses its primary caretaker and perhaps a secondary source of income as well; further, most couples attempt to safeguard the family's future by purchasing life insurance for the primary financial provider but are less likely to do so for a mother not employed outside the home. Silverman and Worden (1992), in a preliminary report from their longitudinal study of

125 children who have lost a parent, found that 4 months after the death mothers were more likely than fathers to encourage their children to talk about their feelings of loss. Widowers with young children at home remarry more quickly than widows (Osterweis et al., 1984; Stroebe & Stroebe, 1987), and in cases of remarriage the new wife and stepmother is asked to take over the functions of mothering (see Chapter 6, where I present Ann Smith, whose mother died when she was 7 and whose father remarried within the year). While a stepmother may find it easy to perform household tasks, even the most generous and mature of stepmothers may find it a psychological struggle to compete with the fresh memories of the recently deceased wife and mother.

Anticipated and Unanticipated Death

An additional stressor accompanying the death of a young parent may be its sudden, unanticipated nature. Stuart Kaplan died of a sudden, unexpected heart attack, a circumstance that has been associated in the clinical and research literature with greater vulnerability to grief that is prolonged and difficult to integrate and resolve (Parkes & Weiss, 1983; Stroebe & Stroebe, 1987). Anticipated death due to chronic illness allows families to prepare for the death by giving them the opportunity both to make practical arrangements for family life afterward and to say good-bye to their loved one. Yet prolonged illness, especially if longer than 6 months in duration, has been associated with its own stressors and strains. The prolonged illness of a parent, such as David Golden's diabetes (described in Chapter 9) or Karen Smith's cardiac illness (described in Chapter 6), requires that a family focus their resources and energy on care of the ill parent, often necessarily putting the needs of well family members, including the children, second. While the family does have an opportunity to prepare for the death under these circumstances, they often describe themselves as living from one day to the next and from one medical crisis to the next. Because of the intensive medical effort to prolong life as long as possible, families may find themselves deeply compelled by the hope of prolonging a loved one's life and at some level surprised when a medical crisis escalates to the point of death. Even with an anticipated death, and even when illness has reached a terminal phase or the dying family member is in deep coma and is no longer in any accessible sense alive to the family, some aspect of the process of mourning is postponed until the moment of actual death. This postponement of grief in cases of chronic illness is often necessary with, for example, cases of cancer, which though at the medical threshold of "terminal" can involve many years of intrusive medical procedures and an ever expanding possibility of cure. But even in situations where an illness is clearly terminal and death is inevitable, some dimension of the full acknowledgment of the reality of the death is postponed until death removes the last opportunity for hope.

With an increase in the survival rates for certain kinds of cancer that were previously considered inevitably fatal and with the occasional miraculous return of a loved one from a deep coma, keeping hope alive can in fact at times seem like a vital factor in enabling a return from near death to life. Yet the work of surviving a potentially fatal illness, especially in instances that require extensive or experimental medical treatment, will require that a family's ongoing development be organized so as to support the ill family member. The sacrifices required by the demands of a chronic life-threatening illness can leave family members feeling depleted, and in some instances relieved, when death finally ends the suffering of a deteriorating member. Chronic terminal illness may also require the mobilization of intensive family attention and enormous resources up to the moment of death, leaving a void after the death in the family routine and in the psychological life of its members. While many adults describe relief at the end of a loved one's prolonged suffering after a long, painful illness, others also feel a looming emptiness in their lives, a void that is often filled by ruminative recollection of the last phase of the illness.

Coping with Life-Threatening Illness: The Donovans' Story. The texture of a grief reaction after a terminal illness and the experiences that live on and that we review and sometimes regret are shaped by the life adjustment responses required by the illness. Sheryl Donovan was a high school junior in individual therapy for depression when her mother, Katherine, was diagnosed as having breast cancer. Katherine, a competent and well-informed nurse, fought her way through the maze of contradictory recommendations and decided on the most radical combination of surgery and chemotherapy; she was determined to have the best chance possible of survival. The Donovans, accustomed to Katherine's taking a great deal of responsibility for the household, had to make an enormous adjustment to her illness. Katherine herself had always been slow to recognize when she was doing too much for others, although she and Sheryl had struggled to determine which household functions Sheryl was capable of assuming.

With her illness, Katherine again assumed a great deal of responsibility for the household, needing desperately to feel the reassurance that her family needed her and could not survive without her. It was part of what she needed to stay alive and keep her will to live strong.

Sheryl and her father, Garth, themselves terrified by the prospect of Katherine's death to cancer, returned to their own previous pattern of expecting a great deal from Katherine, in part as a means of denying the fragility of her health. The family became aware of this regression and of their denial of Katherine's needs during the course of her chemotherapy. Katherine had always done all the cooking for the family, and she insisted on continuing to cook as soon as she was up and around after surgery. Her hair began to fall out, and the family began to complain of finding hair in their food. No matter how extreme her attempts to cover her hair, Katherine could not manage to control the appearance of her hair in the food she prepared.

In a family meeting in which we discussed the family's reaction to Katherine's illness, we realized that the family was having difficulty acknowledging Katherine's heightened need for care from others. At first, Katherine was resentful of what she considered my overly solicitous concern for her health; she retorted angrily, "There's no need to treat me so gently. I am still alive, I'm not dead yet." I was taken aback by her challenge, but I had to honestly admit that part of my concern with her caretaking stance stemmed from my view of her as fragile and potentially dying of her cancer. For Katherine, the important thing was maintaining her will to stay alive; feeling needed and important in her family seemed to her effective in accomplishing this goal. Once Katherine could appreciate that she needed to save her energy for the battle to stay alive and that her family needed to make as much of a contribution as possible to that battle, not only for her well-being but also for their own, she was able to allow Sheryl and Garth to take more responsibility for their own needs and to thus maintain the family's ongoing developmental progression.

Well-publicized clinical lore has suggested that survival rates from cancer are often affected by the patient's belief that he or she will beat the odds and remain alive. While depression and discouragement may in fact interfere with the body's best response to disease, it is a terrible extension of our culture's difficulty with regard to death to blame cancer patients who are dying of their disease for not having believed strongly enough in their own potential cure. Gilda Radner's 1989 biography, *It's Always Something*, documents the painful process she endured as she searched for a treatment of her ovarian cancer that would permit her to regain control over her illness. She struggled with extreme emotional highs and lows as she encountered the contradictory opinions of her highly specialized cancer doctors and her New Age healers. As the causes of cancer and the complex interaction of genetics, the environment, and the immune system become better understood, it will perhaps be possible to treat and support patients without blaming them for causing their own death because they were unable to muster the proper attitude with which to stay alive.

DEATH AND THE MEANING-MAKING PROCESS

The search for the cause of death is a natural part of the meaning-making process by which adults, children, and families try to understand and integrate the death into their lives and to restore a sense of safety and order to their world. As part of that search, both adults and children attempt whenever possible to construct an understanding of the cause of death that restores a sense of the world as being orderly and predictable and a sense of the self as being in control rather than helpless. Most people resort to self-blame as a means of reestablishing a sense of order in the world rather than accept the feeling of helplessness that follows recognition that events are unpredictable and uncontrollable. The restoration of control will often include a painful process of second-guessing, of "what if?" ruminating, and of retracing the steps in decision making in an attempt to determine what might have prevented the death. In both chronic and acute illness the medical decision making will be carefully scrutinized as families try to determine what, if anything, might have preserved the life of their loved one. Families will at times generate the fantasy that medical malpractice was involved because a physician did not respond to an ambiguous symptom as a sign of a potentially fatal illness.

Accidental Death

The most agonizing instances of self-reproach and self-blame are generated in cases of accidental death. Such accidents, which highlight and fix in time a particular sequence in the ordinary flow of events, typically create the impression that a particular act or sequence of acts caused the death even when this sense of cause and effect is illusory or misleading. An accident, by definition, involves an unlucky alignment of elements in an event that with better luck and a slight shift in their configuration might have gone smoothly. I treat a 45-year-old woman whose traumatic childhood has made her a master at figuring out the potential tragic outcome of most human activities. She is hardly able to leave her house. When we reason backward from a traumatic event, it is all too easy, but inaccurate, to simply say that the events preceding it caused it to happen. All of us operate on some measure of automatic pilot some of the time and hope that fate does not bring us an emergency requiring a quick response to avoid a fatal outcome, as most of the time it does not. All of us are guilty of lapses in judgment, from whose consequences we recover and from which we learn, but a fatal accident can elevate what might have been an innocent misjudgment to a "murderous" act.

I remember three sessions of brief therapy with Tom Young, a high school senior who reluctantly came, accompanied by his parents, for an evaluation following a car accident in which he, the driver, had escaped uninjured and in which his best friend, Carl, who had been sitting in the front passenger seat, had been severely injured leaving him in an apparently irreversible coma. Tom had briefly stopped at an intersection and had then proceeded into the flow of traffic, even though his view was obstructed by a parked car; he failed to see an oncoming vehicle, in part because the driver was speeding. Glen and Andrea Young were themselves so burdened with guilt at the injury of this beloved young man, the son of close family friends, that they found it agonizing each time they saw Carl in the hospital or faced his parents, which they as a family did often. Glen and Andrea found it difficult to understand how Tom had managed to cope with his own guilt and wondered if his reaction was normal. Tom had been outraged when he was charged with involuntary manslaughter; as far as he was concerned, he had been guilty only of a sloppy left turn, of the sort most of us execute on a daily basis. I congratulated Tom for figuring out the case in his own defense and for following a line of reasoning that is often difficult after an accident, when most people follow the line of causality toward self-blame no matter what the extenuating circumstances are. At the same time, I warned him that the public or private apportioning of guilt in and of itself would not determine the full range of his feelings about the tragic accident over the course of his life. The most I could tell his parents was that Tom was doing a good job of protecting his own development while remaining in fact devoted to Carl's care and that he would require support in the future as he more fully faced the enormity of his loss and his part in it.

An accident does require a careful weighing of our involvement in it and a true distinguishing of the difference between what Buber (1965) called neurotic guilt and realistic guilt. The adult drunk driver who after a dozen drunk driving violations drives head-on into another vehicle and kills an innocent family surely bears a substantial measure of direct responsibility and differs from the drunk adolescent who commits the same act for the first and only time during the developmental process of mastering impulsivity and learning his or her own realistic limits. Yet another level of responsibility holds when a nighttime driver is reasonably alert but fails to see a runner or bicyclist who abruptly enters the road and is not wearing proper reflecting gear.

Sally Shaw was haunted by the fatal moment during their family bicycle ride when she turned her head to see 7-year-old Laurie's progress on her new three-speed bike; if fate had been kinder, the baby's head would have hit the ground at a different angle and they would have gone on their way after dusting themselves off, after one more fall in the many falls endured by any growing-up family.

It is crucially important to remember that a legalistic weighing of the elements of responsibility often does not take into account the illusion of certain causality generated by reasoning backward from a final act. While involvement in wrongful death litigation can support a family's sense that justice is being served, it can create an artificially one-dimensional frame for the family's understanding of the death and their shared meaning-making process (Rosenblatt, 1983).

It is important to protect families both from a distorted sense of self-blame, which is meant to restore a sense of control, and from the temptation to gloss over true accountability, which can also interfere with a family's ongoing relationships. When Greg Gauditis died in a car accident in which his brother Neal was the driver, his wife, Sheila, could not avoid the thought that Neal should have somehow driven more carefully in order to avert the accident. As the driver, Neal did in fact bear some measure of accountability, although surely not all that Sheila in her acute grief assigned him. The resistance to any exploration of the issue of accountability became an enduring barrier to ongoing relationships in the Gauditis family (see Chapter 9), who became embattled over the grandparents' degree of access to their grandchildren.

Concerns about possible legal liability can interfere with the complex, multidimensional exploration of accountability or guilt in a death. When 11-year-old Alan Jenkins fell to his death during a supervised school outing, his parents, outraged that their son had been so poorly supervised, sued the school for negligence. The school, in part for legal reasons, refused to admit any accountability at all and instead made a case in their own defense by blaming Alan's behavior problems as the reason he had wandered unseen to a dangerous hiking trail. The adversarial legal process made the Jenkins suffer more than they might have if the school had been able or willing to acknowledge their fair share of responsibility.

Murder

In murder, of course, causality is direct and unambiguous, yet families and communities make a distinction between the murder of an innocent bystander and the murder of a gang member who himself was involved in violence. Murder in self-defense, such as the murder of a husband by his battered wife, has come to be recognized in some instances as the only way out of a physically violent relationship. Children who witness the murder of one parent at the hands of the other will have to struggle with the potential loss of both parents, and with the agonizing groping toward an understanding of the event—not just in conjunction with legal proceedings but to some extent independently as well (Eth & Pynoos, 1985). A family's satisfaction with the criminal justice system can substantially help them in their recovery from grief after the murder of a family member (Amick-McMullan et al., 1989; Getzel & Masters, 1984; Poussaint, 1984). However, only communities that have preserved some faith in the criminal justice system will be able to entrust their own need for justice into the time-consuming, drawn-out, and harrowing legal process. African-American communities, in which trust of the police and criminal justice system has been understandably eroded by unjust differential treatment, are less likely to believe in the police and courts as a means of satisfying their need for justice (Spark, 1992). For these families, support from other families who have endured such a loss and involvement in a community response of violence prevention may be more effective means of responding to the overwhelming feelings evoked by the murder of a loved one than is reliance on the criminal justice system.

In addressing issues of responsibility and accountability, I have been highlighting the complex judgments individuals and families make after a violent or accidental death, judgments based on their attempt to reason backward and determine causality as a means of establishing control. As clinicians working with grieving families we need to help members fully explore their feelings and fantasies about the circumstances of a death and determine what realistic action they can take to arrive at justice. The success of this exploration will depend in part on our own capacity to help families establish perspective without unfairly imposing our own need to create a safe universe in which such tragedies do not occur.

TRAUMA AND BEREAVEMENT

The literature on traumatic stress responses contributes to our understanding of the importance of the circumstances of death in structuring family grief reactions. The circumstances of the death create a configuration of stresses to which the family must respond; violent circumstances generate a distinctive grief reaction in which stress and discontinuity make the task of integration even more overwhelming. The trauma literature is itself a newcomer to the mental health field and has not yet been integrated with the literature on individual or family bereavement (Eth & Pynoos, 1985).

Symptoms of Posttraumatic Stress Disorder

The revised third edition of the American Psychiatric Association's (1987) *Diagnostic and Statistical Manual of Mental Disorders (DSM-III-R)* describes posttraumatic stress disorder (PTSD) as a reaction typically following the patient's experience of an event that is outside the range of usual human experience and that would be markedly distressing to almost anyone. Three categories of symptoms typify PTSD: symptoms associated with intrusive remembering, with numbing and avoidance, and with general hyperarousal. Intrusive remembering includes recurrent disturbing dreams, a sense of recurrence or flashback of the event, and heightened responsiveness to symbolic reminders or associative triggers such as anniversaries of the trauma. Persistent avoidance or emotional numbing can include efforts to avoid thoughts, feelings, or activities associated with the trauma; inability to recall an important aspect of the trauma (partial or total psychogenic amnesia); markedly diminished interest in significant activities; feelings of detachment or estrangement from others; a restricted range of affect, such as inability to experience loving feelings; and a foreshortened sense of the future. Persistent symptoms of hyperarousal can include difficulty falling or staying asleep, irritability or outbursts of anger, difficulty concentrating, hypervigilance, exaggerated startle response, and physiologic reactivity upon exposure to events that symbolize or resemble an aspect of the traumatic event.

Posttraumatic stress disorder in a child substantially resembles the adult symptom picture. Traumatized children show intrusive recollection of the event, most often seen in intrusive imagery and nightmares as well as in compulsive, repetitive traumatic play; they show psychic numbing and affective constriction; and they experience increased arousal. Lenore Terr (1990), who has studied many traumatized children, including those buried alive during the Chowchilla school bus kidnapping, describes what she considers unique additional characteristics of childhood reaction to trauma, namely, heightened fear of separation and recurrence of the trauma; hallucination or misperception of the presence of the perpetrators; little or no disavowal or traumatic amnesia, as compared to adults; and apparently permanent personality distortions associated with self-protective coping.

Terr (1990) notes that while a traumatic occurrence prior to age 3 or 4 will succumb to the general forgetting of childhood experiences, a trauma after 3 or 4 is not likely to undergo the massive repression or denial of reality characteristic of some adults. Further, children are more likely to call upon their memories of a traumatic event in conscious fantasy and seem less likely to suffer from intrusive flashbacks of the traumatic event. Eth and Pynoos (1985) suggest that developmental stage further influences the child's response to trauma, determining the means of coping available to the child. PTSD in very young children can be characterized by loss of recently acquired developmental skills, such as bowel and bladder control or language skills.

While the *DSM-III-R* describes PTSD as a response to extraordinary or unexpected life events, the experience of trauma is in fact shockingly common, especially among the powerless or helpless. Among women and children, especially girls, there is emerging evidence (as researchers with sensitivity to the secretiveness of the sexual assault victim conduct more careful and sympathetic studies) that the incidence of sexual abuse and sexual assault is extraordinarily high. For example, Russell (1986) carefully interviewed a random representative sample of adult women in San Francisco after attempting to create conditions of safety and trust that would enable interviewees to disclose experiences of sexual assault; she found that 46% of her respondents had suffered familial or extrafamilial sexual assault. In response to these criticisms, the *DSM-IV* (American Psychiatric Association, 1994) no longer describes traumatic events as "outside of the range of human experience."

The Impact of Trauma

Why is the experience of trauma so devastating to so many aspects of psychological and social functioning? The impact of trauma seems to reverberate at every level of human functioning—the biological; the intrapsychic, involving both cognition and affect; and the social/relational, affecting intimate relationships as well as relationships to those in the wider community. The combination of overwhelming terror and helplessness, with no possibility of either escape or resistance, requires extreme internal and external adaptation. First, the exposure to extreme danger seems almost to reprogram the functioning of the central nervous system, which goes into a perpetual state of hyperarousal (Herman, 1992; van der Kolk, 1990). The trauma survivor's sense of trust or safety in the world is radically altered, with assumptions about how to function in the world shattered, making necessary a state of constant heightened vigilance as a means of warding off danger. The sense of vulnerability is especially heightened in cases of volitional human violence, although it can also persist in cases of PTSD involving accidents.

Experiencing an overwhelming traumatic event seems to so overload our capacity to process both cognitive and emotional information that our usual capacity for integration of experience is disrupted. Most clinicians who work with traumatized patients, whatever the original traumatic event, uniformly describe the fragmentation of ordinarily integrated psychological functions as the most significant feature of traumatization. Traumatic experiences, which are so beyond our ordinary expectations and so violate our assumptions of safety, control, and predictability in the world, compel two simultaneous yet contradictory processes: (1) avoiding, distancing, or dissociating from the event, so as to deny the possibility that such violation could take place, and (2) retrieving and remembering the event, so as to reexperience it and manage a more complete understanding and mastery. Horowitz (1986), in his writing on stress response syndromes, emphasizes the traumatic event's disruption of cognitive or information-processing schemas. He suggests that the event is both avoided, because it provokes painful thoughts and feelings, and repeated, because of a need to develop new schemas that will account for the event. Other writers, such as Bowlby (1980), tend to emphasize the affective component of dissociation and suggest that overwhelming emotions are defended against, isolated, and removed to a parallel psychic system as a means of coping.

The traumatized person's functioning in the social world is also severely disrupted by the experience of trauma. From a systemic developmental perspective, the processes of understanding and integrating our own emotions and perceptions of the world are not simply a private matter but are in fact negotiated between ourselves and those in our family and in our wider culture. A traumatic event shatters our customary patterns of understanding the world, managing emotions, and relating to others and requires that we rebuild those understandings (Herman, 1992; Janoff-Bulman, 1985; Lebowitz & Roth, 1992).

Recovery from Trauma

In describing the recovery process, clinicians uniformly emphasize the importance of social connection and social support as a means of helping the traumatized individual process overwhelming emotions and rebuild a sense of safety. Figley (1989) emphasizes the importance of a family's understanding the nature of PTSD when, for example, a family member has been raped or returns home from war. With information about the nature of PTSD, families can offer support to the traumatized family member while recognizing their own vulnerability to vicarious traumatization and without feeling responsible for the survivor's mood swings or distancing.

Yet isolation from family members often feels necessary to the bereaved, who feel they cannnot tolerate any reminders of the death, including the emotions of other family members. When a family suffers the death of a loved one and shares the task of reestablishing psychological equilibrium, one family member's attempts to isolate or control feelings during a numbing phase may be interfered with by another family member's phase of intrusive repetition. Steve Johnson, who could not bear the pain of loving and parenting his surviving children after his eldest son died, is an extreme example of a bereaved person's need for distance and isolation as a means of managing an overwhelming grief reaction.

Many therapists who treat traumatized patients note that the work of telling a complete, coherent story of the traumatic event, with its associated emotions, is a substantial part of the therapeutic work itself. The trauma literature emphasizes the importance of understanding the traumatic moment in its full violence, and clinicians are advised to elicit the details of the traumatic event as thoroughly and vividly as possible. At the same time, clinicians need to remember that the details of any traumatic event will be subject to substantial dissociation and avoidance, since it is in the details that people relive the full emotional experience of a traumatic event. Further, we clinicians need to be aware that we must exercise constant vigilance against our own need to avoid the reality and helplessness of trauma. The telling of a trauma story can generate dissociation in the therapist, and often the therapist's avoidance of the details of the trauma story takes place at an unconscious level. Patients who have been traumatized are especially sensitized to others' responses to their experience and are very reactive to any communication of distress or disapproval on the therapist's part. Only if we as therapists remain watchful about our all too human capacity for avoidance and denial can we encourage our patients to fully tell their trauma stories without being concerned that they will flood or vicariously traumatize us.

Lifton (1983) suggests that the process of reconstructing traumatic memories requires the reestablishment of three essential elements of psychic functioning: first, a sense of *connection*, or a sense of the organic relationship between past and present; second, a sense of *symbolic integrity*, or a sense of the cohesion and significance of events in one's life, including the traumatic event; and third, a sense of *movement*, or a sense of one's ability to develop and change after the trauma. From a relational developmental perspective, the best chance for restoration of these intrapsychic functions exists when the traumatized individual feels the connection to others who can appreciate the depth of his or her pain and overwhelming sense of disruption has been restored. Trauma survivors' reintegration of emotional experience, restoration of shattered meanings, and reimmersion in the flow of life depends on the capacity of others to hear the whole story and still convey to them the ways they remain connected to the human family. As therapists, we become witnesses to their testimony of brutal fate—and sometimes of even more brutal intentional violence.

Acknowledgment by others of the intrinsic injustice of the trauma survivor's experience, as well as their recognition of any dimension of political or social injustice in the traumatic event, seems further to be an important part of healing. The current traumatic stress literature is likely to discuss the dimension of social justice in cases of survivors of torture who have fled their politically repressive countries (Agger & Buus Jensen, 1990). However, the injustices that characterize our own society and leave a disproportionate number of those who are female, poor, or people of color vulnerable to life-shattering traumatic experiences will similarly need to be addressed in their social as well as personal context in order for healing to occur. Just as family survivors of murder do better when they feel the criminal justice system has functioned effectively in incarcerating the murderer, so too do victims of social injustice find emotional relief in community organization and corrective sociopolitical response.

Combining the Trauma and Bereavement Literatures

While the interweaving of the trauma of the death of a loved one and grief is inevitable, the trauma literature and the bereavement literature have each focused on their own specialty, and their reports frequently obscure the information required in a particular case to distinguish the phenomena associated with grief from those associated with trauma. In their discussion of childhood "traumatic" grief reactions, Eth and Pynoos (1985) note that clinical reports of bereavement cases in general often do not report the circumstances of the death, thus obscuring the possible presence of traumatic events surrounding the death. They note, for example, that the famous study by Glick, Weiss, and Parkes (1974) of widows found that young widows whose husbands died sudden deaths suffered more severe grief reactions and were often unable to visit the cemetery. Eth and Pynoos suggest that in some of these instances the widow may have witnessed a death caused by accident or by deliberately inflicted violence and that her reaction of avoidance may not be the result of denial but, rather, of her attempt to avoid the triggering of traumatic memories. Similarly, reports of traumatic events in the trauma literature often highlight the trauma-inducing violence of an event without reporting, or else reporting in passing, whether the survivor also suffered the death of a family member. The degree of traumatization in surviving a catastrophic event such as a fire or a school yard shooting depends not only on the extent of direct exposure to the violence but also on whether a family member died in the traumatic incident.

Eth and Pynoos (1985), in one of the few discussions specifically addressing the distinctiveness of "traumatic" grief reactions, note that the processing of a traumatic experience takes priority over the processing of the loss. They find that in cases of violent death in which the child has witnessed the physical mutilation of a parent the fear aroused in the child by the violent image may interfere with his or her exploration of reminiscences that would, over the normal course of grief, allow identification with the dead parent. In instances where the murderer is a stranger, the child's sense of safety is significantly disrupted and fear of the murderer on the loose may take priority over other aspects of grieving. When the murderer is another family member, the child suffers conflicts of loyalty as well as rage. Tragically, a child who witnesses the death of one parent at the hands of the other loses one parent to death and the other to incarceration. When a parent commits suicide, the child is likely to suffer intense guilt in addition to resentment, especially if the parent's prior depression or a previous suicide attempt resulted in the child's fantasied—or real—involvement in keeping the parent alive (Lukas & Seiden, 1987).

CONCLUSION

From a family developmental perspective, the specific circumstances of the death create the context for family bereavement, determine the degree of discontinuity the family experiences, and define the conditions for the individual's and family's meaning-making process. Different circumstances generate different constellations of specific stresses with which the family is forced to cope. The literature on traumatic stress, which has not yet been integrated into the bereavement literature, can make an important contribution toward understanding the impact of specific circumstances of death on individual and family bereavement.

PART V

CONCLUSION

CHAPTER 14

Family Development and Grief Therapy

Most grieving families bear their pain and go on with their lives by turning to each other and to their existing family, social, and community networks for support. What can mental health practitioners offer to grieving families that is not already provided by these resources' naturally occurring mechanisms for managing stress? A family developmental model of family bereavement argues that family grief reactions can best be understood as they both interrupt and become interwoven with ongoing family developmental processes. The crisis of grief is not only a crisis of overwhelming emotion but a crisis in the construction of the collaborative self. Therapy after the death of a family member can offer grieving families developmentally formulated interventions that will maximize the family's opportunity to achieve a growth-enhancing adaptation to the crisis. Therapists can help grieving families balance the inevitable stresses with protective supports, the inevitable discontinuities with the most growth-promoting strategies for stability. Systemic developmental grief therapy builds on family strengths, leveraging the family's naturally occurring developmental motion to minimize its use of those stabilizing strategies that are symptomatic or growth-constraining defenses that interfere with the next stage of family development.

We may help grieving families in our professional roles as grief counselors and family therapists or in our social roles as friends, co-workers, and fellow church or synagogue members. Whatever our capacity, we join the pool of community resources that help make the unbearable pain of grieving families eventually more bearable and the torn fabric of family life eventually more whole. In order to be as helpful as possible to the bereaved, we first and foremost need to consider our location in our own family life cycle developmental process, most especially our own personal resonance to the reality, and the possibility, of death and grief in our own lives.

As therapists, our understanding of family bereavement cannot be totally free of cultural assumptions, personal biases, and hypotheses generated by the mental health profession. Our mental health models of bereavement themselves reflect our culture's emphasis on disengagement from the dead and resumption of an unencumbered life. Models of mental health emphasize a psychopathology perspective. A psychopathology perspective can offer therapists protection from full empathy with the anguish of a family's grief experience, as all of us naturally want to be protected from the realization that perfectly ordinary people become overwhelmed by pain in the face of death and loss. As therapists we need to be especially vigilant in guarding against our tendency to pathologize the human extremes that represent the many faces of grief. A systemic developmental perspective that critically examines a community's capacity to provide support for the family bereavement process provides us with a tool for evaluating any family's grief reaction as their own best adaptation to the shattering reality of a family death. With an attitude of critical reflection on our own reactions to the potential vulnerabilities in our own lives, we are better prepared to offer grieving families our support. Grieving families need both our unflinching human presence and our clinical intervention into the configuration of stresses and supports out of which their response to grief is constructed. Grief therapy is itself enormously depleting work, and therapists need to attend to their own working context and those supportive resources that will make the work emotionally tolerable (Lattanzi, 1984; Sanders, 1984, 1989).

A systemic developmental perspective on the family life cycle crisis of bereavement suggests that the developmental course of all families is inevitably altered by the shattering blow of grief. A complex web of historical and current life circumstances contribute to the configuration of stressors and supports that shape a family's initial stable adaptation to the crisis of grief. With close attention to their stresses and available resources, we can help families substantially improve their integration and growth-enhancing adaptation to their shared family grief. The configuration of stresses and supports that contribute to a family's evolving adaptation lends itself to a wide variety of interventions that leverage the family's own developmental momentum to generate new conditions for more successful adaptation.

Most families cope with the crisis of grief without clinical intervention, turning quite naturally to their existing web of relationships in the extended family and community. Medical staff, hospice workers, clergy, and funeral home directors are far more likely than any mental health professional to encounter grieving families in the early stages of acute grief. As therapists we are much more likely to work with grieving families when the circumstances of death are cata-strophic, when a bereavement response has become symptomatic, or when terminal illness and death affect individuals or families already in therapy. The fact that we are more likely to work with clinically referred, symptomatic families makes it tempting to apply the psycho-pathology models to which we have become accustomed. It is pre-cisely these families who are under extraordinary pressures from over-whelming life experiences, including the death, who most benefit from a resource orientation to their developmental struggles.

Any family bereavement reaction, even an apparently pathologi-cal one, must be respectfully appreciated as a family's own best adap-tation within a context of family history, circumstances of the death, family stressors and resources, and cultural beliefs or practices. Symp-toms represent adaptations that are not sufficiently inclusive of the complex, collaborative self because of intrapsychic, interpersonal, or cultural strategies for stability that are barriers to ongoing develop-ment. A respectful therapeutic attitude toward the human extremes in response to the agonies of grief offers us our best opportunity as therapists to help families explore and integrate their grief experience.

In order for individuals and families to achieve optimal integra-tion of their overwhelming feelings and radically discontinuous new life circumstances, they need realistic supports that will clear the way for the psychological work. Our assessments of grieving families need to go far beyond any one individual; we must consider the nested struc-tures within which any individual grief experience unfolds. As clini-cians working from a systemic model of family development, we aim to decrease stressors or risk factors and increase supports or protec-tive factors in the lives of individuals and families. The interlocking systems or nested structures within which families encounter their stresses and marshal their supports include the following:

1. Cultural and religious practices and beliefs
2. Social network of friends, neighbors, fellow workers, and church members
3. Intergenerational and family-of-origin relationships
4. Patterns of mutually adaptive family interaction and shared strategies for stability
5. Personal responses, coping strategies, and images of relation-ships

From the perspective of a systemic developmental model, any change in context changes the organization of adaptation and provides new opportunities for more inclusive integration of previously overwhelming or disturbing experience. The more real-life supports a family can bring to bear in the stressful crisis of death and grief, the more of their emotionally overwhelming experience they will be able to integrate into a coherent, continuous, mutually inclusive sense of self with others. Under circumstances of high stress and high discontinuity without adequate balancing supports, individuals and families are more likely to rely on psychological defenses—individual, familial, or social—as strategies for stabilizing structure. A therapeutic approach that helps a family identify and deal more effectively with the stresses generated by both the real circumstances of the death and the real changes of a transformed life paves the way for the most effective clinical work of emotional and personal integration.

In working with already bereaved families, we cannot change the circumstances of the death, the nature of previous family relationships, or the immediate stresses and discontinuities that result from the death. However, there is a great deal we can do in helping a family recognize and attend to real-life stresses and generate as much support within their wider network of family and community resources. We can also help families understand the strategies for stable adaptation that they established in response to this and other developmental crises so that they can reexplore and better integrate painful or previously overwhelming experiences and re-create more flexible strategies for stability. With support for the considerable real-life distress of their grief experience, family members are in a far better position to listen to each other, to themselves, and to their therapist. Attention to real-life stressors and creation of the safest, most stable conditions possible for them helps grieving families do the psychological work of exploring and bearing their overwhelming feelings of anguish or rage or fear, discovering the psychological strategies for stability in response to the crisis of grief that overly constrain family growth, and generating new strategies for stability that permit greater integration and support of ongoing family development.

Diagnosis of a terminal illness in a family member provides clinicians with the opportunity to support anticipatory grief in ways that will maximize the family's best, most growth-enhancing adaptation to the death. Therapists can provide important support for families in helping them explore both the practical and psychological implications of complex medical decisions, such as those involving treatment, including experimental procedures; the location of treatment facilities; and the consequences of using extreme measures for prolonging life. The pressures of coping with a terminal illness in either a hospital or a hospice setting can become so overwhelming that they are experienced by families as traumatic stress. Such a burden of traumatic stress can interfere with the later work of grieving. Intrusive images of the hospital ordeal and illness can interfere with the family's later attempts to reestablish an accessible image of the dead family member.

Many families exhaust themselves and their resources by focusing on the ill family member, believing that they must devote themselves to a family member they will soon be losing. The demands of caring for a dying family member are inevitably extreme, and it is natural for family members to feel that their time with the dying member is limited while their time for each other and for themselves will come later. In fact, emotional self-care is especially important for grieving adults, who need to preserve their capacity for responsiveness and emotional integration of the death on behalf of surviving family members. Family members can be helped to balance concern for the terminally ill member with self-care and care for each other in ways that will help them feel that they did what they could to safeguard and preserve all the family relationships. This is particularly important with chronic illness, which is especially depleting for families and likely to complicate the subsequent grief reaction (Koocher, 1986; Rando, 1986). Since the children in a family with a dying parent or child are vulnerable to being overlooked by their overwhelmed parents (Rosenheim & Reicher, 1985, 1986), clinicians can help safeguard their ongoing development by enabling families to consider these children's developmental needs.

For families who have already experienced a death, family bereavement work requires sensitivity to the timing of interventions as they interface with the family's unique, complex life circumstances and its configuration of stresses and supports. In the early phases of acute grief children, adults, and families are trying to understand what happened at the same time that they are trying to protect themselves from a full-blown realization of the loss and its implications (Baker et al., 1992; Bowlby, 1980; Weiss, 1988). For this reason, clinical services immediately after the death usually focus on psychoeducational or informational clarification of the circumstances of the death and the expectable reactions of adults and children of different ages. These informational and supportive interventions may be provided by hospital- or school-based therapists, as well as by other participants in the family experience of death, including medical personnel, police, funeral home directors, and clergy (Clark, 1981; Eth, Silverstein, & Pynoos, 1985; Fox, 1979; Miles & Perry, 1985).

While important support services and information about child and family grief reactions can be communicated immediately after a death or in the early weeks or months of the grief reaction, a number of therapists recommend a period of some months for family restabilization before intervening to expand the family process of exploration of the implications and meanings of the death (Baker et al., 1992; Koocher & Kemler, 1992; Sanders, 1989). From a systemic developmental perspective, a family will immediately gather together their existing resources, instrumental and psychological, for restoring stability. Only over the course of developmental time, in the months and even years following the death, will the full implications of these strategies for stability fully unfold. The clinician who attempts to intervene in apparently symptomatic grief reactions will need to assess the role of the symptom in ensuring individual and family stability and will need to offer alternative sources of support that will make the risks of emotional exploration and greater integration tolerable and manageable.

Attention to the family's real-life circumstances paves the way for the most inclusive integration of the experience of death and grief, one that permits the family to resume ongoing family development as fully as possible. A growth-promoting adaptation permits all of the following:

1. Maximum integration of the complex collaborative self, including tolerance of intense emotions and internal conflicts
2. Maximum mutuality of relationships, including tolerance of interpersonal differences and conflicts
3. Restoration of the flow of developmental time for all its members and for the family as a unit, which requires tolerance for the work of reexamining the death and its meanings and flexible responses to evolving family developmental circumstances
4. Restoration of a living, evolving image of the deceased as a supportive resource for ongoing family development
5. Creation of a shared affirming family narrative of the death and its meaning that minimizes self-blame; locates the death in a coherent understanding of past, present, and future; and recognizes the unique private experience of members along with their need for harmonious adaptation to family and culture

The family developmental bereavement process can be enhanced through individual clinical interventions with children and adults that explore the circumstances of the death and its meaning. Grief therapy, whether with children, adults, or families, will inevitably begin with the telling of the story (Baker et al., 1992; Eth & Pynoos, 1985; Koocher & Kemler, 1992; Worden, 1991): What happened, and how did it happen? Immediately upon hearing the story of the death, the therapist begins to listen for the meaning-making process. As therapists we are especially well suited to listen for aspects of the death, its circumstances, and its implications for the collaborative self that seem emotionally overwhelming and are in danger of becoming dissociated or distorted as strategies for regaining stability and coherence.

However, the process of private growth-enhancing understanding and integration is best achieved by understanding individual experience in its systemic context and simultaneously addressing the interlocking systems within which individual experience is structured. Child grief, whether in response to the death of a parent or the death of a sibling, is substantially affected by the child's cognitive developmental stage as well as by the relational developmental processes that characterize the child's developmental moment in time. At a time when their own emotional and instrumental resources are significantly diminished, grieving parents are challenged by the death of a family member to provide their children with the most stable, responsive parenting they are capable of.

Work with grieving children that recognizes a parent's own developmental dilemma and supports the adult grief process is much more likely to help create the continuity and responsiveness of caretaking that children need to achieve their own best developmental efforts at integrating the death and loss. A grieving adult who has attended to his or her own devastating sense of loss and who has marshaled the best supports possible for reestablishing personal continuity is in a far better position to help his or her child grieve. A parent needs to appreciate the child's developmental understandings, and misunderstandings, of the death and its meanings and to support the child's ongoing developmental process of creating a growth-promoting image of the deceased parent or sibling that moves with them through developmental time.

Therapy with adults that enhances their own developmental integration of the grief experience so as to promote their best functioning as parents works just as much for the benefit of the adult as for the benefit of the child. From a systemic developmental perspective, marital and parenting relationships are as central to adult personality organization as are internalized family-of-origin relationships. Grieving adults who find their stable life structures shattered by the out-of-life-cycle death of a spouse or child need desperately to reestablish a sense of stable, successful functioning as a first priority. Once that sense of stability in family functioning is successfully reestablished, adults gain far greater freedom for their own personal integration of the death and its meaning into a relational life structure with a coherent sense of past, present, and future. Individual adult grief work is itself relational. Adult grief precipitates a crisis in the construction of the collaborative self over the course of one's life, a construction that included the deceased family member. Adult grief work requires the emotional reworking of the relationship to make room for the new life circumstances and relational reality created by the death and loss. Adult grief therapy involves helping the bereaved bear the pain of loss in such a way that the relationship with the deceased can be reestablished as a spiritual and psychological resource for ongoing personal and family development.

From a systemic developmental perspective, the family dimension of grief is addressed by any intervention, because family relationships are seen as vital to individual experience and development (Wachtel & Wachtel, 1986). Interventions that involve the family as a unit provide important opportunities for enhancing family bereavement. Family sessions can be either the sole medium of therapy or an adjunct to ongoing child, adult, or parent bereavement work. Family sessions provide an opportunity to bring to light the private realities individual family members bring to the grief experience, as well as the understandings—and misunderstandings—they may have of both the circumstances of the death and its impact on other family members. Family relationships are sources of vital structures for stability, and the death of a family member whose relational presence contributed to family organization and stability initiates a family process of relational transformation in which new patterns of relationship and structures are generated. Because the family has lost its customary patterns of stability at a time when emotional demands are enormously increased, it is more vulnerable to generating new rules or patterns for stable structure that help control or contain its members' overwhelming emotions but that overly constrain their private exploration or public communication.

From a systemic developmental perspective, therapy with grieving families further requires attention to the wider social systems within which a family is embedded. The assessment and enhancement of the wider community of social supports for grieving families is an important aspect of the therapeutic work. Extended family members are themselves burdened by the death of a family member, yet they are a vital resource for the grieving family, who need the support and affirmation of others who appreciate the loss and who can join them in reestablishing a sense of their enduring attachments and relational integrity. For the adult who has lost a spouse or child, adult family relationships can offer emotional support, financial help, and respite from the demands of child care. For the grieving child who has lost a parent, that parent's siblings and parents can extend the child's resources for establishing a growing multidimensional image of the dead parent. It may become important for the clinician to explore the extended family's own responses to the loss and, if necessary, to help the wider family network explore barriers in their own grieving that might interfere with the give and take of emotional and instrumental support for the family in its widest web of relational resources.

For many families, a religious community offers an important source of support following the death of a family member, both in providing instrumental support and in offering a sense of meaning for the place of death and grief in the continuity of life. While therapists tend to emphasize the psychological rather than the spiritual domain in their ongoing work with families, the spiritual component is an especially important one for most families who are grappling with the death of a family member and its meaning. Both children and adults need to maintain some enduring tie to the deceased so as to make that person an ongoing part of their daily life. Some systemic family therapists (Boyd-Franklin, 1989; Walker, 1991) stress the therapist's capacity to join the family's system of meaning-making, including the religious, and to understand the family's religious beliefs as an important tool for creating a family narrative of healing. Immigrant families, already engaged in an attempt to weave a new system of beliefs from their location between cultures, may need help exploring both the mainstream cultural beliefs and their culture-of-origin beliefs as they strive for a coherent understanding of the death and its meaning.

Assessment at the level of social systems also requires that therapists evaluate the social circumstances, and their meanings, associated with a particular death. Acknowledgment of the intrinsic injustice of the experience and recognition of any ethical or sociopolitical dimensions of the traumatic event seem to be important aspects of healing. If the social circumstances of a death involve any of the social injustices of our own society that leave a disproportionate number of women, people of color, and the poor vulnerable to life-shattering traumatic experiences, it will be necessary to be address the social as well as the personal context in order for healing to occur (Spark, 1992). Just as family survivors of murder do better when they feel the criminal justice system has been responsive, so too do grieving family members find emotional relief and help in framing a more satisfying new meaning for their loved one's death when social organizations in the community respond appropriately.

Clinical work with grieving families who have suffered an out-of-

life-cycle death presents us therapists with some of the most emotionally painful work we will ever do. Grieving families also present
a complex interweaving of individual and shared histories and responses, which require assessment and therapy at multiple levels of
intervention. On a personal level, work with grieving families requires
that we face our most fundamental human vulnerabilities. We need
to tolerate the empathic imagining of the wrenching anguish we ourselves would feel with the loss of those relationships we most cherish. In spite of the difficulties, work with grieving families provides
us with the opportunity to join families at moments of their deepest
despair and to help alleviate their loneliness and lighten their overwhelming burden. We can help grieving families identify the resources
within their family relationships and communities as well as within
themselves, resources from which they will gather the strength to
reaffirm the enduring continuity of their family relationships and family
history while rebuilding new family relationships and a renewed sense
of self. By helping families preserve their capacity to grow in response
to the developmental challenge of loss and grief, we inevitably expand
our appreciation of the loving bonds that shape our own lives.

My work toward a clinical and theoretical understanding of family bereavement has been at times disturbing and disrupting, yet it has
also been extraordinarily enriching. It becomes harder to deny the
reality of death when we work with families who know from agonizing experience that none of us is invulnerable. We become familiar
with all the random, unexpected ways illness, accident, or violence
can strike at the most peaceful and stable of lives. We lose our illusion of magical protection from such events. Yet work with the bereaved, our awareness of the impact and presence of death heightened, can help us appreciate life as a gift not to be taken for granted.
It can further help us rediscover our own intergenerational histories,
inevitably bound as they are with the eternal cycles of birth and death,
rejoicing and grief, each affirming the possibility of renewal.

REFERENCES

Agger, I., & Jensen, S. B. (1990). Testimony as ritual and evidence in psychotherapy for political refugees. *Journal of Traumatic Stress, 3*(1), 115–130.

Ainsworth, M., Blehar, M., Waters, E., & Wall, S. (1978). *Patterns of attachment: A psychological study of the strange situation.* Hillsdale, NJ: Erlbaum.

Albee, G. (1992). Powerlessness, politics and prevention: The community mental health approach. In S. Staub & P. Green (Eds.), *Psychology and social responsibility* (pp. 201–220). New York: New York University Press.

Amado, J. (1968). *Dona Flor and her two husbands.* New York: Avon.

American Psychiatric Association. (1987). *Diagnostic and statistical manual of mental disorders* (3rd ed., rev.) (DSM-III-R). Washington, DC: Author.

American Psychiatric Association. (1994). *Diagnostic and statistical manual of mental disorders* (4th ed.) (DSM-IV). Washington, DC: Author.

Amick-McMullan, A., Kilpatrick, D., Veronen, L., & Smith, S. (1989). Family survivors of homicide victims: Theoretical perspectives and an exploratory study. *Journal of Traumatic Stress, 2*(1), 21–36.

Anthony, E. J., & Cohler, B. J. (Eds.). (1987). *The invulnerable child.* New York: Guilford Press.

Aranowitz, S. (1990). Disciplines or punish: Cultural studies and the transformation of legitimate knowledge. *Journal of Urban and Cultural Studies, 1*(1), 39–54.

Bakan, D. (1966). *The duality of human existence.* Boston: Beacon Press.

Baker, J., Sedney, M., & Gross, E. (1992). Psychological tasks for bereaved children. *American Journal of Orthopsychiatry, 62*(1), 105–116.

Bateson, G. (1972). *Steps to an ecology of mind.* New York: Ballantine.

Bateson, G. (1979). *Mind and nature.* New York: Bantam.

Bateson, G. (1992). *Sacred unity: Further steps to an ecology of mind.* New York: Harper Collins.

Beavers, W. (1982). Healthy, midrange, and severely dysfunctional families. In F. Walsh (Ed.), *Normal family processes* (1st ed., pp. 45–66). New York: Guilford Press.

Beavers, W. (1977). *Psychotherapy and growth.* New York: Brunner/Mazel.

Becker, E. (1973). *The denial of death.* New York: Free Press.

Beckwith, B., Beckwith, S., Gray, T., Micsko, M., Holm, J., Plummer, V., & Flaa, S. (1990). Identification of spouses at high risk during bereavement: A preliminary assessment of Parkes and Weiss' Risk Index. *The Hospice Journal, 6*(3), 35–46.

Beebe, B., & Lachmann, F. (1988). The contribution of mother–infant mutual influence to the origins of self and object representations. *Psychoanalytic Psychology, 5*(4), 305–337.

Belle, D. (1988). Gender differences in the social moderators of stress. In R. Barnett, L. Beiner, & G. Baruch (Eds.), *Gender and stress* (pp. 257–277). New York: Free Press.

Belle, D. (1989). *Children's social networks and social supports.* New York: Wiley.

Belsky, J., & Isabella, R. (1985). Marital and parent–child relationships in family of origin and marital change following the birth of a baby: A retrospective analysis. *Child Development, 56*(2), 342–349.

Belsky, J., & Vondra, J. (1989). Lessons from child abuse: The determinants of parenting. In D. Cicchetti & V. Carlson (Eds.), *Child maltreatment: Theory and research on the causes and consequences of child abuse and neglect* (pp. 153–202). Cambridge, England: Cambridge University Press.

Benjamin, J. (1988). *The bonds of love: Psychoanalysis, feminism, and the problem of domination.* New York: Pantheon.

Ben-Sira, Z. (1983). Loss, stress and readjustment: The structure of coping with bereavement and disability. *Social Science and Medicine, 17*(21), 1619–1632.

Bepko, C. (1980). Disorders of power: Women and addiction in the family. In M. McGoldrick, C. Anderson, & F. Walsh (Eds.), *Women in families* (pp. 406–426). New York: Norton.

Bernard, J. (1972). *The future of marriage.* New Haven, CT: Yale University Press.

Bluebond-Langner, M. (1978). *The private worlds of dying children.* Princeton, NJ: Princeton University Press.

Bollas, C. (1987). *The shadow of the object: Psychoanalysis of the unthought known.* New York: Columbia University Press.

Boszormenyi-Nagy, I., & Krasner, B. (1986). *Between give and take: A clinical guide to contextual therapy.* New York: Brunner/Mazel.

Boszormenyi-Nagy, I., & Spark, G. (1973). *Invisible loyalties.* New York: Harper & Row.

Bowen, M. (1976). Family reaction to death. In P. Guerin (Ed.), *Family therapy* (pp. 335–348). New York: Gardner.

Bowen, M. (1978). *Family therapy in clinical practice.* New York: Aronson.

Bowlby, J. (1969). *Attachment and loss: Vol. 1. Attachment.* New York: Basic Books.

Bowlby, J. (1973). *Attachment and loss: Vol. 2. Separation.* New York: Basic Books.

Bowlby, J. (1979). *The making and breaking of affectional bonds*. London: Tavistock Publications.

Bowlby, J. (1980). *Attachment and loss: Vol. 3. Loss*. New York: Basic Books.

Bowlby-West, L. (1983). The impact of death on the family system. *Journal of Family Therapy, 5*, 279-294.

Boyd-Franklin, N. (1989). *Black families in therapy: A multisystems approach*. New York: Guilford Press.

Bretherton, I., & Waters, E. (Eds.). (1985). Growing points in attachment theory and research. *Monographs of the Society for Research in Child Development, 50* (1-2, Serial No. 209).

Bronfenbrenner, U. (1979). *Ecology of human development*. Cambridge, MA: Harvard University Press.

Brown, G., Harris, T., & Bifulco, A. (1986). Long-term effects of early loss of parent. In M. Rutter, C. Izard, & P. Read (Eds.), *Depression in young people: Developmental and clinical perspectives*. New York: Guilford Press.

Buber, M. (1965). *The knowledge of man*. New York: Harper & Row.

Buber, M. (1970). *I and thou*. New York: Scribner.

Buckley, N. (1986). *Essential papers on object relations*. New York: New York University Press.

Burgess, A. (1975). Family reaction to homicide. *American Journal of Orthopsychiatry, 45*, 391-398.

Cain, A., & Fast, I. (1966). Children's disturbed reactions to parent suicide. *American Journal of Orthopsychiatry, 5*, 873-880.

Caplan, G. (1964). *Principles of preventive psychiatry*. New York: Basic Books.

Carter, B., & McGoldrick, M. (Eds.). (1989). *The changing family life cycle: A framework for family therapy* (2nd ed.). Boston: Allyn & Bacon.

Cicchetti, D. (1989). How research on child maltreatment has informed the study of child development: Perspectives from developmental psychopathology. In D. Cicchetti & V. Carlson (Eds.), *Child maltreatment: Theory and research on the causes and consequences of child abuse and neglect* (pp. 377-431). Cambridge, England: Cambridge University Press.

Cicchetti, D., & Carlson, V. (Eds.). (1989). *Child maltreatment: Theory and research on the causes and consequences of child abuse and neglect*. Cambridge, England: Cambridge University Press.

Clark, D. (1981). Death in the family: Providing consultation to the police on the psychological aspects of suicide and accidental death. *Death Education, 5*(2), 143-155.

Cohen, S., & Syme, S. (1985). *Social support and health*. New York: Academic Press.

Combrinck-Graham, L. (1985). A model for family development. *Family Process, 24*, 139-150.

Cook, J. (1984). Influence of gender on the problems of parents of fatally ill children. *Journal of Psychosocial Oncology, 2*(1), 71-91.

Cook, J., & Cohler, B. (1986). Reciprocal socialization and the care of off-spring with cancer and schizophrenia. In N. Datan, A. Greene, & H. Reese (Eds.), *Life-span developmental psychology: Intergenerational relations* (pp. 223–244). Hillsdale, NJ: Erlbaum.

Cook, J., & Wimberley, D. (1983). If I should die before I wake: Religious commitment and adjustment to the death of a child. *Journal for the Scientific Study of Religion, 22*(3), 222–238.

Crosby, J., & Jose, N. (1983). Death: Family adjustment to loss. In C. Figley & H. McCubbin (Eds.), *Stress and the family: Vol. 2. Coping with catastrophe* (pp. 76–89). New York: Brunner/Mazel.

Cushman, P. (1990). Why the self is empty: Toward a historically situated psychology. *American Psychologist, 45*, 599–611.

Darder, A. (1991). *Culture and power in the classroom: A critical foundation for bicultural education.* New York: Bergin & Garvey.

Demi, A. (1984). Social adjustment of widows after a sudden death: Suicide and non-suicide survivors. *Death Education, 8*, 91–111.

Dicks, H. (1967). *Marital tensions.* New York: Basic Books.

Dinnerstein, D. (1978). *The mermaid and the minotaur.* New York: Harper & Row.

Doi, T. (1973). *The anatomy of dependence.* Tokyo: Kodansha International.

Doolittle, H. (1956). *Tribute to Freud.* New York: McGraw-Hill.

Dunne, E., McIntosh, J., & Dunne-Maxim, K. (1988). *Suicide and its aftermath: Understanding and counseling the survivors.* New York: Norton.

Dunst, C., & Trivette, C. (1990). Assessment of social support in early intervention programs. In S. Meisels & J. Shonkoff (Eds.), *Handbook of early childhood intervention* (pp. 326–349). Cambridge, England: Cambridge University Press.

Egeland, B., & Erickson, M. (1990, December). Rising above the past: Strategies for helping new mothers break the cycle of abuse and neglect. *Zero to Three*, 29–35.

Eisenbruch, M. (1984a). Cross-cultural aspects of bereavement. 1: A conceptual framework for comparative analysis. *Culture, Medicine and Psychiatry, 8*, 283–309.

Eisenbruch, M. (1984b). Cross-cultural aspects of bereavement. 2: Ethnic and cultural variations in the development of bereavement practices. *Culture, Medicine and Psychiatry, 8*, 315–347.

Erikson, E. (1950). *Childhood and society.* New York: Norton.

Erikson, E. (1968). *Identity, youth and crisis.* New York: Norton.

Eth, S., & Pynoos, R. (1985). Interaction of trauma and grief in childhood. In S. Eth & R. Pynoos (Eds.), *Post-traumatic stress disorder in children* (pp. 171–186). Washington, DC: American Psychiatric Press.

Eth, S., Silverstein, S., & Pynoos, R. (1985). Mental health consultation to a pre-school following the murder of a mother and child. *Hospital and Community Psychiatry, 36*(1), 73–76.

References

291

Falicov, C. J. (Ed.). (1988). Family transitions: Continuity and change over the life cycle. New York: Guilford Press.
Fenichel, O. (1945). The psychoanalytic theory of neurosis. New York: Norton.
Ferenczi, S. (1955). Confusion of tongues between parent and child: The language of tenderness and of passion. In Final contributions to the problems and methods of psychoanalysis (pp. 155–167). New York: Basic Books. (Original work published 1932)
Figley, C. (1989). Helping traumatized families. San Francisco: Jossey-Bass.
Figley, C., & McCubbin, H. (1983). Stress and the family: Vol. 1. Coping with normative transitions; Vol 2. Coping with catastrophe. New York: Brunner/Mazel.
Fisch, R., Weakland, J., & Segal, L. (1982). The tactics of change. San Francisco: Jossey-Bass.
Fleming, J., & Altschul, S. (1963). Activation of mourning and growth by psychoanalysis. International Journal of Psycho-Analysis, 44, 419–431.
Fox, S. S. (1979). The Family Support Center: Helping families cope with death and grief. Unpublished manuscript, Judge Baker Children's Center.
Fox, S. S. (1984). Children's anniversary reactions to the death of a family member. Omega, 15, 291–305.
Framo, J. (1982). Explorations in marital and family therapy: Selected papers of James L. Framo. New York: Springer.
Frankiel, R. (1994). Essential papers on object loss. New York: New York University Press.
Freire, P. (1985). The politics of education: Culture, power and liberation. New York: Bergin & Garvey.
Freire, P. (1990). Pedagogy of the oppressed. New York: Continuum. (Original work published 1970)
Freud, S. (1957a). Mourning and melancholia. In J. Strachey (Ed. & Trans.), The standard edition of the complete psychological works of Sigmund Freud (Vol. 14, pp. 239–260). New York: Norton. (Original work published 1917)
Freud, S. (1957b). The ego and the id. In J. Strachey (Ed. & Trans.), The standard edition of the complete psychological works of Sigmund Freud (Vol. 19, pp. 1–66). New York: Norton. (Original work published 1923)
Fromm, E. (1961). Marx's concept of man. New York: Continuum.
Fromm, E. (1970). The crisis of psychoanalysis. New York: Holt.
Furman, E. (1974). A child's parent dies: Studies in childhood bereavement. New Haven, CT: Yale University Press.
Garbarino, J. (1990). The human ecology of early risk. In S. Meisels & J. Shonkoff (Eds.), Handbook of early childhood intervention (pp. 79–86). Cambridge, England: Cambridge University Press.

Garbarino, J., Dubrow, N., Kostelny, K., & Pardo, C. (1992). *Children in danger: Coping with the consequences of community violence.* San Francisco: Jossey-Bass.

Garmezy, N. (1987). Stress, competence and development: Continuities in the study of schizophrenic adults, children vulnerable to psychopathology, and the search for stress-resistant children. *American Journal of Orthopsychiatry, 57,* 159–185.

Gay, P. (1988). *Freud: A life for our time.* New York: Norton.

Gelcer, E. (1983). Mourning is a family affair. *Family Process, 22*(4), 501–516.

Getzel, G., & Masters, R. (1984). Serving families who survive homicide victims. *Social Casework, 65*(3), 138–144.

Glick, I., Weiss, R., & Parkes, C. (1974). *The first year of bereavement.* New York: Wiley.

Goldberg, A. (Ed.). (1980). *Advances in self psychology: Part 1. Self psychology and development; Part 2. Self-psychology and the concept of health.* New York: International Universities Press.

Goldner, V. (1989). Generation and gender: Normative and covert hierarchies. In M. McGoldrick, C. Anderson, & F. Walsh (Eds.), *Women in families: A framework for family therapy* (pp. 42–60). New York: Norton.

Gore, S., & Eckenrode, J. (1994). Context and process in research on risk and resilience. In R. J. Hagerty, N. Garmezy, M. Rutter, L. R. Sherrod (Eds.), Stress, risk, and resilience in children and adolescents: Processes, mechanisms, and interventions (pp. 19–63). Cambridge, England: Cambridge University Press.

Gottlieb, B. (1988). *Social stress and social support.* Beverly Hills: Sage.

Greenberg, J. (1991). *Beyond Oedipus: Psychoanalytic theory in clinical practice.* Cambridge, MA: Harvard University Press.

Greenberg, J., & Mitchell, S. (1983). *Object relations in psychoanalytic theory.* Cambridge, MA: Harvard University Press.

Guntrip, H. (1973). *Psychoanalytic theory, therapy and the self: A basic guide to the human personality in Freud, Erikson, Klein, Sullivan, Fairbairn, Hartmann, Jacobson, and Winnicott.* New York: Basic Books.

Haley, J. (1973). *Uncommon therapy.* New York: Norton.

Hare-Mustin, R. (1979). Family therapy following the death of a child. *Journal of Marital and Family Therapy, 5,* 51–60.

Hare-Mustin, R. (1988). The meaning of difference. *American Psychologist, 43,* 455–464.

Harwood, A. (1981). *Ethnicity and medical care.* Cambridge, MA: Harvard University Press.

Held, D. (1980). *Introduction to critical theory.* Berkeley: University of California Press.

Herman, J. (1992). *Trauma and recovery.* Boston: Beacon Press.

Herz, F. (1980). The impact of death and serious illness on the family life cycle. In E. Carter & M. McGoldrick (Eds.), *The family life cycle: A framework for family therapy* (pp. 223–240). New York: Gardner.

Herz, F. (1989). The impact of death and serious illness on the family life cycle. In B. Carter & M. McGoldrick (Eds.), *The changing family life cycle: A framework for family therapy* (2nd ed., pp. 457–482). Boston: Allyn & Bacon.

Hofer, M. (1984). Relationships as regulators: A psychobiologic perspective on bereavement. *Psychosomatic Medicine, 46*(3), 183–197.

Hoffman, L. (1981). *Foundations of family therapy.* New York: Basic Books.

Hoffman, L. (1990). Constructing realities: An art of lenses. *Family Process, 29,* 1–12.

Hogan, N., & Balk, D. (1990). Adolescent reactions to sibling death: Perceptions of mothers, fathers and teenagers. *Nursing Research, 39*(2), 103–106.

Horney, K. (1967). *Feminine psychology.* New York: Norton.

Horowitz, M. (1986). *Stress response syndromes.* New York: Aronson.

Horowitz, M. (1988). *Introduction to psychodynamics.* New York: Basic Books.

Horowitz, M., Wilner, N., Marmar, C., & Krupnick, J. (1980). Pathological grief and the activation of latent self-images. *American Journal of Psychiatry, 137,* 1157–1162.

Humphry, D. (1991). *Final exit.* Eugene, OR: The Hemlock Society.

Huntington, R., & Metcalf, P. (1979). *Celebrations of death: The anthropology of mortuary rituals.* Cambridge, England: Cambridge University Press.

Ianni, F. (1989). *The search for structure.* New York: Free Press.

Imber-Black, E. (1991). Rituals and the healing process. In F. Walsh & F. McGoldrick (Eds.) *Living beyond loss* (pp. 207–213). New York: Norton.

Isabella, R., & Belsky, J. (1985). Marital change during the transition to parenthood and security of infant–parent attachment. *Journal of Family Issues, 6*(4), 505–522.

Janoff-Bulman, R. (1985). The aftermath of victimization: Rebuilding shattered assumptions. In C. Figley (Ed.), *Trauma and its wake* (pp. 15–35). New York: Brunner/Mazel.

Jay, M. (1973). *The dialectical imagination: A history of the Frankfurt School and the Institute of Social Research, 1923–1950.* Boston: Little, Brown.

Jordan, J. (1990). *An integrative model of family development: Part 1. The transformation of attachments; Part 2. The impact of loss.* Working paper, Family Loss Project, Framingham, MA.

Jordan, J. V., Kaplan, A. G., Miller, J. B., Stiver, I. P., & Surrey, J. L. (1991). *Women's growth in connection: Writings from the Stone Center.* New York: Guilford Press.

Keeney, B. P. (1983). *Aesthetics of change.* New York: Guilford Press.

Keeney, B. P., & Thomas, F. N. (1986). Cybernetic foundations of family therapy. In F. Piercy, D. H. Sprenkle, & Associates, *Family therapy sourcebook* (pp. 262–287). New York: Guilford Press.

Kerr, M., & Bowen, M. (1988). *Family evaluation*. New York: Norton.

Klass, D. (1988). *Parental grief: Solace and resolution*. New York: Springer.

Kliman, A. (1986). *Crisis: Psychological first aid for recovery and growth* (2nd ed.). New York: Aronson.

Kohon, G. (1986). *The British school of object relations: The independent tradition*. New Haven, CT: Yale University Press.

Kohut, H. (1971). *The analysis of the self*. New York: International Universities Press.

Kohut, H. (1977). *The restoration of the self*. New York: International Universities Press.

Koocher, G. (1974). Talking with children about death. *American Journal of Orthopsychiatry, 44*, 404–411.

Koocher, G. (1986). Coping with a death from cancer. *Journal of Consulting and Clinical Psychology, 54*, 623–631.

Koocher, G., & Kemler, B. (1992, May). Death of a child: A family treatment approach. In *Crisis and opportunity: Facilitating grief and recovery for individuals, families and communities*. Conference held at Children's Hospital, Boston.

Krell, R., & Rabkin, L. (1979). The effects of sibling death on the surviving child: A family perspective. *Family Process, 18*, 471–477.

Kübler-Ross, E. (1969). *On death and dying*. New York: Macmillan.

Laird, J. (1989). Women and stories: Restorying women's self-constructions. In M. McGoldrick, C. Anderson, & F. Walsh (Eds.), *Women in families* (pp. 427–450). New York: Norton.

Lattanzi, M. (1984). Professional stress: Adaptation, coping and meaning. *Family Therapy Collections, 8*, 95–106.

Leavitt, J. (1986). *Brought to bed: Childbearing in America, 1750–1950*. New York: Oxford University Press.

Lebowitz, L., & Roth, S. (1992, October). *The sociocultural context and women's response to being raped*. Paper presented at the International Society for Traumatic Stress Studies, New Orleans.

Leenars, A. (1991). *Life span perspectives of suicide*. New York: Plenum.

Lehman, D., Wortman, C., & Williams, A. (1987). Long-term effects of losing a spouse or child in a motor vehicle crash. *Journal of Personality and Social Psychology, 52*, 218–231.

Leon, I. (1990). *When a baby dies: Psychotherapy for pregnancy and newborn loss*. New Haven, CT: Yale University Press.

Leon, I. (1992). Perinatal loss: Choreographing grief on the obstetric unit. *American Journal of Orthopsychiatry, 62*(1), 7–8.

Lerner, M. (1986). *Surplus powerlessness*. Oakland, CA: Institute for Labor and Mental Health.

Levin, D. (1987). *Pathologies of the modern self.* New York: New York University Press.

Levinson, D. (1986). A conception of adult development. *American Psychologist, 41,* 3-13.

Lifton, R. (1983). *The broken connection: On death and the continuity of life.* New York: Basic Books.

Lindemann, E. (1944). Symptomatology and management of acute grief. *American Journal of Psychiatry, 101,* 141-148.

Loevinger, J., with Blasi, A. (1976). *Ego development.* San Francisco: Jossey-Bass.

Lovell, A. (1983). Some questions of identity: Late miscarriage, stillbirth, and perinatal loss. *Social Science and Medicine, 17*(11), 755-761.

Lukas, C., & Seiden, H. (1987). *Silent grief: Living in the wake of suicide.* New York: Scribner.

Madanes, C., & Haley, J. (1977). Dimensions of family therapy. *Journal of Nervous and Mental Disease, 165,* 88-98.

Main, M., & Goldwyn, R. (1984). Predicting rejection of her infant from mother's representation of her own experiences: Implications for the abused-abusing intergenerational cycle. *Child Abuse and Neglect, 8,* 203-217.

Marcus, G., & Fischer, M. (1986). *Anthropology as cultural critique.* Chicago: University of Chicago Press.

Martinson, I., Nesbit, M., & Kersey, M. (1984). Home care for the child with cancer. In A. Christ & K. Flomenhaft (Eds.), *Childhood cancer: Impact on the family* (pp. 177-198). New York: Plenum.

Masson, J. (1984). *The assault on truth: Freud's suppression of the seduction theory.* New York: Farrar, Straus & Giroux.

Masson, J. (1985). *The complete letters of Sigmund Freud to Wilhelm Fliess.* Cambridge, MA: Harvard University Press.

Masud-Khan, M. (1988). *The long wait and other psychoanalytic narratives.* New York: Summitt.

McGoldrick, M., Almeida, R., Moore Hines, P., Rosen, E., Garcia-Preto, N., & Lee, E. (1991). Mourning in different cultures. In F. Walsh & M. McGoldrick (Eds.), *Living beyond loss* (pp. 176-206). New York: Norton.

McGoldrick, M., Anderson, C., & Walsh, F. (Eds.). (1989). *Women in families.* New York: Norton.

McGoldrick, M., & Gerson, R. (1985). *Genograms in family assessment.* New York: Norton.

Miles, M., & Perry, K. (1985). Parental responses to sudden accidental death of a child. *Critical Care Quarterly, 8*(1), 73-84.

Miller, A. (1984). *For your own good: Hidden cruelty in childrearing and the roots of violence.* New York: Farrar, Straus & Giroux.

Miller, J. (1986). *Toward a new psychology of women* (2nd ed.). Boston: Beacon Press.

Minuchin, P. (1985). Families and individual development: Provocations from the field of family therapy. *Child Development, 56,* 289–302.

Minuchin, S. (1974). *Families and family therapy.* Cambridge, MA: Harvard University Press.

Minuchin, S., & Fishman, H. (1981). *Family therapy techniques.* Cambridge, MA: Harvard University Press.

Mitchell, J. (1992, April). *Thinking about hysteria.* Paper presented at the annual meeting of the American Psychological Association, Division 39, Psychoanalytic Psychology, Philadelphia.

Mitchell, S. (1988). *Relational concepts in psychoanalysis.* Cambridge, MA: Harvard University Press.

Moss, M., & Moss, S. (1984–1985). Some aspects of the elderly widower's persistent tie with the deceased spouse. *Omega, 15*(3), 195–206.

Mulhern, R., Lauer, M., & Hoffmann, R. (1983). Death of a child at home or in the hospital: Subsequent psychological adjustment of the family. *Pediatrics, 71,* 743–747.

Nieto, S. (1992). *Affirming diversity: The sociopolitical context of multicultural education.* New York: Longman.

Nobles, W. (1978). Toward an empirical and theoretical framework for defining black families. *Journal of Marriage and the Family, 40,* 679–688.

Olson, D. (1988). Family types, family stress, and family satisfaction: A family developmental perspective. In C. J. Falicov (Ed.), *Family transitions: Continuity and change over the life cycle* (pp. 55–80). New York: Guilford Press.

Olson, D., McCubbin, H., Barnes, H., Larsen, A., Muxen, M., & Wilson, M. (1983). *Families: What makes them work.* Newbury Park, CA: Sage.

Osterweis, M., Solomon, F., & Green, M. (1984). *Bereavement: Reactions, consequences, and care.* Washington, DC: National Academy Press.

Parkes, C. (1972). *Bereavement: Studies of grief in adult life.* New York: International Universities Press.

Parkes, C., & Weiss, R. (1983). *Recovery from bereavement.* New York: Basic Books.

Paul, N. (1974). The use of empathy in the resolution of grief. In J. Ellard (Ed.), *Normal and pathological responses to bereavement.* New York: MSS Information Corporation.

Paul, N., & Grosser, G. (1965). Operational mourning and its role in conjoint family therapy. *Community Mental Health Journal, 1*(4), 339–345.

Paul, N., & Paul, B. (1989). *A marital puzzle.* Boston: Allyn & Bacon.

Piaget, J. (1954). *The construction of reality in the child.* New York: Basic Books.

Piercy, F. P., & Sprenkle, D. H., & Associates. (1986). *Family therapy sourcebook*. New York: Guilford Press.

Pincus, L. (1974). *Death and the family: The importance of mourning*. New York: Pantheon.

Pinderhughes, E. (1989). *Understanding race, ethnicity and power*. New York: Free Press.

Pine, V., & Brauer, C. (1986). Parental grief: A synthesis of theory, research and intervention. In T. Rando (Ed.), *Parental loss of a child* (pp. 59–96). Champaign, IL: Research Press.

Plotkin, D. (1983). Children's anniversary reactions following the death of a family member. *Canada's Mental Health*, 13–15.

Polak, P., Egan, D., Vanderbergh, R., & Williams, W. (1975). Prevention in mental health: A controlled study. *American Journal of Psychiatry*, *132*, 146–149.

Pollock, G. (1961). Mourning and adaptation. *International Journal of Psycho-Analysis*, *42*, 341–361.

Pope, K., & Johnson, P. (1987). Psychological and psychiatric diagnosis: Theoretical foundations, empirical research, and clinical practice. In D. Levin (Ed.), *Pathologies of the modern self* (pp. 385–404). New York: New York University Press.

Poussaint, A. (1984, August). *The grief response following a homicide*. Paper presented at a symposium, "Models of early intervention with bereaved children and families," at the American Psychological Association, Toronto.

Prilleltensky, I. (1989). Psychology and the status quo. *American Psychologist*, *44*, 795–802.

Prilleltensky, I. (1990). Enhancing the social ethics of psychology: Toward a psychology at the service of social change. *Canadian Psychology*, *31*(4), 310–319.

Radner, G. (1989). *It's always something*. New York: Simon & Schuster.

Rando, T. (1983). An investigation of grief and adaptation in parents whose children have died from cancer. *Journal of Pediatric Psychology*, *8*(1), 3–20.

Rando, T. (1985). Bereaved parents: Particular difficulties, unique factors, and treatment issues. *Social Work*, *30*(1), 19–23.

Rando, T. (Ed.). (1986). *Parental loss of a child*. Champaign, IL: Research Press.

Raphael, B. (1977). Preventive intervention with the recently bereaved. *Archives of General Psychiatry*, *34*(12), 1450–1454.

Raphael, B. (1983). *The anatomy of bereavement*. New York: Basic Books.

Reiss, D. (1981). *The family's construction of reality*. Cambridge, MA: Harvard University Press.

Riegel, K. (1976). The dialectics of human development. *American Psychologist*, *31*, 689–700.

Rolf, J., Masten, A., Cicchetti, D., Nuechterlein, K., & Weintraub, S. (1990).

Risk and protective factors in the development of psychopathology.
Cambridge, England: Cambridge University Press.

Rolland, J. (1987). Chronic illness and the life cycle: A conceptual framework. *Family Process, 26*(2), 203–221.

Rolland, J. (1991). Helping families with anticipatory loss. In F. Walsh & M. McGoldrick (Eds.), *Living beyond loss* (pp. 144–163). New York: Norton.

Rosaldo, R. (1989). Grief and a headhunter's rage. In *Culture and truth: The remaking of social analysis* (pp. 1–21). New York: Beacon Press.

Rosen, E. (1989). Family therapy in cases of interminable grief for the loss of a child. *Omega, 19*(3), 187–202.

Rosenblatt, P. (1983). Grief and involvement in wrongful death litigation. *Law and Human Behavior, 7*(4), 351–359.

Rosenheim, E., and Reicher, R. (1985). Informing children about a parent's terminal illness. *Journal of Child Psychology and Psychiatry, 6*, 995–998.

Rosenheim, E., & Reicher, R. (1986). Children in anticipatory grief: The lonely predicament. *Journal of Clinical Child Psychology, 15*(2), 115–119.

Rosenthal, P. (1980). Short-term family therapy and pathological grief resolution with children and adolescents. *Family Process, 19*, 151–159.

Rossi, A., & Rossi, P. (1990). *Of human bonding: Parent–child relations across the life course.* New York: Aldine de Gruyter.

Rubin, S. (1981). A two-track model of bereavement: Theory and application in research. *American Journal of Orthopsychiatry, 51*(1), 101–109.

Rubin, S. (1984). Mourning distinct from melancholia: The resolution of bereavement. *British Journal of Medical Psychology, 57*, 339–345.

Rubin, S. (1984–1985). Maternal attachment and child death: On adjustment, relationship and resolution. *Omega, 15*(4), 347–352.

Rubin, S. (1985). The resolution of bereavement: A clinical focus on the relationship to the deceased. *Psychotherapy: Theory, Research, Training and Practice, 22*, 231–235.

Russell, D. (1986). *The secret trauma: Incest in the lives of girls and women.* New York: Basic Books.

Rutter, M., & Garmezy, N. (1983). Developmental psychopathology. In P. Mussen (Ed.), *Handbook of child psychology* (Vol. 4, pp. 775–911). New York: Wiley.

Rynearson, E. (1984). Bereavement after homicide: A descriptive study. *American Journal of Psychiatry, 14*(11), 1452–1454.

Sameroff, A., & Emde, R. (1989). *Relational disturbances in early childhood.* New York: Basic Books.

Sanders, C. (1984). Therapists, too, need to grieve. *Death Education, 8*, 27–35.

Sanders, C. (1989). *Grief: The mourning after.* New York: Wiley.

Santostefano, S. (1984–1985). Metaphor in development. *Imagination, Cognition and Personality, 4*(2), 127–145.

Schachtel, E. (1958). *Metamorphosis*. New York: Basic Books.

Scheper-Hughes, N. (1990). Mother love and child death in northeast Brazil. In J. Stigler, R. Shweder, & G. Herdt (Eds.), *Cultural psychology: Essays on comparative human development* (pp. 542–565). Cambridge, England: Cambridge University Press.

Scheper-Hughes, N. (1992). *Death without weeping: The violence of everyday life in Brazil*. Berkeley: University of California Press.

Schorr, L., & Schorr, D. (1988). *Within our reach*. New York: Doubleday.

Schuchter, S., & Zizook, S. (1986). Treatment of spousal bereavement: A multi-dimensional approach. *Psychiatric Annals, 16*(5), 295–305.

Schultz, L., & Selman, R. (1989). Bridging the gap between interpersonal thought and action in early adolescence: The role of psychodynamic process. *Developmental Psychopathology, 1*, 133–152.

Schumacher, D. (1984). Helping children cope with a sibling's death. *Family Therapy Collections, 8*, 82–94.

Seedat, M., & Nell, V. (1990). Third world or one world: Mysticism, pragmatism and pain in family therapy in South Africa. *South African Journal of Psychology, 20*(3), 141–149.

Sekaer, C. (1987). Toward a definition of "childhood mourning." *American Journal of Psychotherapy, 41*, 201–219.

Selman, R. (1980). *The growth of interpersonal understanding: Clinical and developmental analyses*. New York: Academic Press.

Selman, R. (1990). *Making friends in youth*. Chicago: University of Chicago Press.

Selvini-Palazzoli, M., Boscolo, L., Cecchin, G., & Prata, G. (1978). *Paradox and counterparadox*. New York: Aronson.

Selvini-Palazzoli, M., Boscolo, L., Cecchin, G., & Prata, G. (1981). The treatment of children through grief therapy of their parents. In R. Green & J. Franco (Eds.), *Family therapy: Major contributions* (pp. 529–550). New York: International Universities Press.

Shanfield, S. (1983). Predicting bereavement outcome: Marital factors. *Family Systems Medicine, 1*(1), 40–66.

Shanfield, S., Benjamin, A., & Swain, B. (1984). Parents' reactions to the death of an adult child from cancer. *American Journal of Psychiatry, 14*(9), 1092–1094.

Shanfield, S., & Swain, B. (1984). Death of adult children in traffic accidents. *Journal of Nervous and Mental Disease, 172*(9), 533–538.

Shapiro, E. (1975, August). *Social network groups as action research: Method, data and prospects*. Paper presented at the annual meeting of the American Psychological Association, Chicago.

Shapiro, E. (1986, January). *Transition to parenthood*. Paper presented at the Massachusetts Association for Psychoanalytic Psychology, Boston.

Shapiro, E. (1988). Individual change and family development: Individuation as a family process. In C. J. Falicov (Ed.), *Family transitions: Continuity and changes over the life cycle* (pp. 159–180). New York: Guilford Press.

Shapiro, E. (1990). The future of psychoanalytic education: Intergenerational conflict and the balance of tradition and innovation. In M. Meisels & E. Shapiro (Eds.), *Tradition and innovation in psychoanalytic education: Clark Conference on Psychoanalytic Training for Psychologists* (pp. 261–288). Hillsdale, NJ: Erlbaum.

Shapiro, E. (1994). On finding what had been lost in plainview. *Michigan Quarterly Review 33*(3), 579–590.

Siegel, K., Mesagno, F., & Christ, G. (1990). A prevention program for bereaved children. *American Journal of Orthopsychiatry, 60*(2), 168–175.

Silverman, P. (1986). *Widow to widow*. New York: Springer.

Silverman, P. (1987). In search of new selves: Accommodating to widowhood. In L. Bond (Ed.), *Families in transition: Primary prevention programs that work* (pp. 200–220). Beverly Hills, CA: Sage.

Silverman, S., & Silverman, P. (1978). Parent–child communication in widowed families. *American Journal of Psychotherapy, 33*, 428–441.

Silverman, P., & Worden, W. (1992). Children's reactions in the early months after the death of a parent. *American Journal of Orthopsychiatry, 62*(1), 93–104.

Slavin, M. O., & Kriegman, D. (1992). *The adaptive design of the human psyche: Psychoanalysis, evolutionary biology, and the therapeutic process*. New York: Guilford Press.

Spark, E. (1992, June). The Life After Murder Program. In *Responding creatively to children and violence: Psychology and human rights*, conference by the Mental Health Committee, Boston College.

Stanley, L. (1990). *Feminist praxis: Research, theory and epistemology in feminist sociology*. London: Routledge.

Stephenson, J. (1985). *Death, grief and mourning: Individual and social realities*. New York: Free Press.

Stern, D. (1985). *The interpersonal world of the infant: A view from psychoanalysis and developmental psychology*. New York: Basic Books.

Stierlin, H. (1977). *Psychoanalysis and family therapy*. New York: Aronson.

Stigler, J., Shweder, R., & Herdt, G. (1990). *Cultural psychology: Essays on comparative human development*. Cambridge, England: Cambridge University Press.

Stolorow, R., & Lachmann, F. (1980). *Psychoanalysis of developmental arrests*. New York: International Universities Press.

Stroebe, M., & Stroebe, W. (1983). Who suffers more? Sex differences in health risks of the widowed. *Psychological Bulletin, 93*(2), 279–301.

Stroebe, W., & Stroebe, M. (1987). *Bereavement and health*. New York: Cambridge University Press.

Stroebe, M., & Stroebe, W. (1991). Does "grief work" work? *Journal of Consulting and Clinical Psychology, 59*(3), 479–482.

Sugarman, S. (1986). *The interface of individual and family therapy.* Rockville, MD: Aspen.

Sullivan, H. (1953). *The interpersonal theory of psychiatry.* New York: Norton.

Taylor, C. (1989). *Sources of the self.* Cambridge, MA: Harvard University Press.

Taylor, S. (1983). Adjustment to threatening events: A theory of cognitive adaptation. *American Psychologist, 38,* 1161–1173.

Terr, L. (1990). *Too scared to cry.* New York: Harper & Row.

Tronick, E. (1989). Infant development and mother/infant interaction. *American Psychologist, 44*(2), 112–119.

Tyler, F., Brome, D., & Williams, J. (1991). *Ethnic validity, ecology, and psychotherapy.* New York: Plenum.

Vachon, M., Sheldon, A., Lancee, W., Lyall, W., Rogers, J., & Freeman, S. (1982). Correlates of enduring distress patterns following bereavement: Social network, life situation and personality. *Psychological Medicine, 12,* 783–788.

Vaillant, G. (1985). Loss as a metaphor for attachment. *American Journal of Psychoanalysis, 45*(1), 59–67.

van der Kolk, B. (1987). *Psychological trauma.* Washington, DC: American Psychiatric Press.

Vida, S., & Grizenko, N. (1989). *DSM-III-R* and the phenomenology of childhood bereavement: A review. *Canadian Journal of Psychiatry, 34,* 148–154.

Videka-Sherman, L. (1982). Coping with the death of a child: A study over time. *American Journal of Orthopsychiatry, 52,* 688–698.

Videka-Sherman, L., & Lieberman, M. (1985). Effects of self-help groups and psychotherapy after a child dies: The limits of recovery. *American Journal of Orthopsychiatry, 55,* 70–82.

Volkan, V. (1981). *Linking objects and linking phenomena.* New York: International Universities Press.

Vollman, R., Ganzert, A., Picher, L., & Williams, W. (1971). The reactions of family systems to sudden and unexpected death. *Omega, 2,* 101–106.

Wachtel, E. F., & Wachtel, P. L. (1985). *Family dynamics in individual psychotherapy: A guide to clinical strategies.* New York: Guilford Press.

Walker, G. (1991). *In the midst of winter: Systemic therapy with families, couples and individuals with AIDS infection.* New York: Norton.

Walsh, F. (1978). Concurrent grandparent death and birth of schizophrenic offspring: An intriguing finding. *Family Process, 17,* 457–463.

Walsh, F. (Ed.). (1982). *Normal family processes* (1st ed.). New York: Guilford Press.

Walsh, F., & McGoldrick, M. (Eds.). (1991). *Living beyond loss.* New York: Norton.

Walters, M., Carter, B., Papp, P., & Silverstein, O. (1988). *The invisible web: Gender patterns in family relationships*. New York: Guilford Press.

Wass, H., & Corr, C. (Eds.). (1984). *Childhood and death*. New York: Hemisphere.

Weiss, R. (1988). Loss and recovery. *Journal of Social Issues, 44*(3), 37-52.

Weber, J., & Fournier, D. (1985). Family support and a child's adjustment to death. *Family Relations, 34*, 43-49.

Werner, E. (1990). Protective factors and individual resilience. In S. Meisels & J. Shonkoff (Eds.), *Handbook of early childhood intervention* (pp. 97-115). Cambridge, MA: Cambridge University Press.

Werner, H. (1948). *Comparative psychology of mental development*. New York: International Universities Press.

Westkott, M. (1988). *The feminist legacy of Karen Horney*. New Haven, CT: Yale University Press.

White, L., & Booth, A. (1985). The transition to parenthood and marital quality. *Journal of Family Issues, 6*(4), 435-450.

Williamson, D. (1978). New life at the graveyard: A method of therapy for individuation from a dead former parent. *Journal of Marriage and Family Counseling, 4*, 93-101.

Winnicott, D. W. (1965). *The maturational process and the facilitating environment*. New York: International Universities Press.

Winnicott, D. W. (1971). The transitional object. In *Playing and reality* (pp. 1-30). Harmondsworth, England: Penguin Books.

Winnicott, D. W. (1975). *Through pediatrics to psychoanalysis*. New York: Basic Books.

Wolfenstein, M. (1966). How is mourning possible? *Psychoanalytic Study of the Child, 21*, 93-123.

Worden, W. (1991). *Grief counseling and grief therapy: A handbook for the mental health practitioner* (2nd ed.). New York: Springer.

Wortman, C., & Silver, R. (1989). The myths of coping with loss. *Journal of Consulting and Clinical Psychology, 57*, 349-357.

Yates, T., & Bannard, J. (1988). The haunted child: Grief, hallucinations and family dynamics. *Journal American Academy of Child and Adolescent Psychiatry, 27*(5), 573-581.

Accidental death, 264-266
Accommodation in family context,
    155-156
Acculturation, tension of, 233-236
Adaptation, 77, 177-180
    to grief crisis and family
        development, 141-158
Adolescence and family grief, 201-211
Adolescent grief, 113-119. *See also*
        Adult grief; Childhood grief;
        Family grief; Grief
    identity development in, 117-119
Adult development, effect of death of
        child, 185-213
Adult grief, 21-43. *See also* Childhood
        grief; Family grief; Grief
    and death of child, 39
    and death of spouse, 23, 44-70
    dissociation in, 22
    life structure and parental grief,
        190-200
    management of, 14
    methodological problems in
        resolution, 24
    models of, 25-39
    and parenting, 79-81
    recovery in, 23-24
    stressors in, 258-259
    as systemic developmental process,
        21-25
AIDS deaths, 259
Anger component of grief, 225-227
Anticipated death, 261-264
Assimilation in family context, 155-156
Attachment theory, 25-26, 34-36, 40,
        224
    in childhood grief, 90
    and social role theory, 35
Autonomous self, 142
Avoidance, 160-161
    in childhood grief, 106-112

Bakan, David, 152
Belief and ritual, diversity of, 224-227
Bereavement. *See* Grief
Body metaphors, 91
Boszormenyi-Nagy, I., 168
Bowen, M., 130-132
Bowlby, J., 34-36, 224, 270
    on childhood grief, 73-74, 76
Bowlby-West, L., 135
Buber, M., 156, 157, 265
Burgess, Ann, 255

Caplan, Gerald, 33-34
Caretaking environment, in childhood
        grief, 78-85, 93
Causality, in childhood grief, 102-103
Cebollero, Ana Margarita, 232
Childhood grief, 71-86. *See also* Adult
        grief; Family grief; Grief
    in adolescence, 113-119
    attachment in, 90
    avoidance in, 106-112
    Bowlby on, 73-74, 76
    caretaking environment in, 78-85, 93
    causality in, 102-103
    chronic illness and, 112-113
    cognitive-developmental influence
        on, 74-75
    collaborative construction of
        relational self in, 76-77
    concrete operational state in, 105
    concrete thinking in, 102-103
    cultural influences on, 83-85
    developmental psychopathology in,
        75-78
    and developmental stages, 88-89
    family developmental context in,
        119-122
    and family responsibility, 168-170
    father's death in, 80, 115-117

Childhood grief (*continued*)
  in infancy, 87–98
  management of, 14
  mother's death in, 79
  parental influences on, 81–85
  and parenting by grieving adults,
    79–81
  preoperational stage in, 99–100
  and preschool child, 98–105
  and preverbal children, 91–92
  psychoanalytic thought on, 72–75
  and reality of death, 82–83
  stressors in, 257–258
  symptoms and family functioning
    in, 135–136
  toddlers in, 91–92
A Child's Parent Dies, 257
Chronic illness and childhood grief,
    112–113
Coconstructing new family narrative,
    138, 180–183
Cognitive–developmental influence
    on childhood grief, 74–75
Cognitive information processing
    theory and object relations
    theory, 37
Collaborative construction of
    relational self, in childhood
    grief, 76–77
Complex self
  defense and constriction of, 149–
    153
  and family development principles,
    147–148
  rediscovering aspects of, 67–70
Complicated grief, 10
Concrete operational stage in
    childhood grief, 105
Concrete thinking in childhood grief,
    102–103
Connection, 271
Control of family change and power
    asymmetries, 156–158
Coping theories, 33–34
Couples' therapy with dead, 56–62
Crisis theory, 33–34
Cross-cultural perspective on grief,
    222–224
Cultural anthropology on grief,
    222–223

Cultural perspective
  on childhood grief, 83–85
  on death of child, 228–230
  on grief, 23
  in grieving families, 219–239

Daughter's grief, 240–251
Dead, changing image of, 62–67
Death
  circumstances of, 252–273
  importance of in families, 132
  and meaning-making process, 264–267
  and relinquishment process, 27–28
  stressors in, 254–264
Death of child
  on adult development, 185–213
  and adult grief, 39
  cultural influence on, 228–230
Death of spouse, 23, 44–70
Defense and constriction of complex
    self, 149–153
Delayed grief in intergenerational
    family therapy, 129–130
Development, family. *See* Family
    development
Developmental psychopathology, in
    childhood grief, 75–77
Developmental stages and childhood
    grief, 88–89
Developmental stress, managing, 153–
    158
Developmental theories
  integration, 77–78
  self-regulation through relational
    adaptation, 77
  symbolic representation, 77
Dicks, H., 37
Differentiation of self
  and family grief, 170–177
  and intergenerational family
    therapy, 130–133
Discontinuity, in developmental
    stress, 153–158
Dissociation, 49, 77
  in adult grief, 22
Durkheim, Emile, 227

The Ego and the Id (Freud), 31
Eisenbruch, M., 224, 227, 229, 235

Emotional avoidance as stability strategy, 160-161
Emotional equilibrium, establishing, 159-164
Eth, S., 273

Families
  death in, importance of, 132
  grief reaction in, 132-134
  shared adaptation of, 177-180
  sources of stability, 16
  structures of, 279
Family cut-off, 175-177
Family development, 146-153
  and adaptation to grief crisis, 141-158
  childhood grief in, 119-122
  and grief therapy, 277-286
  integrating complex self, 147-148
  model of, 142-143
  and pathological grief, 141-146
Family grief
  and differentiation of self, 170-177
  and early adolescence, 201-211
  and family systems theory, 125-140
  helping, 159-184
  and stressors, 259-264
  systemic developmental approach, 9-18
Family narratives, coconstructing, 138, 180-183
Family systems
  child symptoms and family function, 135-136
  disruptions of homeostasis, 134-135
  and grief, 134-135, 138
  structural change in grieving families, 136-137
  terminal illness and family grief, 137
  theory, 125-140
Family triangles, 164-168
Father's death
  in adolescence, 115-117
  in childhood, 80
Father's grief, 193-198
Figley, C., 270
Freire, P., 158
Freud, S.
  The Ego and the Id (Freud), 31

on grief, 26-28
"Mourning and Melancholia," 27
personal grief of, 29-32
Funerals, 132, 225
Furman, E., 73, 257-258

Gelcer, E., 136
Gender effects and object relations theory, 38-39
Goodness of fit, 220
Grief. *See also* Adult grief; Childhood grief; Family grief
  in adulthood, 21-43
  anger component of, 225-227
  as cultural criticism, 3-8
  and differentiation of self, 130-133
  and family choreography, 9-12
  and family narratives, 138
  and family systems, 134-135
  Freud on, 26-28
  management of, 14
  and post traumatic stress disorder, 268-269
  reaction in families, 132-134
  relational aspects of, 39-42
  ritual and belief, diversity of, 224-227
  sharing, 15
  as social transition, 227-228
  sociocultural context of, 217-239
  structure of, 252-273
  and tension of acculturation, 233-236
  therapy, 277-286
  and trauma, 267-273
Grief crisis, adaptation to, 141-158
"Grief and a Headhunter's Rage," 225

Herz, F., 132
High technology medicine, impact of, 231-233
Homeostasis
  in family systems, 126, 134-135
Horowitz, M., 270

Ideal developmental process, 148-149
Identity development and adolescent grief, 117-119
Ilongot people, 225-227

Individuation, 142
Information processing theory and
    object relations theory, 37
Integration, developmental theories,
    77-78
Integration of complex self, 147-148
Intergenerational family therapy
    delayed grief in, 129-130
    family systems theory, 128-134
    grief and differentiation of self, 130-
    133
    operational mourning, 129-130
Interpersonal object relational
    perspective, 36-39
It's Always Something, 263

Jordan, J., 134-135

Koocher, G., 81

Lifton, R., 271
Liminality, 49-50, 227-228
Lindemann, Erich, 32-33

Masson, J., 29
McGoldrick, M., 125, 134
Meaning-making process and death,
    264-267
Melancholia, 27
Mental health limitations on grief,
    236-239
Metamorphosis, 152
Mitchell, J., 29
Morphogenesis, in family systems,
    126
Mother's death in childhood, 79, 93
Mother's grief, 198-200
"Mourning and Melancholia," 27, 29
Movement, 271
Murder, 266-267
"The Myths of Coping With Loss,"
    237

Narratives, family, 138, 180-183
Nell, V., 235

Object relations theory, 36
    and cognitive information
    processing theory, 37
    and gender effects, 38-39
    and spousal grief, 38-39
Oedipal stage, 99
Operational mourning, 179-180
    and intergenerational family
    therapy, 129-130

Parentification, 168-170
Parenting by grieving adults, 79-81
Parents
    distortion of death, 82
    grief of and adult life structure,
    190-200
    in different cultures, 229
    influences on childhood grief, 81-85
Pathological grief, 27-28
    and family development, 141-146
Paul, N., 129-130
Piaget, J., 155-156
    and childhood grief, 90, 99
Pincus, L., 21
Polak, P., 236
Positioned subject, 226
Posttraumatic stress disorder (PTSD),
    268-269
Power asymmetries and control of
    family change, 156-158
Preoperational stage in childhood, 99-
    100
Preschool child and grief, 98-105
Preverbal children and grief, 91-92
Psychoanalytic thought
    adult grief and, 27-39
    childhood grief and, 72-74, 75
Pynoos, R., 273

Radner, Gilda, 263
Rando, T., 186
Reality of death, 82-83
Recovery in adult grief, 23-24
Reiss, D., 137
Relational adaptation, 77
Relational aspects of grief, 39-42
Relational self, 76-77
Religious community as support, 285

Relinquishment process of death, 27–28
Replacement child, 161–162
Riegel, K., 147, 148
Ritual and belief, diversity of, 224–227
Rolland, J., 137, 259
Rosaldo, Renato, 225–226
Rosen, E., 136
Rubin, S., 36

Schemas in childhood grief, 90
Scheper-Hughes, N., 229–230
School-age children, grief in, 105–113
Seedat, M., 235
Self, transformation of, 56–62
Self-regulation through relational adaptation, 77
Shachtel, E., 152
Shared adaptation of families, 177–180
Silver, R., 237
Silverman, P., 237, 260
Social isolation of grief, 221–222
Social role theory and attachment theory, 35
Sociocultural context of grief, 217–239
Spousal grief and object relations theory, 38–39
Stability
  in family systems, 126
  sources of, 16
Stress, developmental, 153–158
Stressors
  in adult grief, 258–259
  in childhood grief, 257–258
  and family grief, 259–264
  specific to circumstances of death, 254–264
Stroebe, M., 24, 237
Stroebe, W., 24, 237
Structure of families, 161
  change in, 136–137

Structure of grief, 252–273
Suicide deaths, 259
Support groups for grief, 238, 285
Symbolic integrity, 271
Symbolic representation, in developmental theories, 77
Systemic developmental approach
  adult grief as, 21–25
  family grief, 9–18
  framework of, 17–18

Tension of acculturation and grief, 233–236
Terminal illness
  coping with, 262–264
  and family systems, 137
Terr, Lenore, 268–269
Toddlers, grief in, 91–92
Transformation of self, 56–62
Transformational mechanisms, in family systems, 126
Trauma
  and grief, 267–273
  impact of, 269–272
  recovery from, 270–272
Traumatic death, 255–256
Triangulation of dead, 164–168

Unanticipated death, 261–264
Universality of death, 224–227
U.S. grief practices, sociocultural perspective of, 231–236

Walker, G., 138
Walsh, F., 125, 129, 143
Weiss, R., 24
Werner, H., 148
Winnicott, D. W., 41
Worden, W., 237, 260
Wortman, C., 237